Some Techniques and Procedures in

Small Animal SURGERY

3rd Edition

Some Techniques and Procedures in

Small Animal SURGERY

3rd Edition

Reprinted from vm sac

VETERINARY MEDICINE & SMALL ANIMAL CLINICIAN

Articles selected by

Robert L. Leighton, V.M.D.

Published by

V. M. Publishing Company, 690 South 4th, Edwardsville, Kansas 66113

1982

PREFACE

Truly the ancient sage was right in saying that one picture is worth ten thousand words. The illustrated surgical article often reveals much more than the words of the author. In addition to surgical techniques, draping and aseptic procedures, instrumentation, and anesthesia are demonstrated. The scope and variety reveal current interests and capabilities, excellent indicators of contemporary and relevant advances.

The willingness to share one's knowledge and to help the other guy says something about veterinarians.

The articles are not all the polished results of skilled writers or basic researchers, but they do reflect the state of the art and the rapid progress of the practitioner. They will be then of immediate interest as an instructive sharing of knowledge, observation or technique.

The selection was made from those articles published during the last five years, which were thought to be suitable by reason of subject material, photographic excellence and general informative appeal. The idea was to select the most helpful article for the everyday veterinary surgeon in a number of surgical areas. In such an endeavor, there will undoubtedly be omissions and due apologies are offered to those whose works are quite equally meritorious, but were not included.

Robert L. Leighton, VMD

ISBN 0-935078-21-5

Library of Congress Catalog No. 82-060417

CONTENTS

G. GENITO — URINARY

H. OPTIC

Small Animal Surgery

HEAD & NECK

Correction of Traumatic

Avulsion of the Upper Lip in Two Dogs

(A Photographic Essay)

Marvin L. Olmstead, DVM, MS
Veterinary Hospital
Ohio State University
Columbus, Ohio 43201

David R. Stoloff, DVM
Colleen M. O'Keefe, DVM
Department of Surgery and Medicine
Kansas State University
Manhattan, Kansas 66506

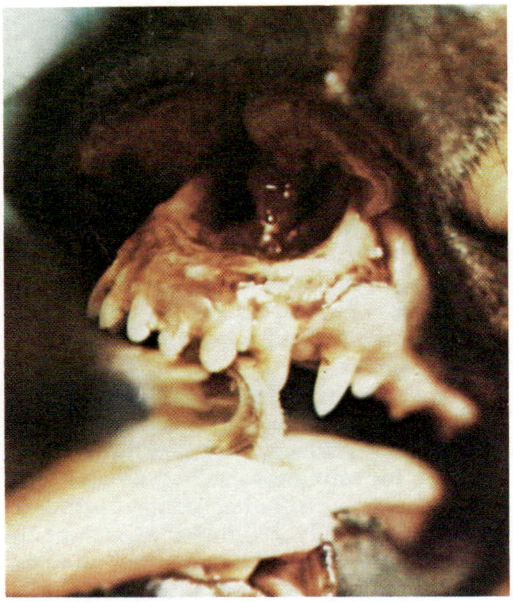

Figure 1—Case 1. Extensive traumatic avulsion of the upper lip and alar fold. Proximal maxillary gingival tissue was inadequate to hold sutures.

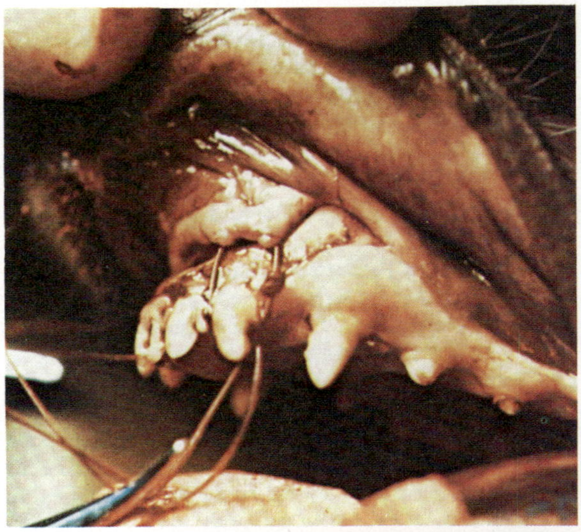

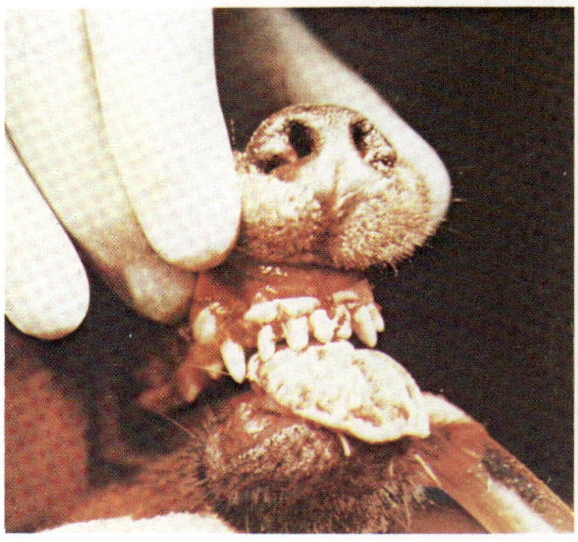

Figure 2 (*right, top*)—Using 2-0 chromic catgut, a mattress suture was placed from the anterior border of the gingival flap around the left upper corner incisor.

Figure 3 (*right*)—Two additional mattress sutures were placed similarly to the suture shown in Figure 2, anchoring the upper lip.

MOST TRAUMATIC avulsions of the lip seen at Dykstra Veterinary Hospital, Kansas State University, have been in cats and have involved the lower lip at the interior portion of the mandible. But recently two dogs were presented with varying degrees of traumatic avulsion of the upper lip at the anterior maxilla. Both cases are illustrated (*Figures 1-7*).

The location of the avulsions presented special problems in reapposing tissue edges, because the gingiva over the maxilla is thin and tightly adherent. Thus, suturing at this site without tearing the tissues is difficult. An alternative method of placing sutures was used to overcome this problem. The sutures were anchored around the incisors.

In one case (*Figures 1-5*) total avulsion of the alar fold accompanied the tear in the lip. No attempt was made to repair the fold.

Healing in both cases was uneventful. ■

Figure 4 (*below, top*)—One week postoperatively, when the sutures were removed, tissue was healing normally.

Figure 5 (*below, bottom*)—Satisfactory apposition of the involved tissue resulted in a normal facial profile.

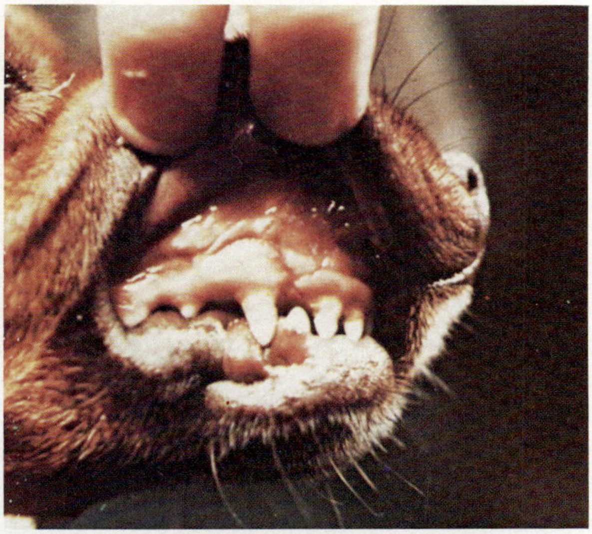

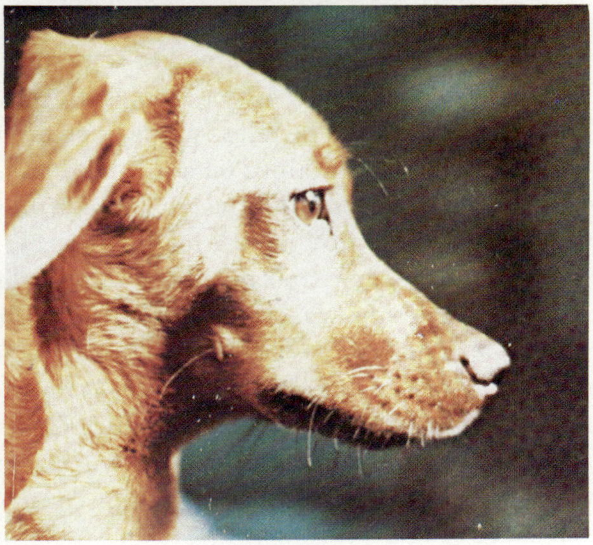

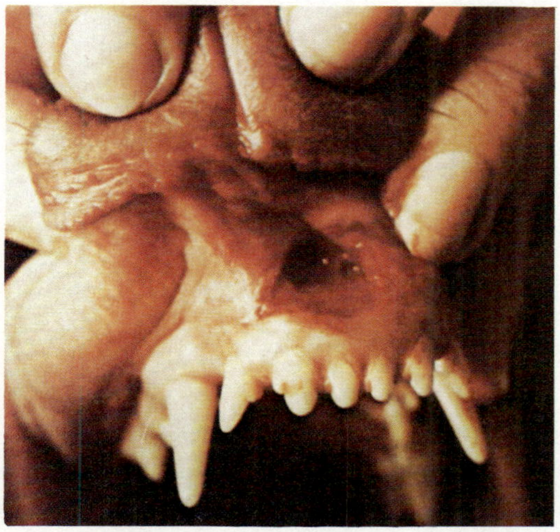

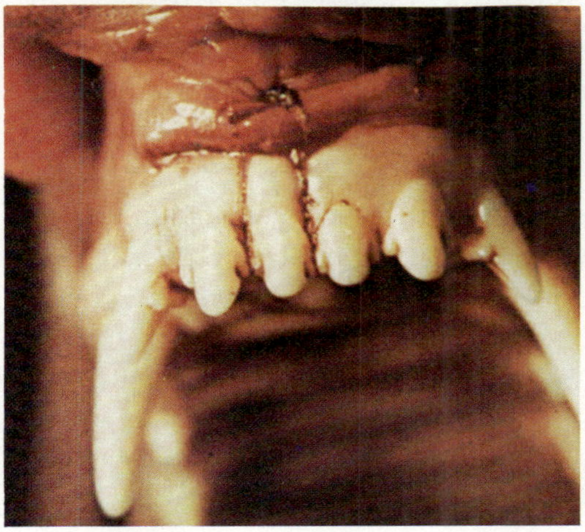

Figure 6 (*top*)—Case 2. The avulsion was less extensive than in Case 1.

Figure 7—As in Case 1, the sutures were anchored to the incisors to hold the tissues in place. Healing was satisfactory.

OSTEOSARCOMA

of the hard palate in a dog

(a case report)

Donald R. Howard, DVM, PhD
John J. Lammerding, VMD
David F. Merkley, DVM, MS
Mark S. Bloomberg, DVM, MS
Dept. of Small Animal Surgery & Medicine
College of Veterinary Medicine
Michigan State University
East Lansing, Michigan 48824

IN THIS paper we cite the successful removal of a circumscribed mass from the hard palate in a dog. Closure was accomplished using a two-stage grafting technique: a pedicle-based flap of soft palate followed six months later by a mucoperiosteal flap of hard-palate mucoperiosteum.

Case history

On January 15, 1975, a 5-year-old male Beagle was referred to the Michigan State University Veterinary Clinic for surgical evaluation of a growth in the mouth. Upon initial examination, a hard-tissue swelling, 2 cm in diameter, was seen in the center of the hard palate at the level of the upper molars. The lesion extended approximately 0.5 cm into the oral cavity. Abnormal respiratory and swallowing signs had been present for eight months before the dog was admitted.

Radiographic evidence was supportive of a dense, bony mass consistent with the findings of the physical examination. Lateral radiographs indicated an invasive advancement of the tumor into the nasal sinus (*Figure 1*). The ventrodorsal radiograph taken with the patient's mouth open defined the lateral limits of the growth (*Figure 2*).

Presurgical radiographic evaluation of the chest was negative for metastatic disease. The hemograms were well within normal limits.

Excision of the growth was performed with the dog under halothane-oxygen anesthesia. A 3-mm osteotome was used for total excision of the mucoperiosteal, nasal, and bony tissue. The resultant oral-nasal fistula was closed with a pedicle graft from a bisected piece of adjacent soft palate (*Figure 3*).

The pedicle graft was secured in position with 10 interrupted sutures of 5-0 polyglycolic acid. An area at the extreme distal portion of the graft tissue appeared ischemic. Several days later a small dehiscence of the wound developed at that site. The tissue was submitted for histopathologic examination and was found to be a low-grade osteosarcoma.

The dog was maintained on a soft-food diet and water for 10 days postoperatively. Tetracycline antibiotics were given by mouth for three weeks.

When the dog was examined six weeks later, the dehisced lesion was about 3 mm in diameter (*Figure 4*). This lesion was observed for six months and then closed using a mucoperiosteal flap technique similar to that previously described for repair of cleft palate.[1] Closure of the lesion was complete and no radiographic evidence of tumor recurrence was noted (*Figure 5*).

Discussion

The incidence of osteosarcoma has been listed elsewhere.[2-5] In one study of 86 cases osteosarcoma was found on the skull 20 times.[6] According to this survey, 98% of all bone neoplasms were found to be malignant.[6] Of these, 85% were osteosarcomas. Osteosarcomas occur at numerous sites but may have some predilection for the pectoral limb.[5,6] The incidence of osteosarcoma reported to occur in the skull varies from 11% to 19%.[7] Thus, it can be said that osteosarcoma of the skull occurs infrequently.

It may be possible that early extirpation of osteosarcomas of the skull gives more favorable results than does removal of affected limbs when the tumor involves the long bones. At least one other case report may support this view.[3]

ACKNOWLEDGMENTS

The authors recognize and thank the following persons for their assistance: Dr. Colin Carrig for radiography, Dr. Roger Cook for the histopathologic work-up, and Ms. Nancy Lee for surgical and technical assistance.

REFERENCES

1. Howard, D.R. *et al*: Mucoperiosteal Flap Repair for Cleft Palate in the Puppy. *JAVMA 165*(4):352-355; 1974.
2. Brodey, R.S.: Surgical Treatment of Canine Cancer. *JAVMA 157*(4):467-470; 1970.
3. Frank, G. *et al*: Bone Neoplasm Sterilization—Case Report. *VM/SAC 67*:161-164; Feb. 1972.
4. Ling, G.V. *et al*: Primary Bone Tumors in the Dog: A Combined Clinical, Radiographic, and Histologic Approach to Early Diagnosis. *JAVMA 165*(1):55-78; 1974.
5. Moulton, J.E.: *Tumors in Domestic Animals.* University of California Press, Berkeley, Calif., 1961.
6. Brodey, R.S. *et al*: Canine Bone Neoplasms. *JAVMA 143*(5):471-495; 1963.
7. Jubb, R.V.F.; Kennedy, D.C.: *Pathology of Domestic Animals.* Academic Press, New York, N.Y., 1963.

Figure 1—Ventrodorsal radiograph of a 5-year-old male Beagle. Arrows indicate the extent of a tumorous mass.

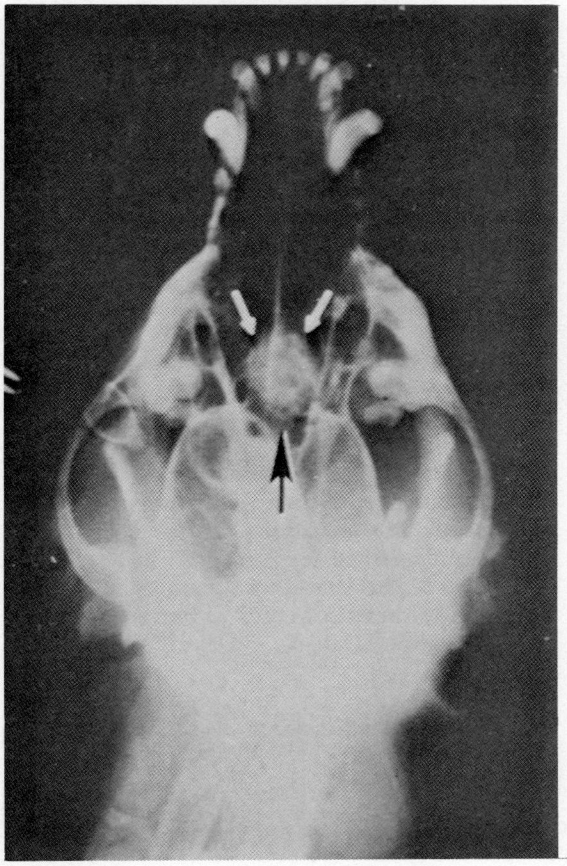

Figure 2—A lateral radiograph of the same dog. Arrows indicate the limits of a tumorous mass.

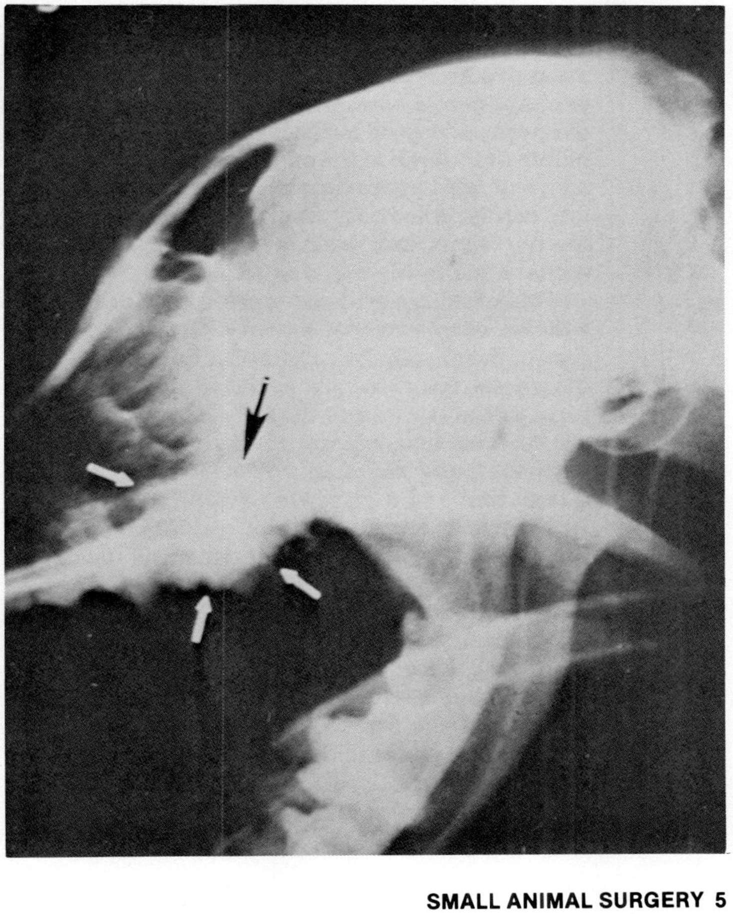

Figure 3—Appearance of the hard palate one day after pedicle grafting. White arrows point to the sutured graft and black arrows to the bed site. The bed site in the soft palate granulated very well. Notice the bisected soft-palate bed site.

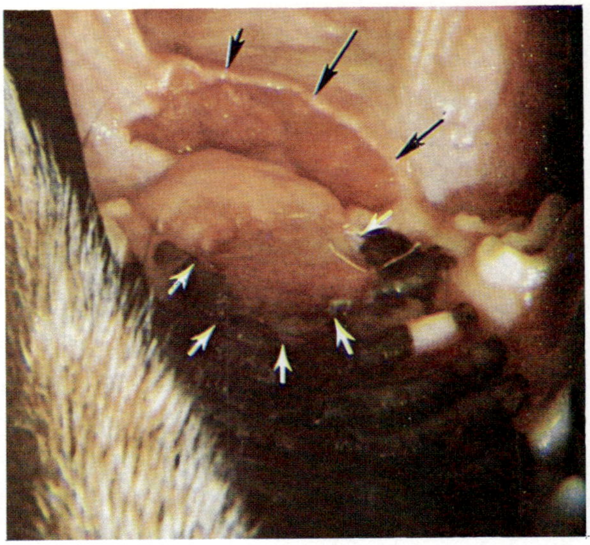

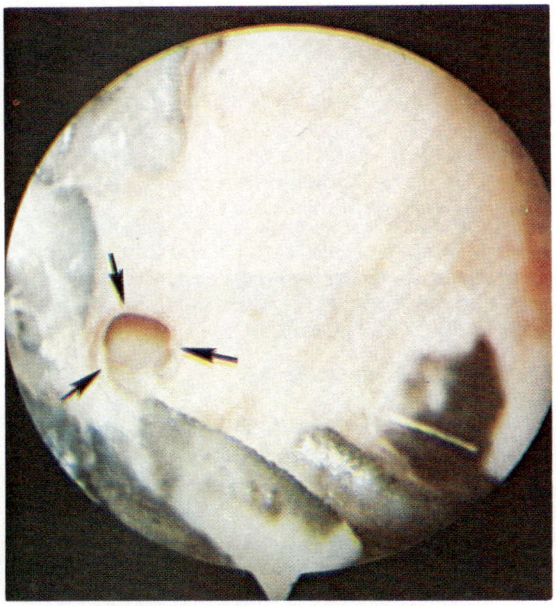

Figure 4—A Small (3 mm) dehisced lesion at the cranial end of the graft site. This lesion was subsequently closed without postoperative problems.

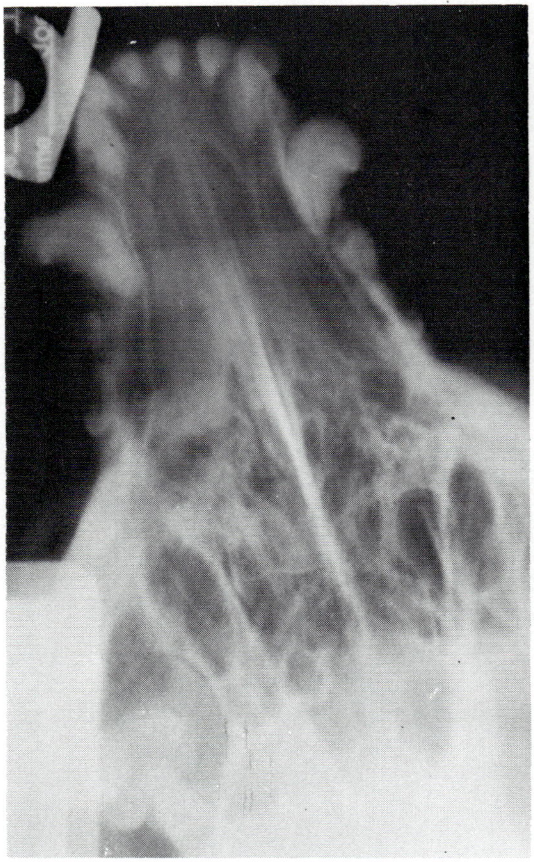

Figure 5—Radiograph taken six months postoperatively shows no evidence of regrowth of the tumor.

PSEUDO-SARCOMATOUS FASCIITIS

of the upper lip of a cat

William B. Kemp, DDS
Asst. Professor of Endodontics
Louis M. Abbey, DMD, MS
Asst. Professor of Oral Pathology
School of Dentistry
Medical College of Virginia
Richmond, Virginia 23298

Locke A. Taylor, DVM
Veterinary Practitioner
Richmond, Virginia 23298

One of a group of farm cats was presented to the veterinary hospital for euthanasia because of a large growth on the upper lip that made eating difficult. The size of the lesion probably hampered the cat's ability to compete for food and contributed to its moderately emaciated state.

In lieu of euthanasia, surgical excision of the tumor was elected.

The spherical lesion (*Figures 1-3*) measured 35 mm in diameter and had a pedunculated base derived from the mucocutaneous border near the midline of the upper lip. Portions of the tumor were covered with a crusty material, imbedded with foreign matter, and had numerous lacerations. A presumptive diagnosis of eosinophilic granuloma was made.

Surgical Procedure

Anesthesia was induced by intravenous administration of 3% thiamylal sodium (Surital® —Parke-Davis) and maintained with oxygen and methoxyflurane (Metofane™ —Pitman-Moore) administered via endotracheal intubation in an open system.

After routine preparation of the surgical site, a through-and-through wedge incision was made which included margins of normal tissue. After removal of the lesion, the incision sites were closed with multiple interrupted 4-0 black silk sutures. The prehensile papillae were removed from the dorsal surface of the tongue to reduce the possibility of the cat dislodging the sutures (*Figure 4*).

A specimen of the lesion was fixed in 10% neutral buffered formalin for examination microscopically.

Pathology

The mass was gray and almost round. The largest diameter measured 3.5 centimeter. The exterior surface glistened. Cut sections had a hard, fibrous, light-tan surface.

Serial sections of the lesion revealed a large, circumscribed, unencapsulated, hemisected mass

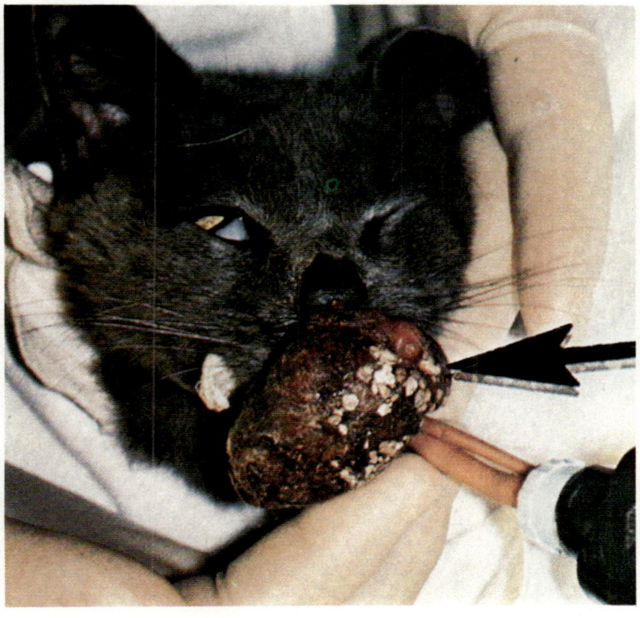

Figure 1—Anterior view of lesion showing the foreign debris attached.

composed primarily of interlacing bundles of fibrocollagenous connective tissue. This appearance was uniform throughout the sections except on one surface, where ulceration, attending surface fibrin and debris were noted.

The predominant cells were fibroblastic in appearance (*Figure* 5), with elongated, indistinct, eosinophilic cytoplasmic processes and round-to-oval vesicular nuclei, which were basophilic and varied moderately in size. In some areas, a storiform appearance was noticeable. A uniform chronic inflammatory cell infiltrate was noted throughout the specimen. Occasional giant cells and mitotic figures were visible. The periphery of the lesion was marked by numerous capillaries and infiltrating inflammatory cells.

These findings led to a diagnosis of pseudosarcomatous (nodular) fasciitis.

Discussion

A veterinary pathology textbook makes no mention of nodular fasciitis is animals,[1] but the lesion in man is well known. It was first described in 1955.[2] The lesion is benign; some think it is not even neoplastic. These lesions in man have attained a size of 10.5 centimeter. The favored location is the upper extremities,[3] but the lesion has been found in most soft-tissue areas of the human body.

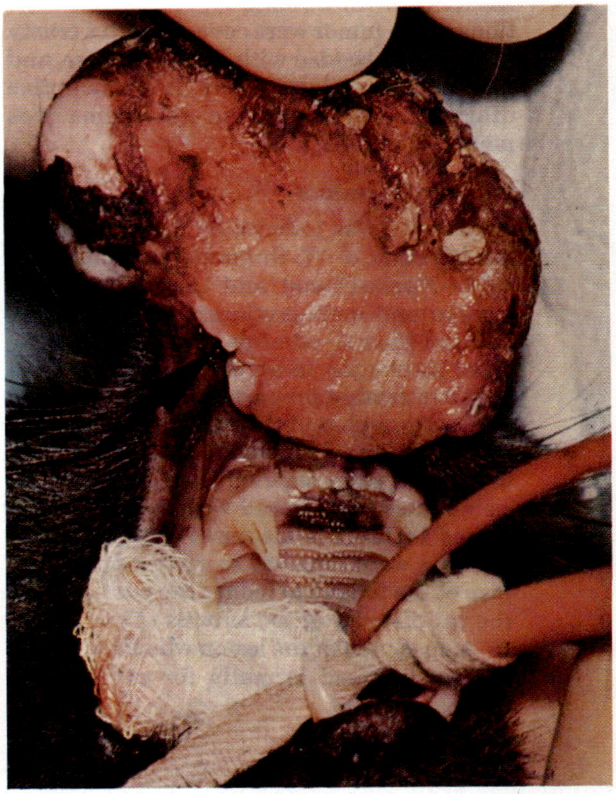

Figure 3—Inferior aspect of the lesion which appeared to be mucosal tissue.

Figure 2—Lateral view of the lesion.

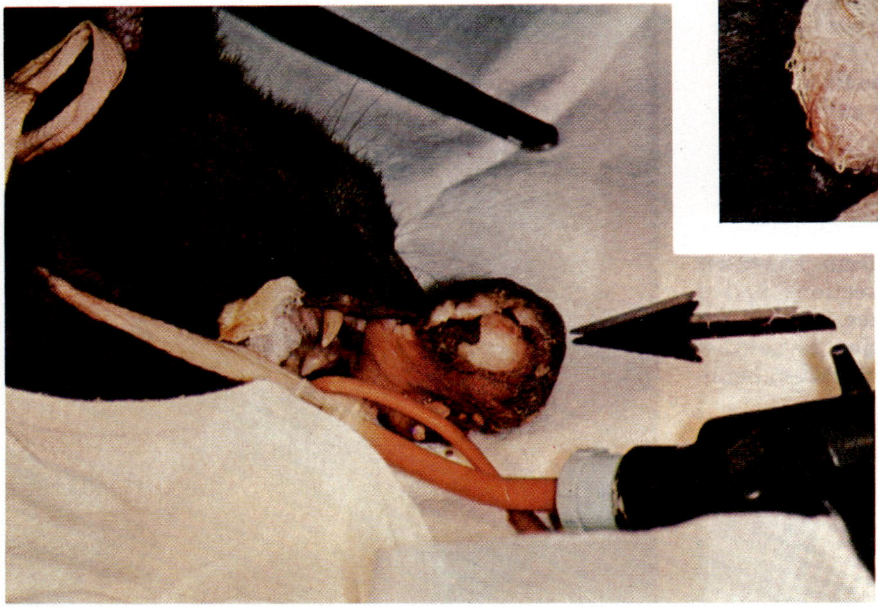

Clinically, this lesion usually appears suddenly as a single, discrete nodule. It grows rapidly, reaching maximum size in a short time. Tenderness, but not severe pain, usually accompanies its development.

Histologically, nodular fasciitis can be differentiated from the pseudosarcomatous dermatofibroma. The latter lesion, also benign, is usually characterized by pleomorphic, bizarre, sarcoma-like fibroblasts, in addition to bizarre multinucleated giant cells. This lesion suggests a non-metastasizing fibrosarcoma of the skin, but an unequivocal primary fibrosarcoma of the superficial tissues would be uncommon.

REFERENCES

1. Smith, H.A. *et al: Veterinary Pathology*, 4th ed. Lea & Febiger, Philadelphia, Pa., 1972.
2. Konwaller, B.E. *et al*: Subcutaneous Pseudosarcomatous Fibromatosis (Fasciitis). Report of 8 Cases. *Am. J. Clin. Path.* 25:241-252; 1955.
3. Stout, A.P.; Lattes, R.: Tumors of the Soft Tissues. In *Atlas of Tumor Pathology*, 2nd Series. Fasicle 1; AFIP Washington, D.C., 1967.

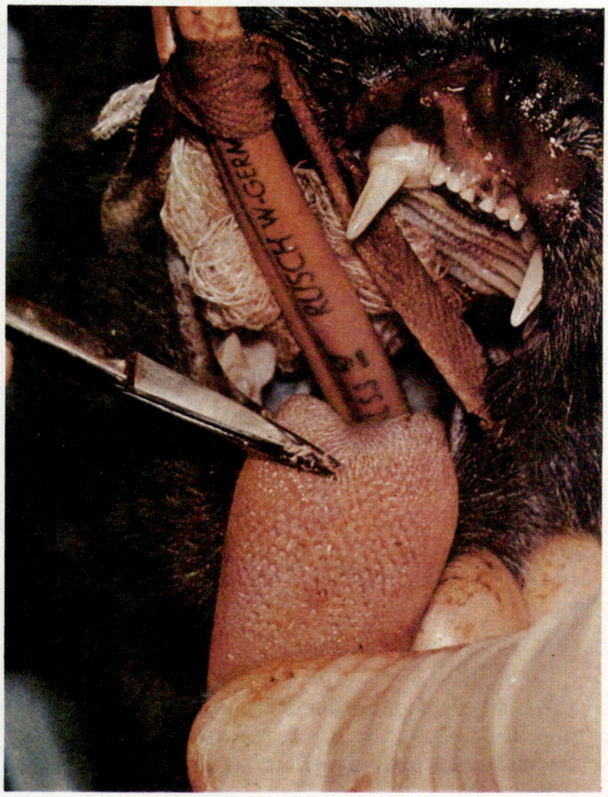

Figure 4—Following excision of the lesion, prehensile papillae were removed from the dorsal surface of the tongue.

Figure 5—Microscopic section of the lesion (*H&E X40*).

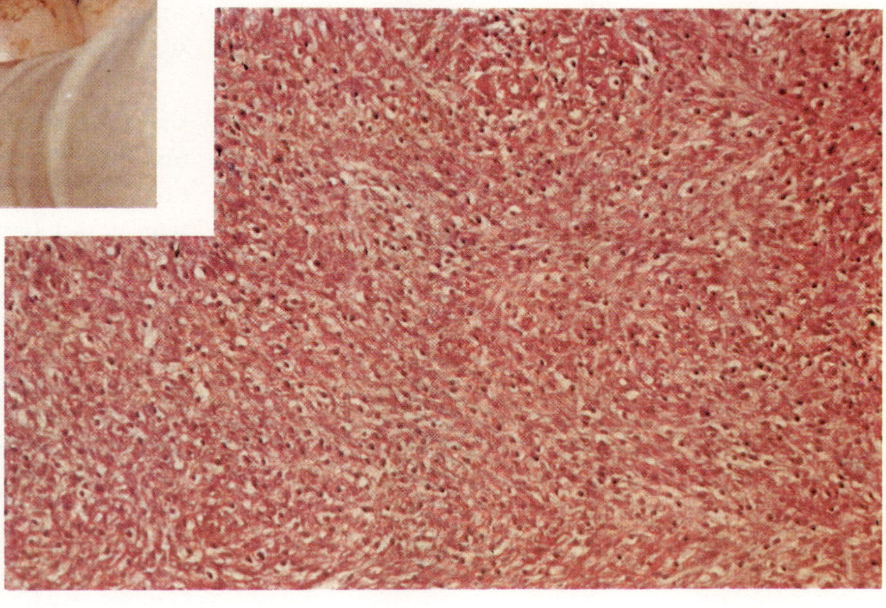

surgical correction of *Prognathous Inferior* in a dog

Robert L. Leighton, VMD
School of Veterinary Medicine
University of California
Davis, California 95616

PROGNATHISM is the term used to designate marked projection of the jaw. The part of the jaw affected is specified as *superior* (upper) or *inferior* (lower). The common terms are *overshot jaw* (prognathous superior) and *undershot jaw* (prognathous inferior).

Prognathism is a hereditary anomaly which in most cases does no harm. However, it is a defect in appearance. When the condition is not a desired characteristic (as it is in the English Bulldog), the animal is unacceptable for showing and should not be used for breeding. If prognathism is severe enough to cause chronic irritation to the gums, surgical correction may be requested.

Case report

On May 23, 1976, a 7-month-old, male, brown and white Tibetan Terrier with prognathous inferior was presented at the Veterinary Medical Teaching Hospital. The dog's upper canine teeth were causing chronic irritation where they contacted the lower mandibles. Except for being quite thin, the dog was in excellent health.

The mandible was found to be 1 cm longer than the maxilla. Dentition was complete, but the fourth lower premolar angled somewhat caudally, contacting the first lower molar. A slight loss of bone was noted between these two teeth. Radiographs (*Figure 1 & 2*) delineated the problem.

On May 25, surgery was performed to correct the condition.

Surgical procedure

An approach was made through the skin and subcutaneous tissue over the ventral surface of the mandible on each side. Tissues down to the periosteum and the muscles on the glossal side were retracted to expose the bone. Starting 7 mm caudal to

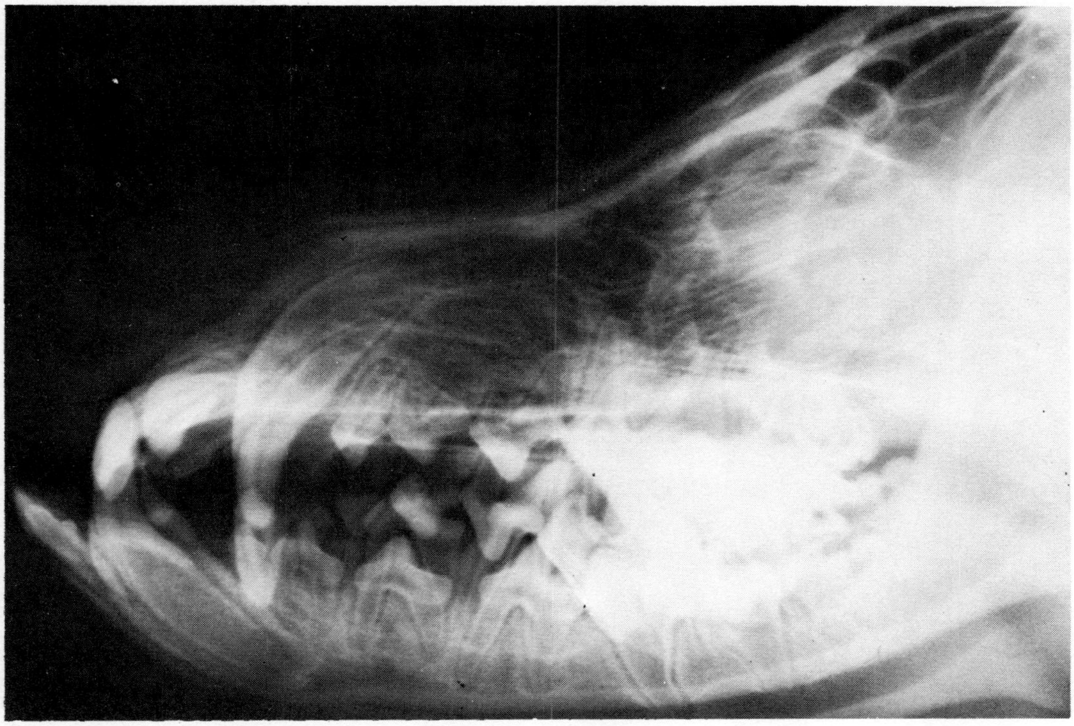

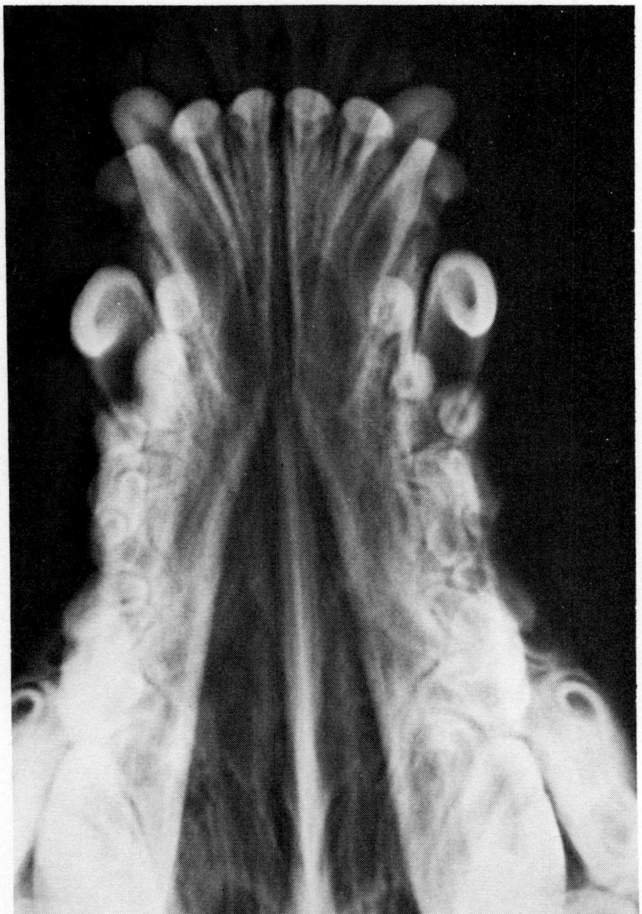

Figures 1 & 2—Lateral and dorsoventral radiographs showing the prognathous extension of the lower jaw of a 7-month-old Tibetan Terrier.

the mandibular foramen, a block of bone approximately 1 cm long was removed. The transverse cuts were made with a Hall air drill. The nerve, artery, and vein were preserved. Removal of the involved fourth lower premolar involved cutting the gum around the tooth and an entry into the oral cavity.

A portion of the mandibular canal was cut out of both the caudal and rostral fragments to accept the nerve, artery, and vein when the fragments were apposed. With the fragments in apposition, the lower canine teeth assumed their normal position just rostral to the upper canine teeth. Small, four-hole bone plates were applied across each bone cut. The screw holes were drilled, measured, and tapped, and the bone screws set firmly.

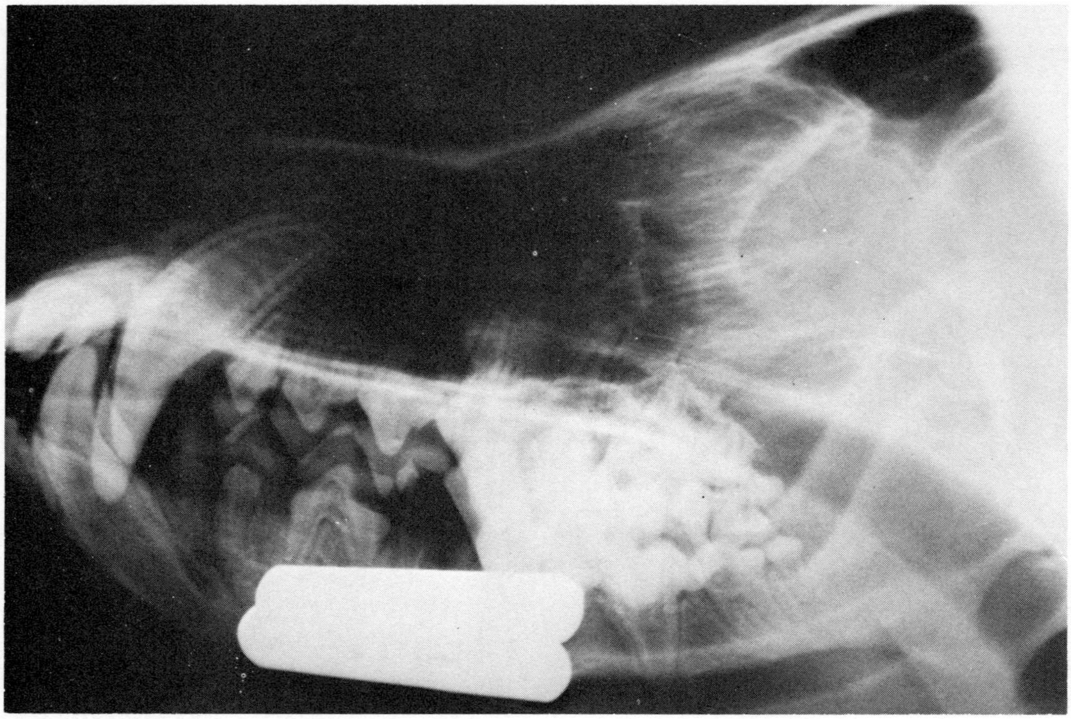

Figures 3 & 4—Lateral and dorsoventral radiographs of the head taken immediately after surgery. The overly long mandible has been shortened by osteotomies of the horizontal rami. Stabilization was achieved with short, four-hole bone plates (Compare to *Figures 1 & 2*).

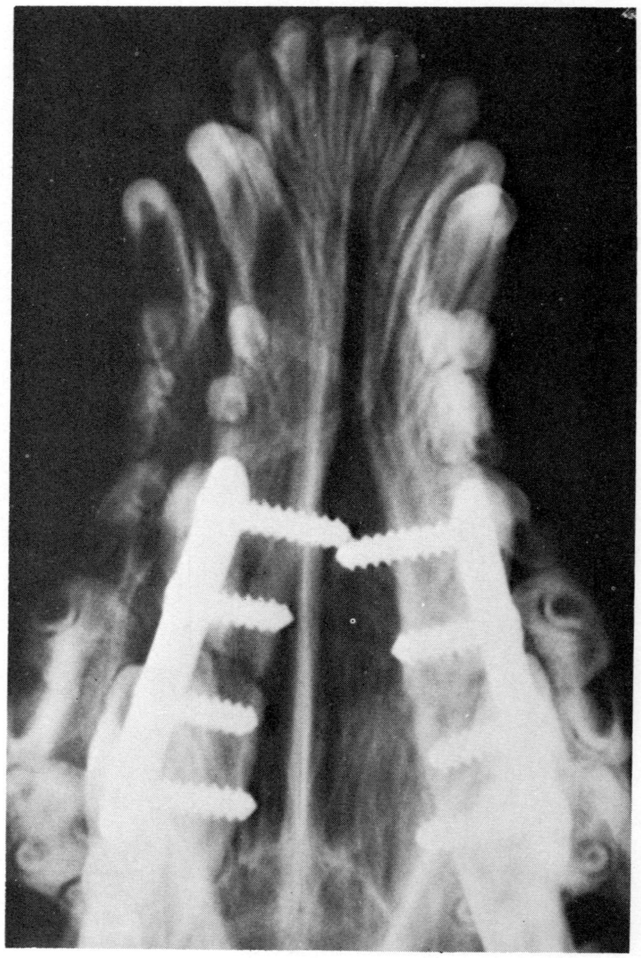

Closure of the incisions was made with 2-0 chromic catgut in the fascia and subcutaneous tissue. Number 30 Vetafil® (S. Jackson) was used in the skin and the gums.

Aftercare

No muzzle was used. The dog's diet during hospitalization consisted of milk and Prescription Diet p/d® (Hill's Division, Riviana Foods) blended to a creamy consistency. Ampicillin (250 mg) was given intramuscularly three times a day until May 31, when the patient was released from the hospital.

Results

Radiographs taken immediately after surgery (*Figures 3 & 4*) showed shortening of the overly long mandible by about 1 cm. Fixation of the osteotomies with short bone plates led to slight dorsal angulation of the right ramus and slight ventral angulation of the left ramus.

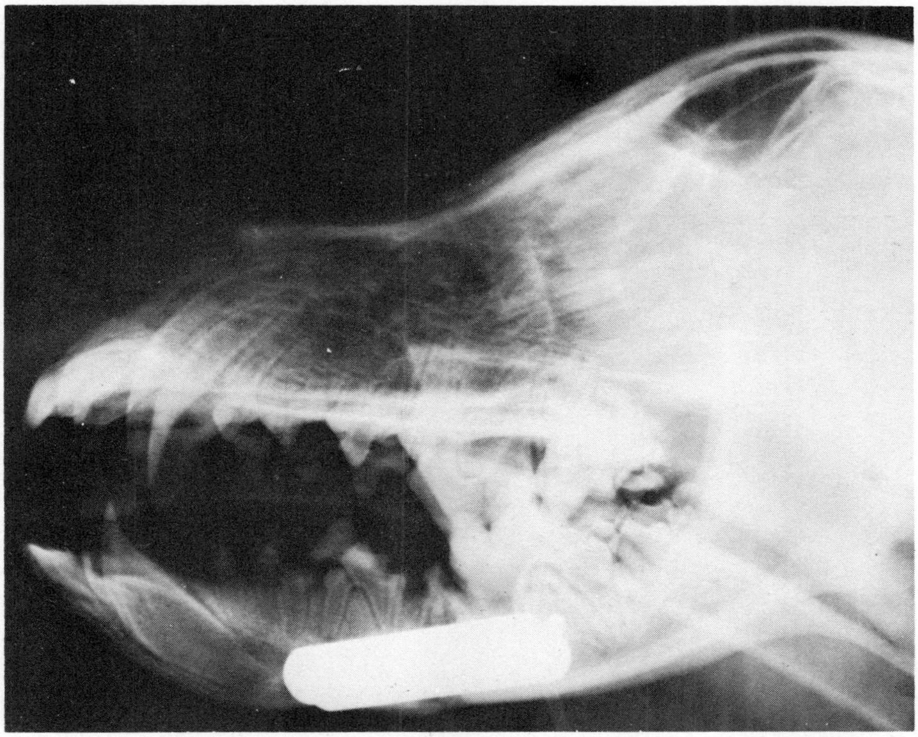

Figures 5, 6 & 7—Lateral and dorsoventral radiographs taken about six weeks after surgery to check progress of healing. Healing and dental occlusion are good.

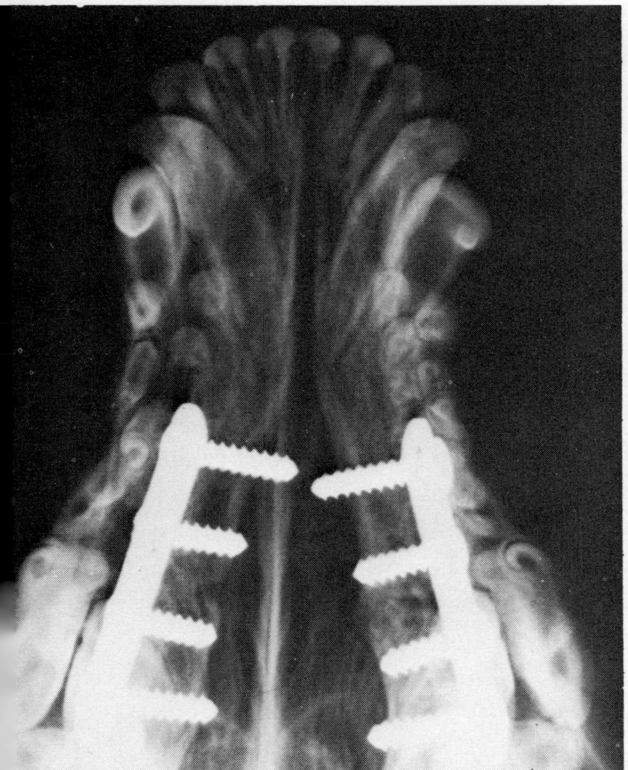

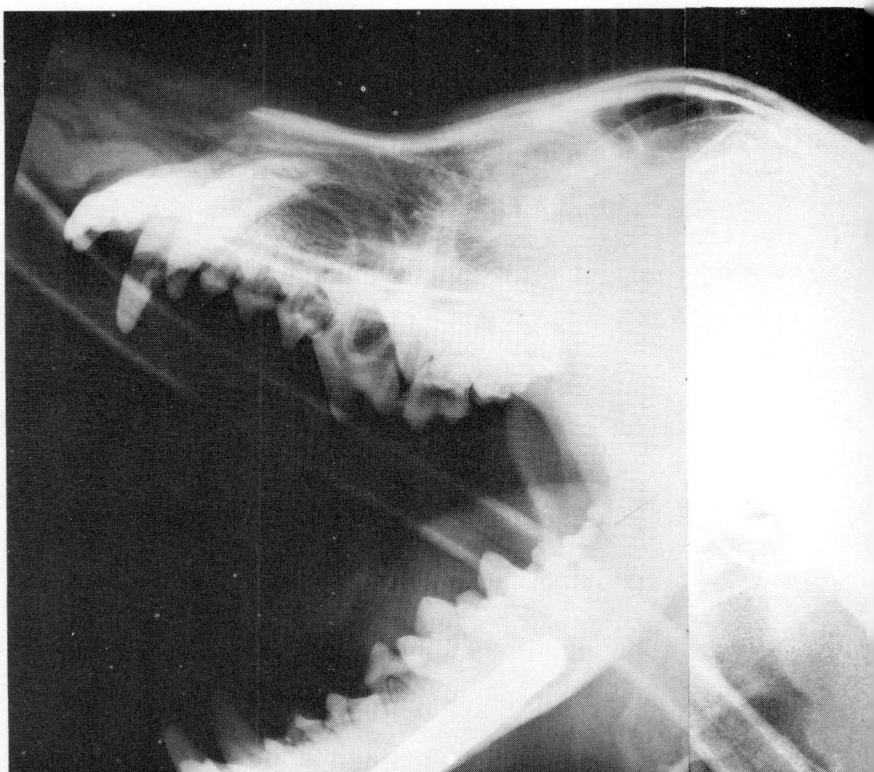

Figure 8—Approximately six weeks after surgery, the bite was remarkably good.

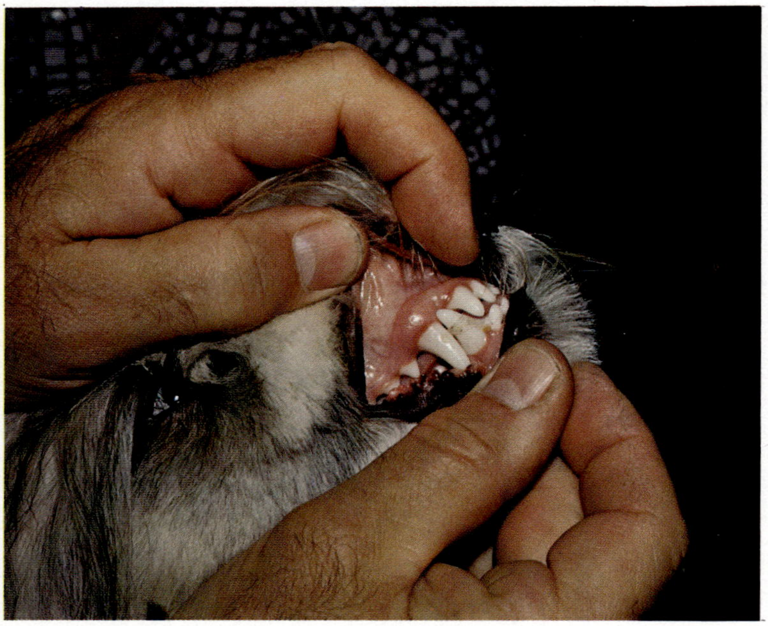

Good healing was seen on radiographs taken on July 6 (*Figures 5-7*) to check the progress of the patient. The bite was remarkably good at that time (*Figure 8*).

On October 12 the right plate was found to be loose and was removed.

The patient's progress has been good, and no untoward effects of the surgery have been observed.

Comment

Opportunity to perform the surgery described here is rare. Further, the ethical considerations related to the breeding of an animal on which the surgery has been performed requires excellent rapport between the owner and the veterinarian. In the case reported here, we felt the procedure was justified by the dog's discomfort and the need to improve its appearance and well being. ■

EAR CROPPING:
a technique

Thomas J. Rogers, VMD
Twinbrook Veterinary Hospital, Inc.
5065 Buffalo Road
Erie, Pennsylvania 16510

THE ETHICS of ear cropping have been debated for many years. Adversaries argue that the surgery is bloody, painful, and, as a whole, barbarous, and disfiguring. However, when done properly the surgery is not only humane; it also contributes to the animal's beauty and well-being. Also, infections, wounds, and hematomas in the ears are encountered much more frequently in dogs with drooping ears than in dogs with prick or cropped ears.

Adversaries of ear cropping say that most ear croppings are poorly done. Therefore, successful techniques must be employed to negate this argument. In this article I describe a procedure for successful and cosmetic ear cropping. It is not a rigid technique; practitioners can vary it according to their needs.

Materials and Methods

The dog is preanesthetized with acepromazine maleate (Ayerst), Innovar™-Vet (Pitman-Moore), and atropine. Surgical anesthesia is induced with thiamylal sodium (Surital® —Parke-Davis) and maintained with a colatile anesthetic.

Before surgery, an ear splint is made of sheet aluminum. The splint is covered with adhesive tape and measured to fit the patient (*Figures 1 & 2*).

Figures 1 & 2—Aluminum sheet metal, to serve as a splint, is measured to fit the patient and a strip of tape is applied to it.

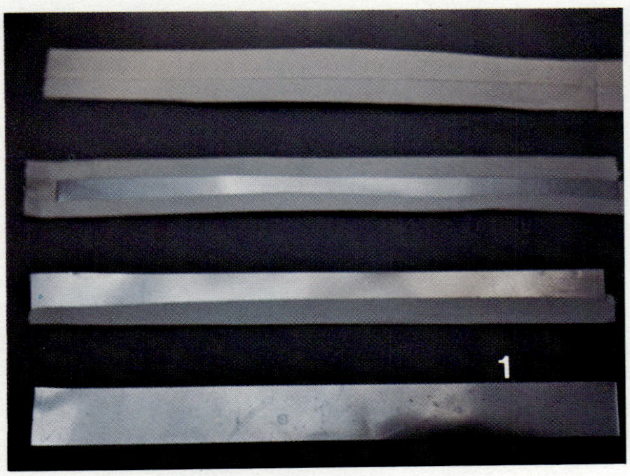

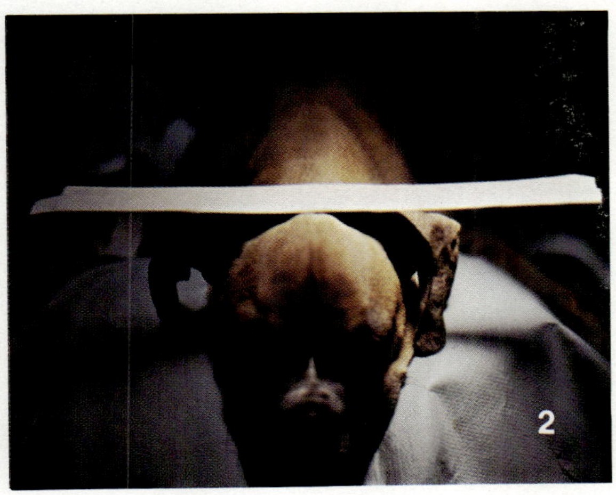

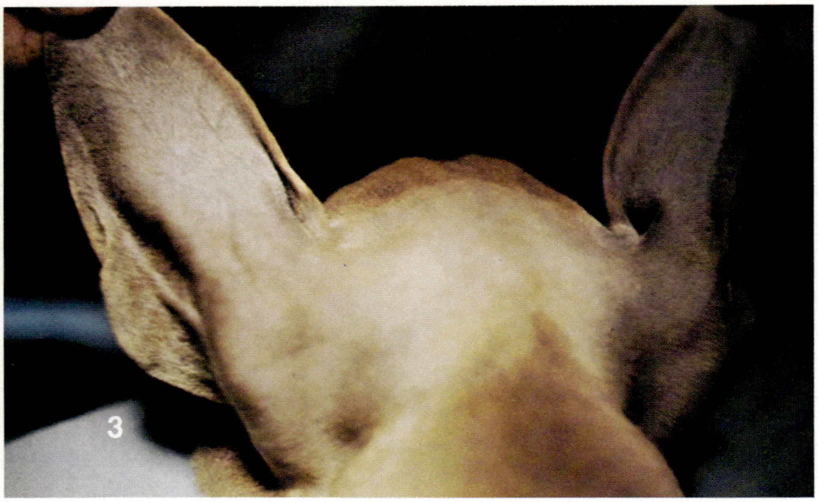

Figure 3
The surgical area is clipped.

Figure 4
Marks on the ear indicate short cut and long cut. Marks are placed with reference to the lateral canthus (short cut) and medial canthus (long cut).

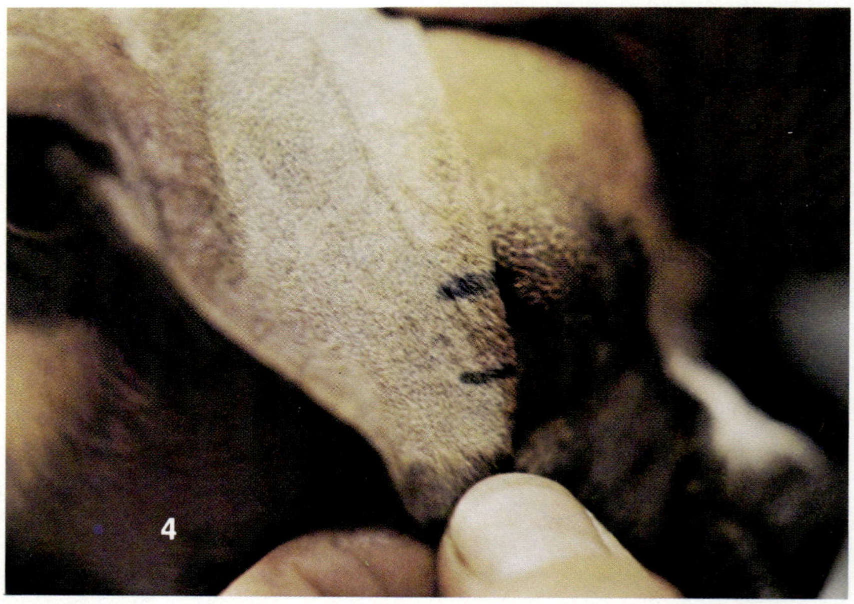

The hair on both surfaces of the pinnae is clipped, as is the hair on the area between the ears to below the opening of the external canal (*Figure 3*).

With the patient in sternal recumbency, the length to which the ear is to be cropped is determined by stretching the ear over to the canthus of the eye (*Figure 4*). A short cut is measured to the lateral canthus and a long cut to the medial canthus. The shape of the ear flap is then marked freehand with indelible ink on the inside of the ear (*Figure 5*). The crop is made to conform to the dog's head and to the owner's wishes.

The pinna is held erect while the top lateral third is removed with Mayo scissors (*Figure 6*). The remainder is removed using electrocautery, set for cutting (*Figure 7*). Cautery should not be used on the upper third of the pinna because it can cause

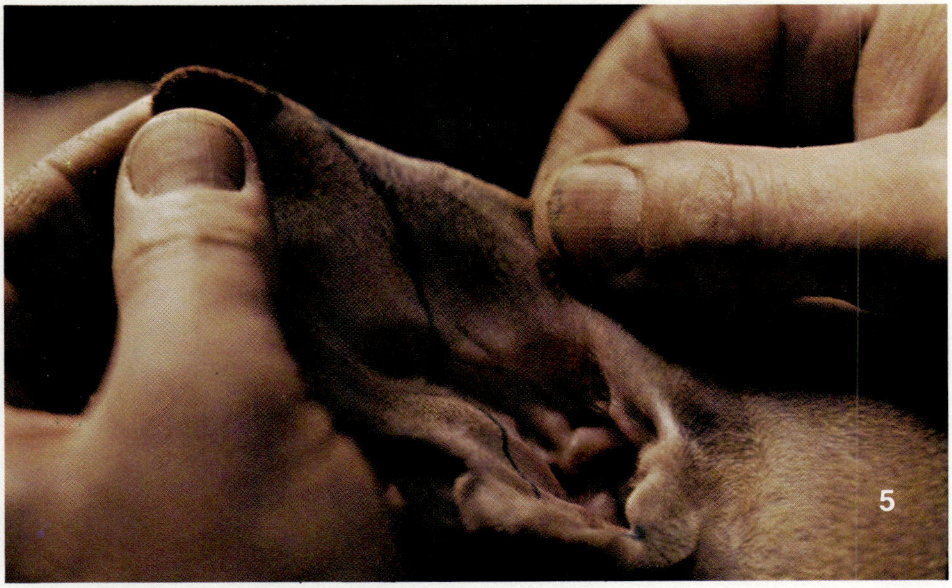

Figure 5
The shape of the ear crop is drawn with indelible ink on the inside of the ear.

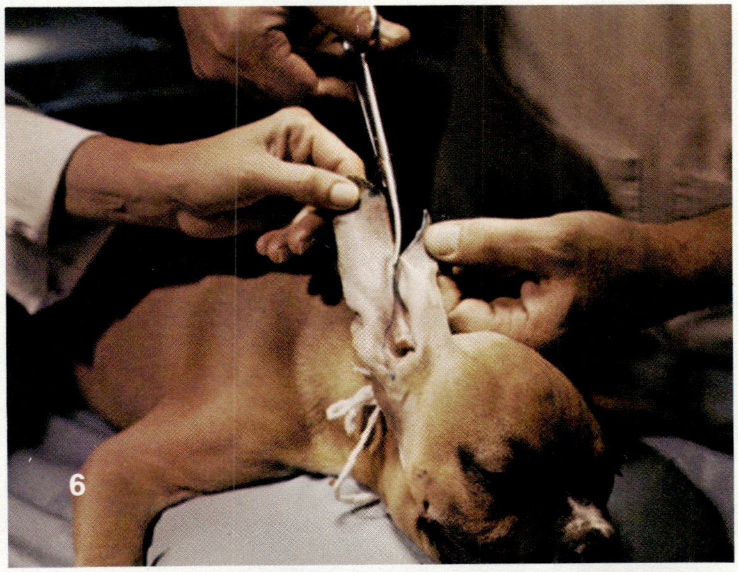

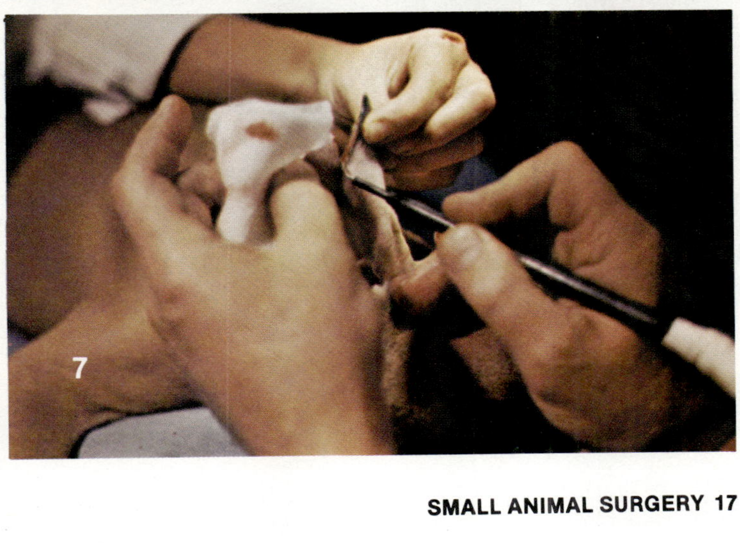

Figures 6 & 7
The upper third of the pinna is cut with Mayo scissors. The cut is completed with electrocautery.

Figures 8-10
Electrocoagulation is used to control hemorrhage.

Figures 11-14
To prepare the second ear the portion removed from the other ear is aligned against it and secured with staples. Cropping proceeds as for the first ear, using the piece from the first ear as a pattern.

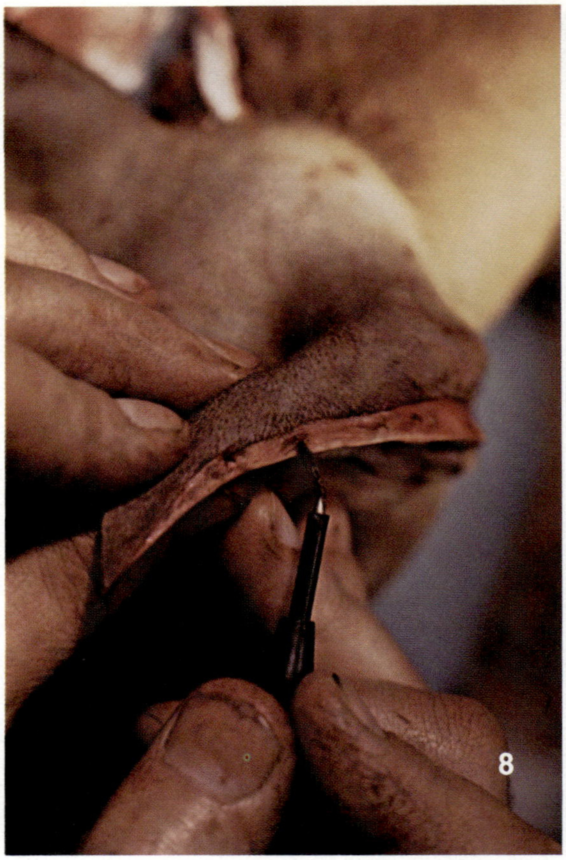
8

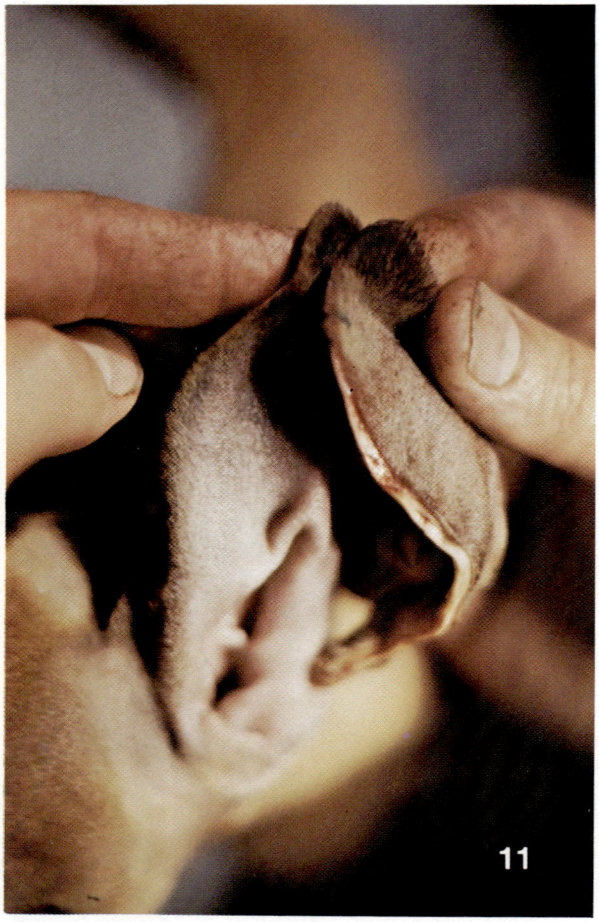
11

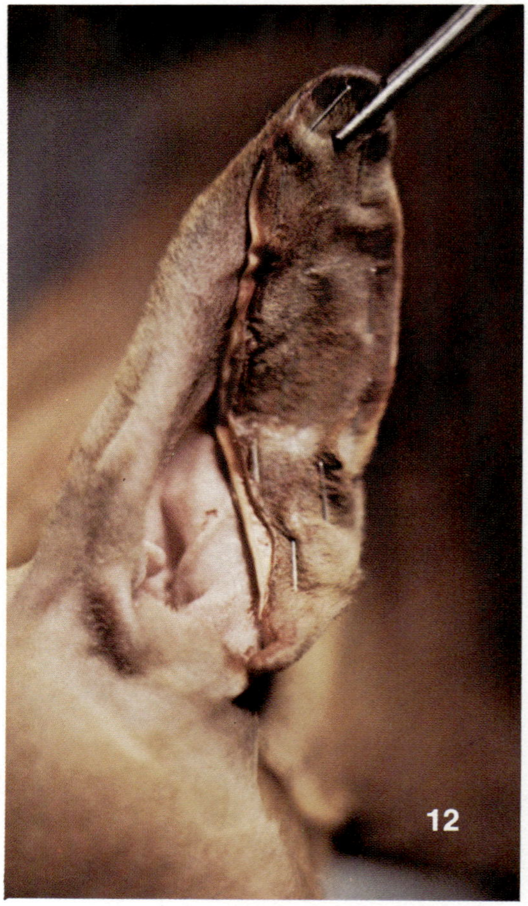
12

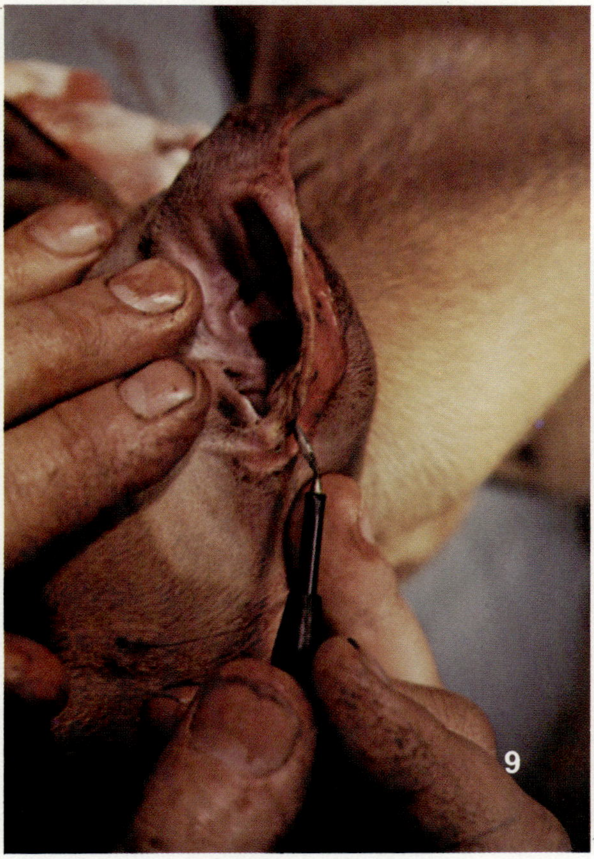

9

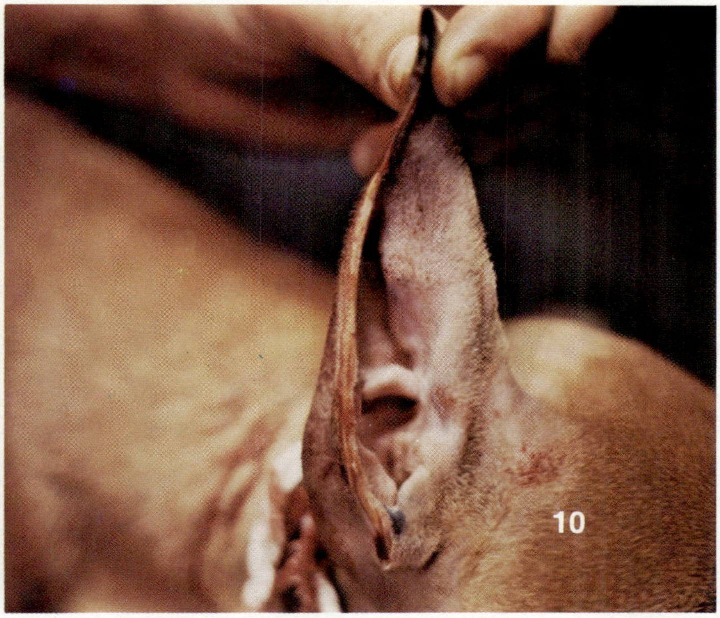

10

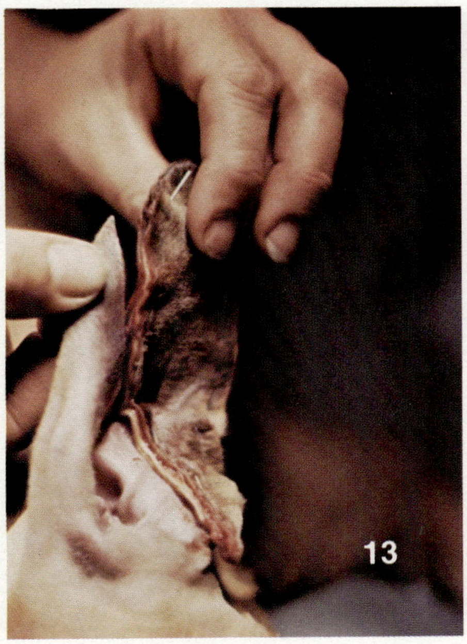

13

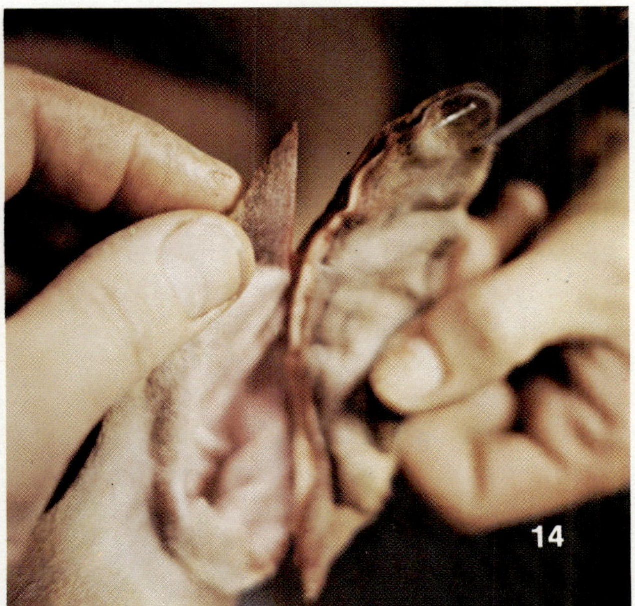

14

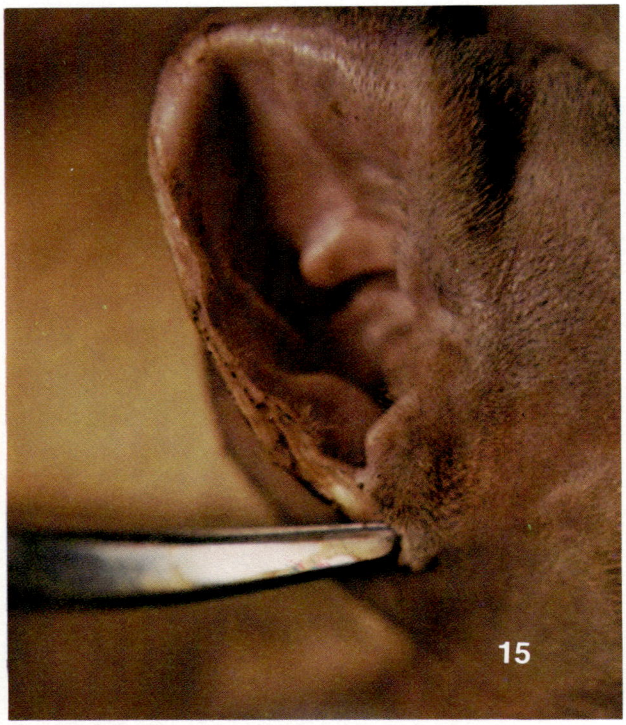

Figure 15—The auricular cartilage at the base of the ear is trimmed to blend into the head.

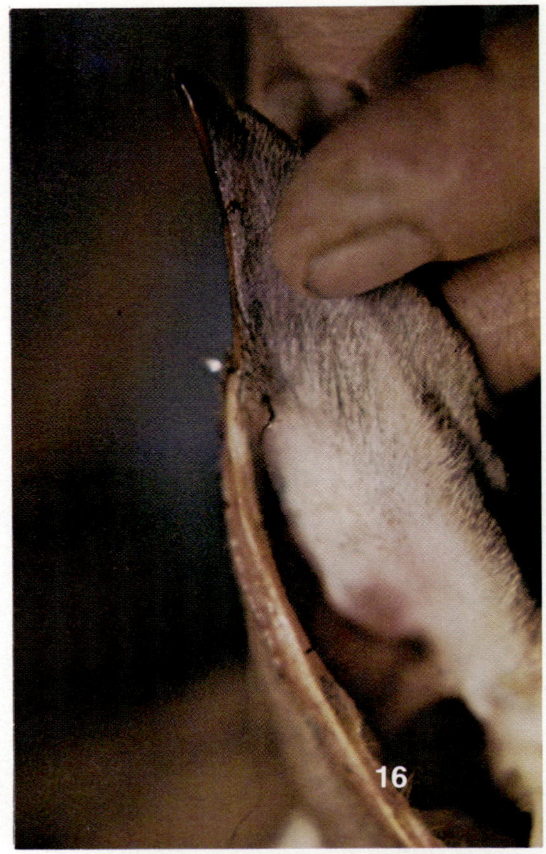

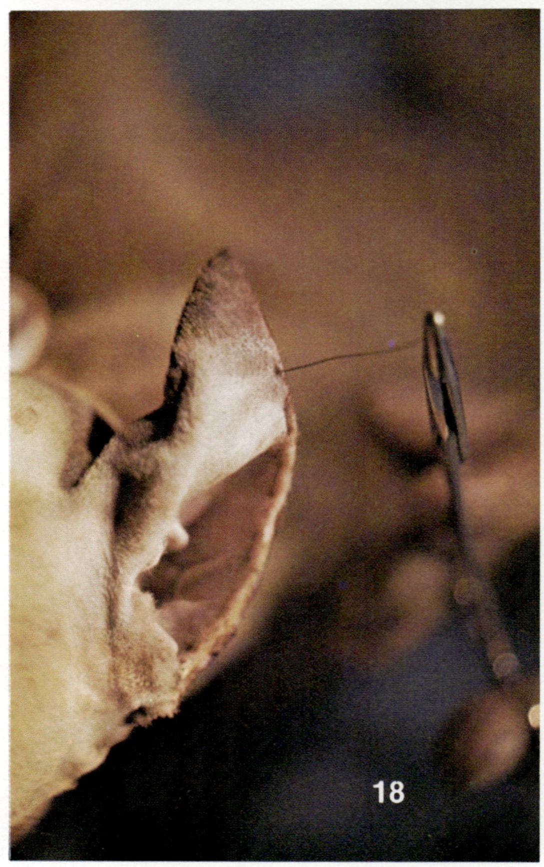

excessive destruction of the normal tissue. This often results in curling of the ear tip during the final stages of healing.

Hemorrhage, usually from the lateral, intermediate, and medial branches of the caudal auricular artery on the outer edge of the ear, is controlled carefully by electrocoagulation (*Figures 8-10*).

The second ear is prepared by aligning against it the portion removed from the other ear and securing it with staples (*Figures 11 & 12*). The ear is then cropped and hemostasis achieved in exactly the same way as for the first crop (*Figures 13 & 14*).

The auricular cartilage at the base of the ear flaps is trimmed to blend smoothly into the head (*Figure 15*).

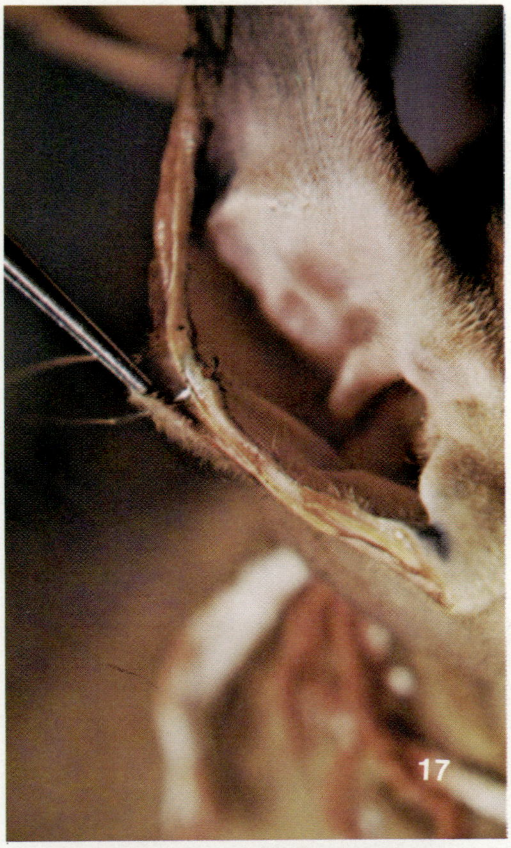

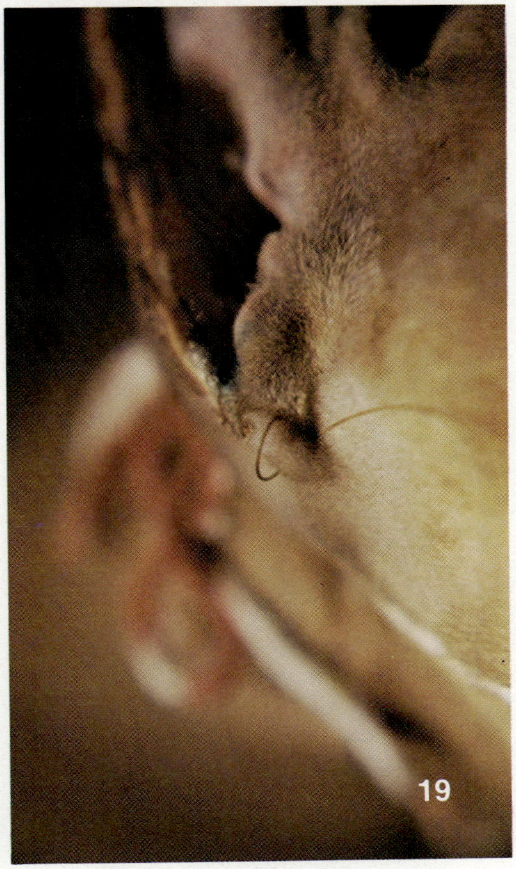

Figures 16-19—The pinnae are sutured. Sutures are not placed in the top third of the ear tip, nor are they knotted. About 2 cm is left at the end of the suture.

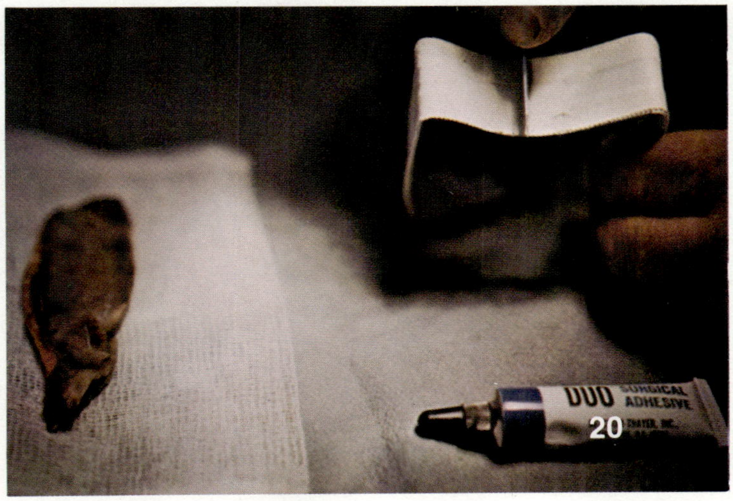

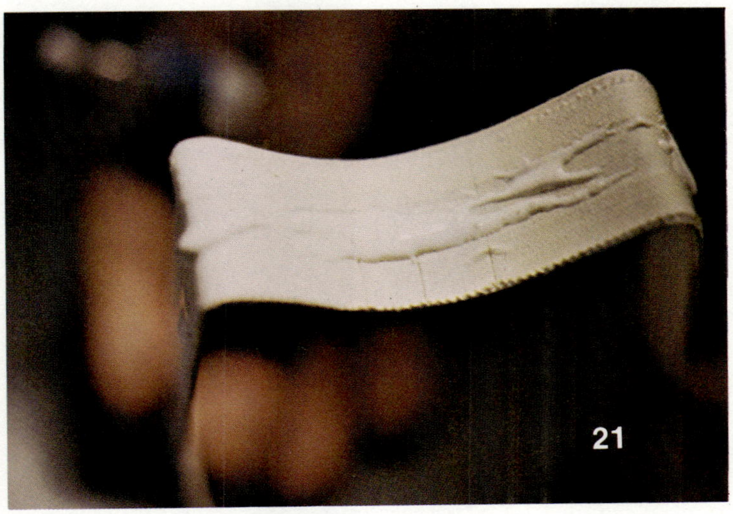

Figures 20 & 21—The ear splint is bent and notched, and surgical adhesive is applied.

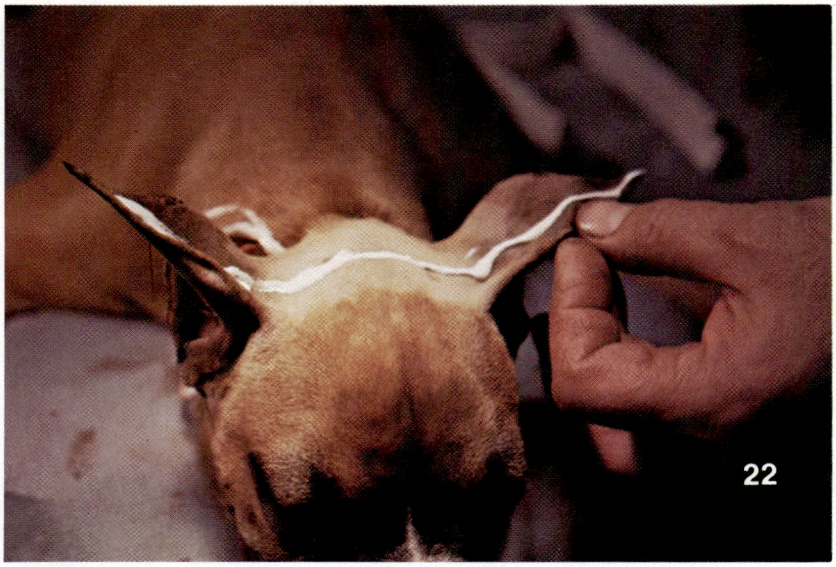

Figures 22-26

The adhesive is allowed to dry partially before the ear splint is applied.

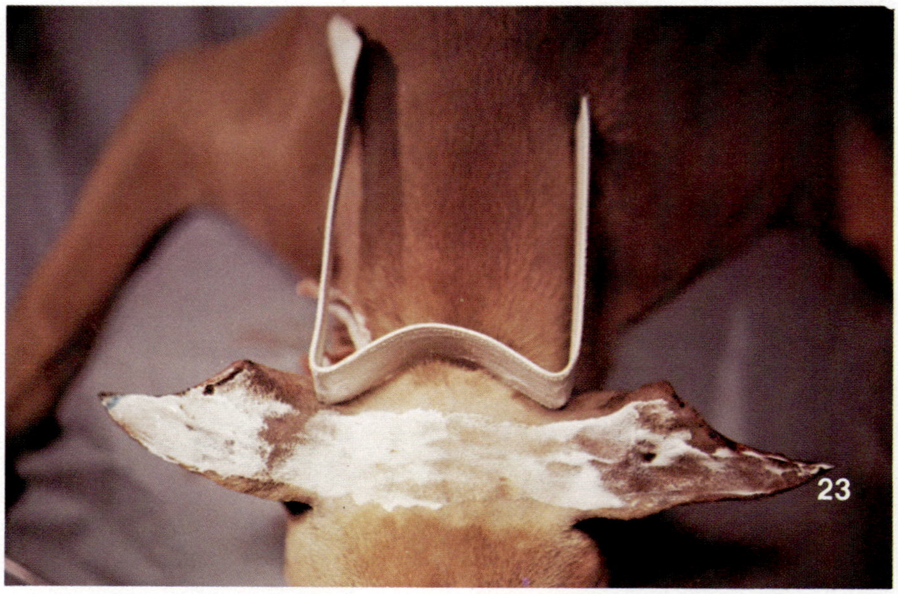

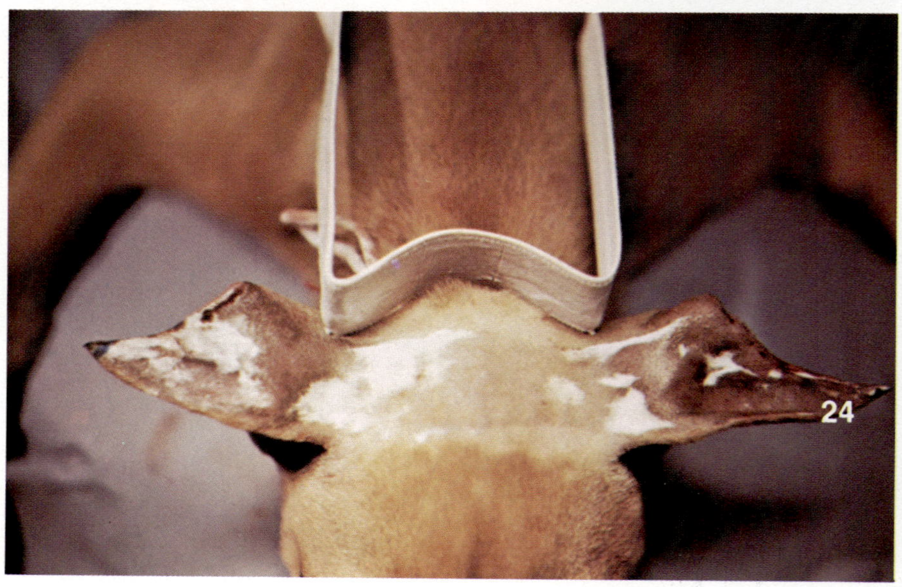

The skin edges of the lower two-thirds of the cropped ear are sutured with 000 chromic gut and a cutting needle, using a simple continuous through-and-through pattern. About 2 cm is left at each end of the suture. These ends are not knotted (*Figures 16-19*). No skin sutures are put in the top third of the crop; this area heals entirely by granulation.

The ear splint is bent to conform to the shape of the top of the head, notched on its concave surface with a scalpel, and coated with surgical adhesive (*Figures 20 & 21*). Surgical adhesive is also spread on top of the dog's head and the top surfaces of the ear flaps. The adhesive is allowed to dry partially before the splint is applied (*Figures 22-26*).

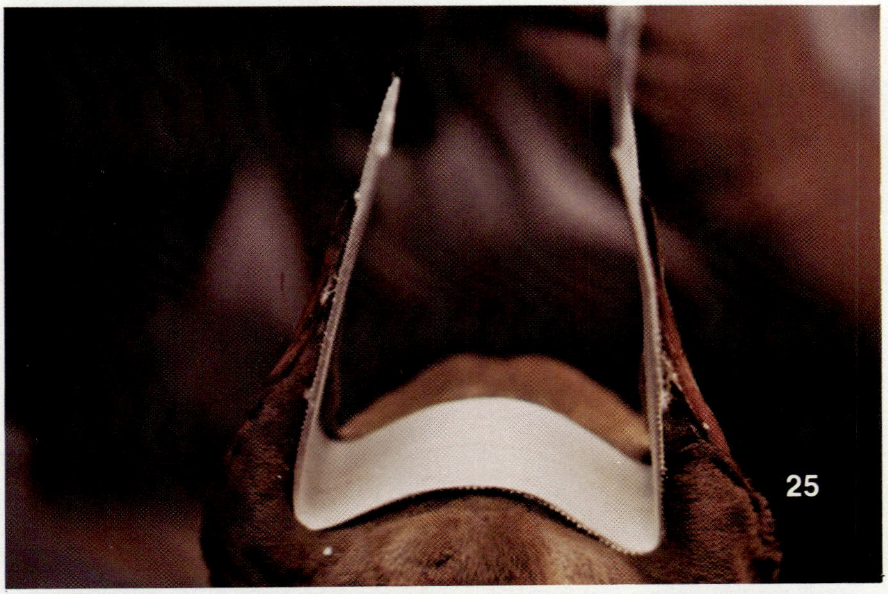

25

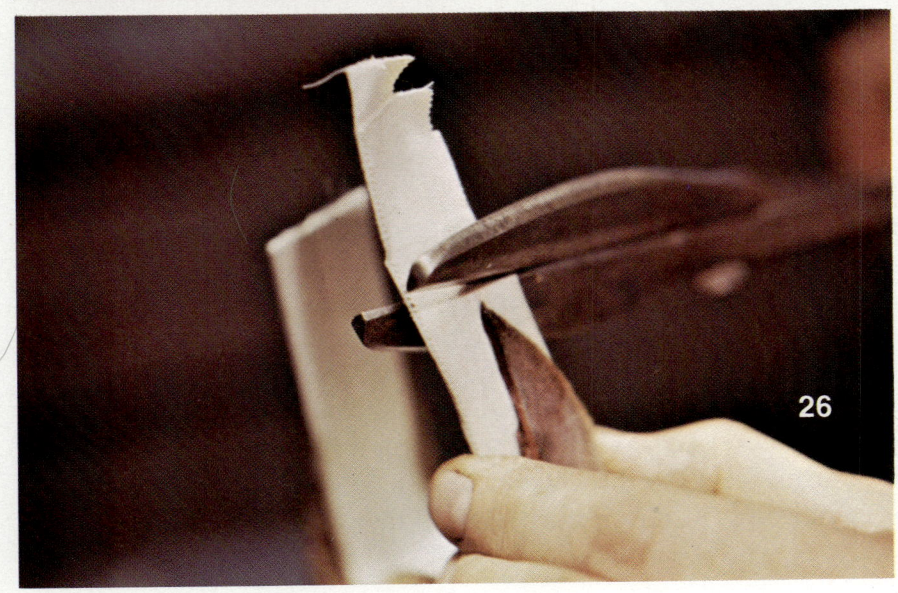

26

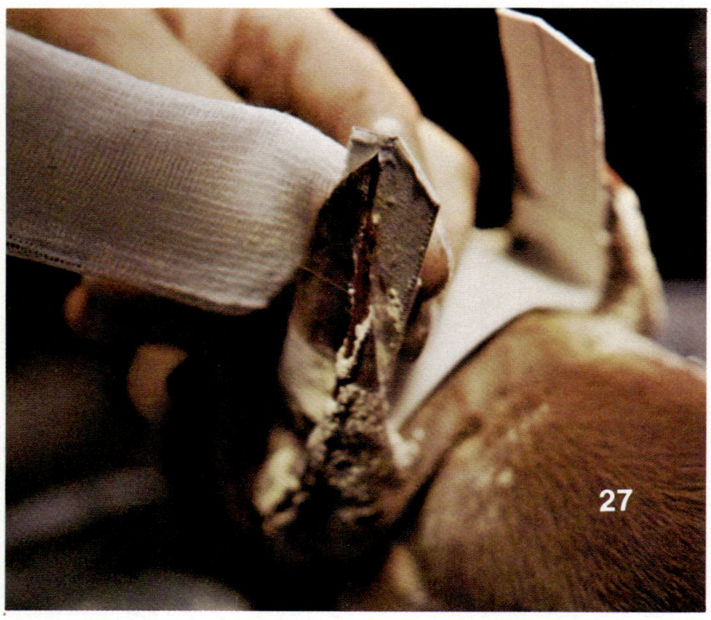

Figure 27
The uncut surface of the ear is taped to the splint.

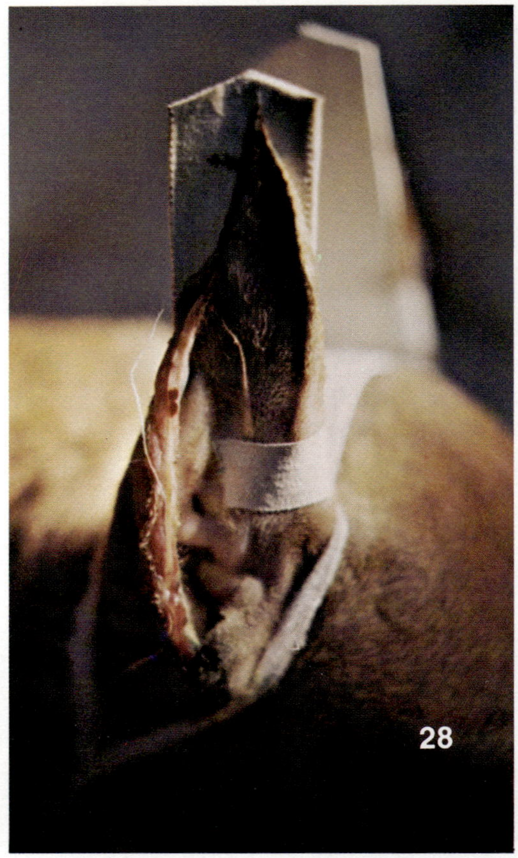

Figure 28
Gauze is wrapped from the uncut to the cut surface.

The erect uncut surface of each ear is taped to the splint. Tape must not be placed over any cut surfaces (*Figure 27*). A temporary gauze bandage is used to secure the pinnae to the splint. The gauze is wrapped from uncut to cut surface (*Figure 28*). A gauze head band is then placed around the base of each ear and secured under the chin (*Figures 29 & 30*). This head band stabilizes the splint during the dog's normal activities until healing is complete.

Postoperative care

Postoperative care consists of administering systemic antibiotics and applying topical nitrofurazone powder (Furacin® —Eaton) to the edges of the ears. If the dog begins scratching its ears, the feet are hobbled to prevent hemorrhage, disruption of the suture line, and destruction of the splint.

Ideally, the splint is left in place for at least two to three weeks until it falls off. If the splint comes off prematurely and the ears are not standing suffi-

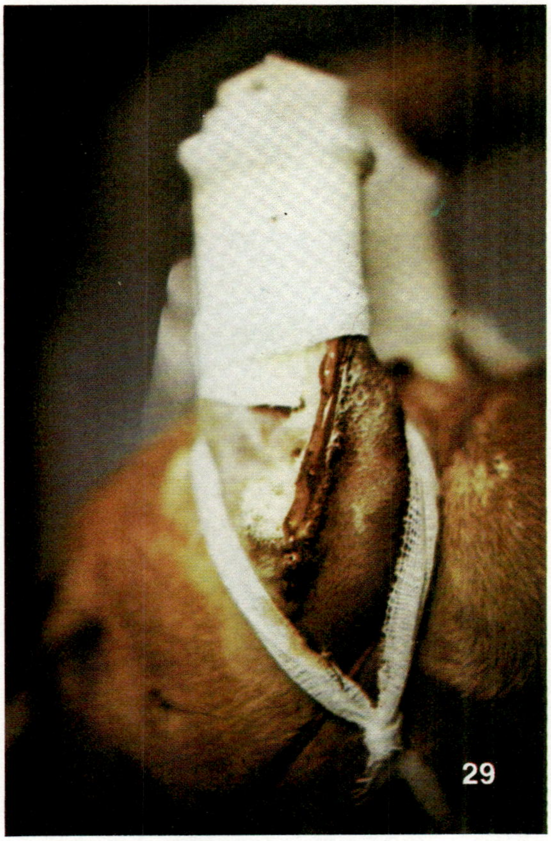

Figures 29 & 30

A gauze strip is attached to the base of the ears and fastened under the chin.

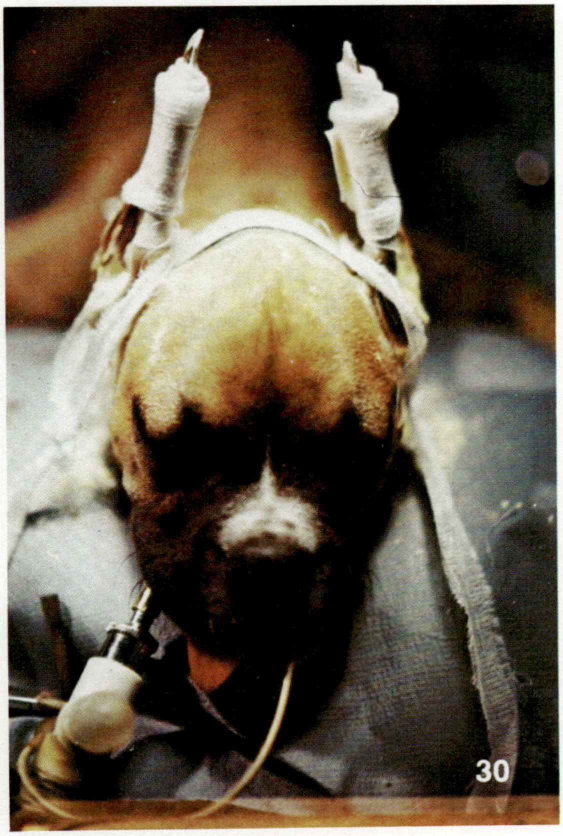

ciently, the splint should be reapplied as previously described. The time required for an ear to stand varies according to breed, conformation, age at cropping, and individual.

The ideal age for cropping puppie's ears is 8 to 11 weeks. Cropping of older dogs usually requires more vigorous postoperative efforts to achieve standing. Cropped ears should be supported until maximal standing has been achieved. Within two weeks the cut edges will heal. Standing may then be aided by instructing the client to stretch the pinnae upward daily.

After this, the client should place a styrofoam cup upside down on the dog's head between the ears and tape the ears to the cup. Since the edges of the ear will have healed, tape may cover the edges without danger of adverse effect.

When the ears are standing unaided, the client may discontinue these measures.

ACKNOWLEDGMENT

The author thanks Donna King and Robin Rogers-Bollinger for their excellent technical assistance.

Resection and anastomosis of the trachea for removal of an intraluminal foreign body

C. Dave Richards, DVM
2905 Bemiss Road
Valdosta, Georgia 31601
W.W. Kallenback, DVM
Cortez Animal Clinic
422 Cortez Road
Bradenton, Florida 33507

TRACHEAL RESECTION AND ANASTOMOSIS is an uncommon surgical procedure in veterinary practice. However, situations arise in which this procedure could be the only means of alleviating a problem.

In this article we describe and depict the removal of a foreign body and associated granulomatous tissue from the trachea of a dog. As the surgical procedure progressed we became convinced that the condition could not be corrected without tracheal resection and anastomosis.

Case History

On December 9, 1976, an 8-month-old mongrel dog, with previous history unknown, was admitted to Veterinary Services at Moody Air Force Base. The presenting complaint was a superficial skin abrasion circling the dog's neck. The new owner assumed the abrasion was caused by a collar fastened too tightly.

During the physical examination, intermittent small draining abscesses were found along the lesion. All other physical findings were normal. The owners were believed to be correct in their assumption regarding the cause of the lesion.

Chloromycetin® (Parke-Davis) was given for seven days. Recovery was uneventful.

On January 20, 1977, the dog was readmitted because of dyspnea and small draining abscesses at the same sites as before. The patient was referred to us for radiography.

When presented, the dog was exhibiting open-mouth breathing with its head and neck in extension. On radiographs, a linear soft-tissue density could be seen crossing the trachea (*Figure 1*).

(Continued on next page)

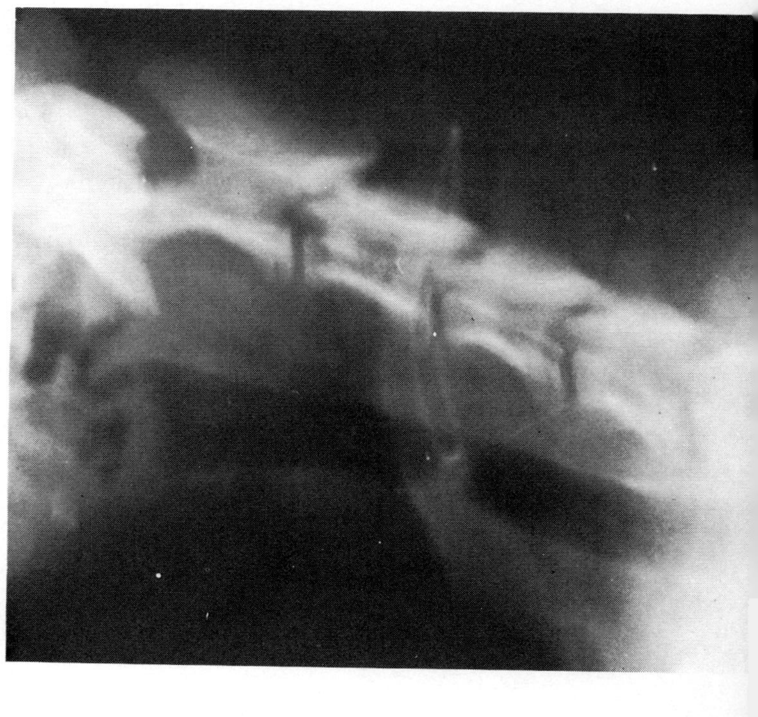

Figure 1—A linear, soft-tissue density interrupts the trachea. Because it contains a small amount of lead, the foreign object (a rubber band) is very apparent on the radiograph.

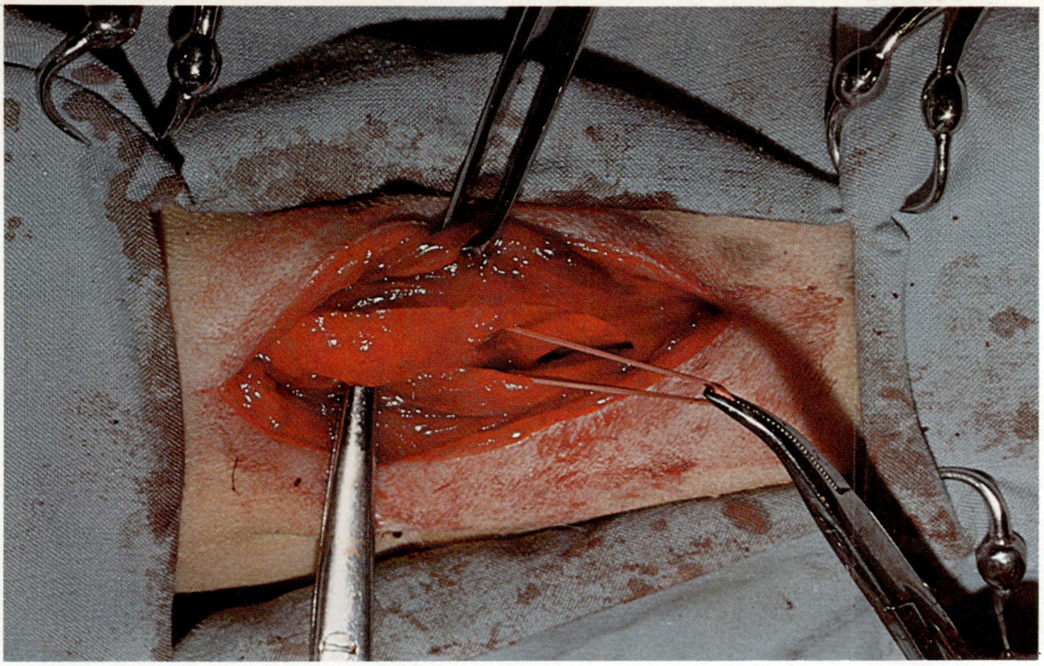

Figure 2
The rubber band is stretched to demonstrate its presence in the lumen of the trachea.

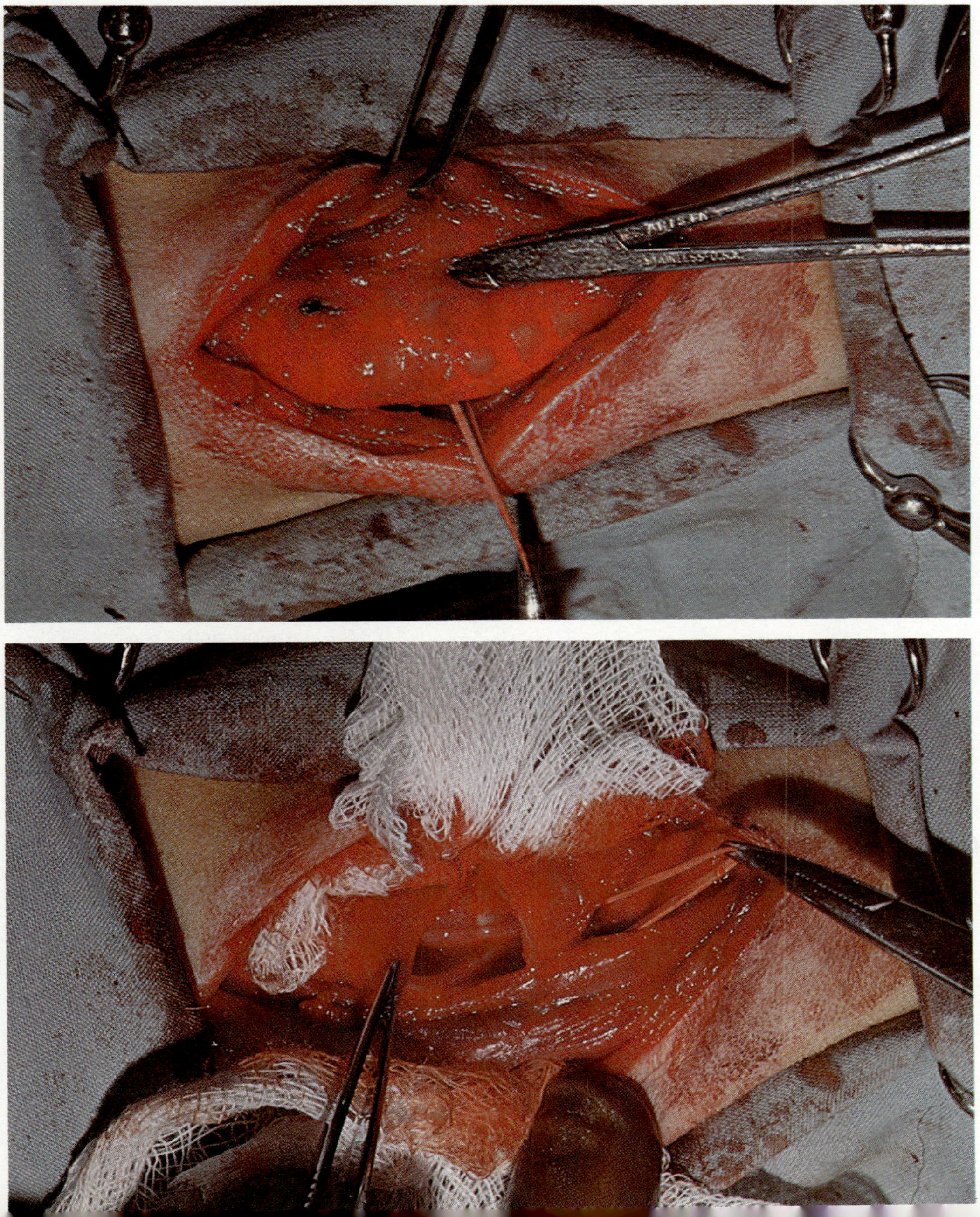

Figures 3 & 4
By blunt dissection the granulomatous tissue is being freed from the normal tissue around the trachea.

After routine induction of preanesthesia, surgical anesthesia was maintained with methoxyflurane (Metofane® —Pitman-Moore). The conventional approach to the ventral aspect of the neck was made. Because of the excessive granulation tissue in the region, the recurrent laryngeal nerve was never isolated.

The granulomatous mass encircling the trachea was bluntly dissected, revealing a rubber band that had perforated the space between two tracheal rings (*Figure 2*). The lumen of the trachea was partially filled with the foreign body and granulomatous tissue. The foreign body and three tracheal rings were removed and the cut ends of the trachea were anastomosed (*Figures 3-10*). Closure was routine. Antibiotics were administered during the recuperative period.

On the return visit to the office for removal of the sutures, the owner complained that the dog

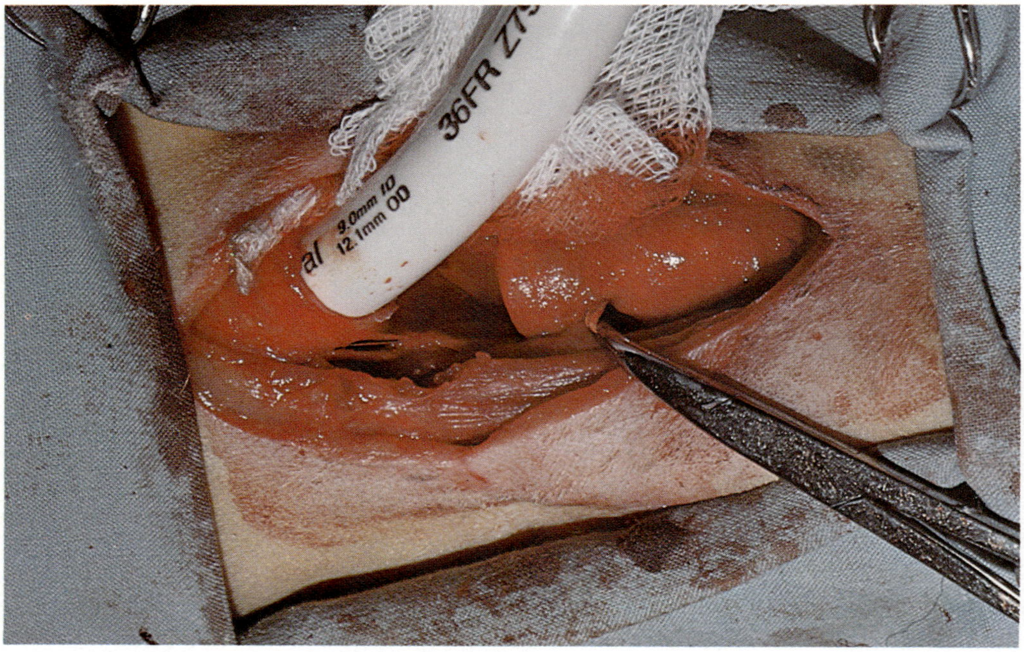

Figure 5
The endotracheal tube has been pulled cranially. The trachea is resected distal to the occlusion and a sterile endotracheal tube is inserted into the distal trachea. This second tube is attached to the anesthesia machine.

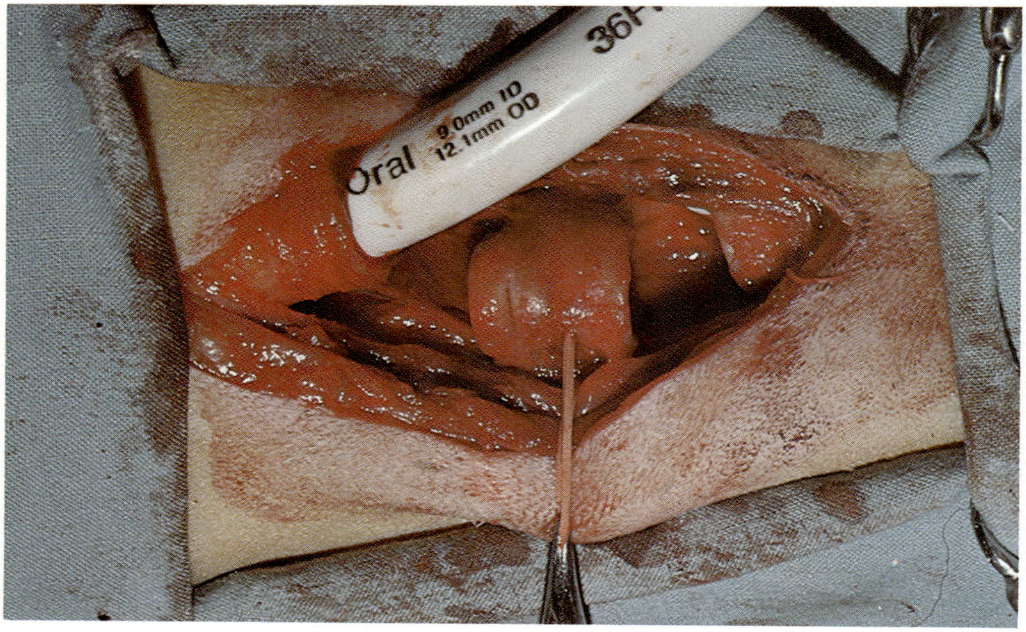

Figure 6
Resection of the affected three tracheal rings has been completed.

constantly made a wheezing noise when inhaling. Radiographs showed no evidence of an air leak at the site of the anastomosis. Increased density in the cardiac lobes of the lung was noted. The decision was made to take no action until the dog had been given more time to recuperate.

Six weeks postoperatively the dog was reexamined and found to be physically normal. The owner reported that the wheezing sound stopped 10 days

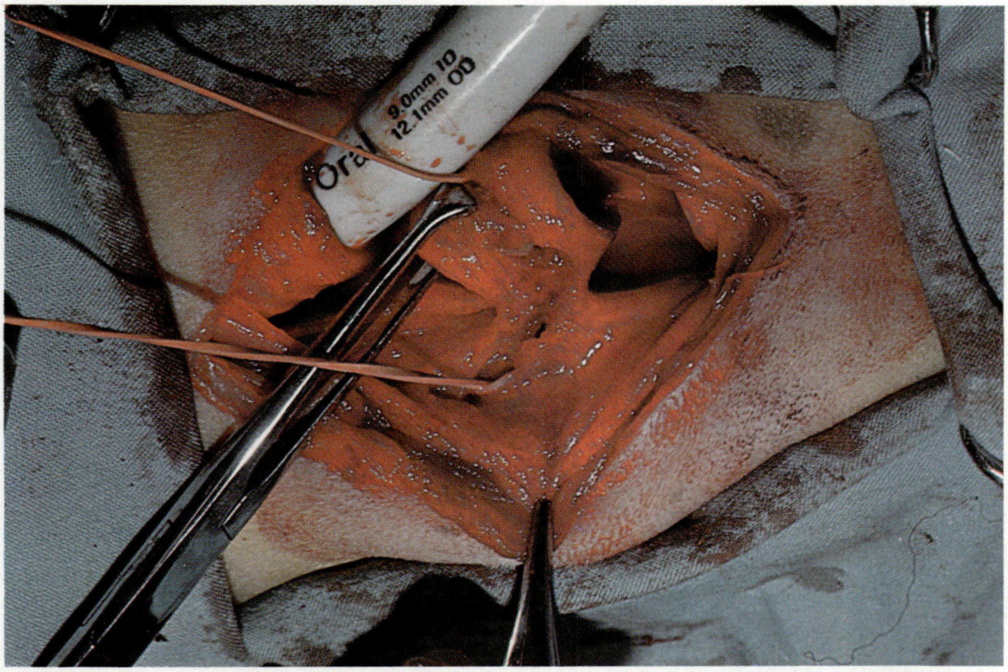

Figure 7
The resected portion of the trachea with the associated foreign body is removed from the surgical field.

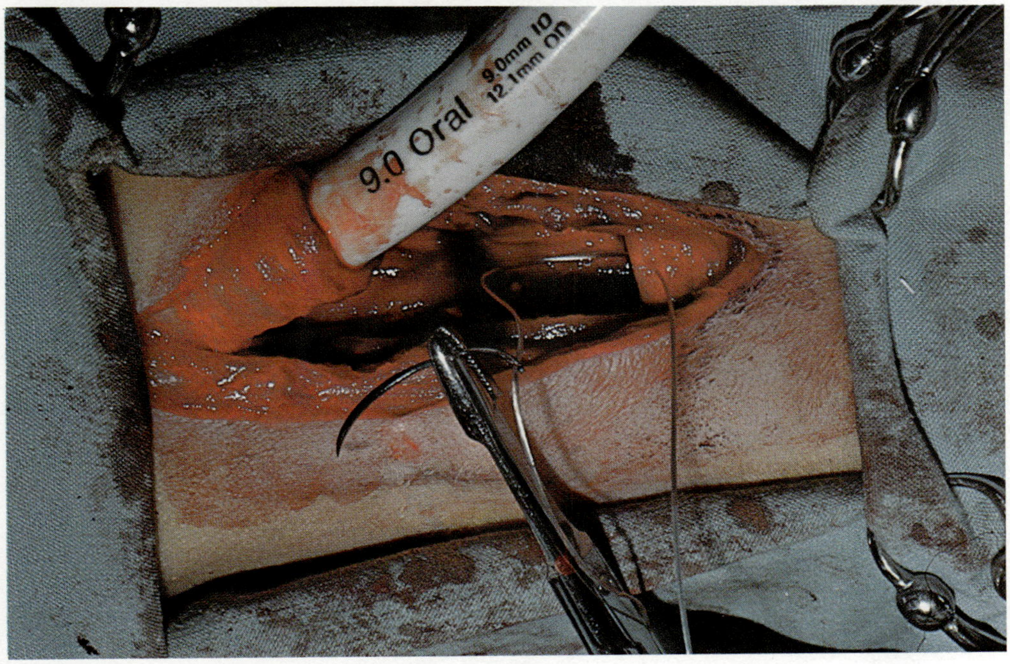

Figure 8
Sutures are placed through and through the cartilage of each apposing end of the trachea.

after the previous visit (20 days after surgery).

At the present time the dog is thriving and appears clinically normal.

Discussion

We were surprised at the lack of readily available information on tracheal resection and anastomosis in the veterinary literature. We were aware of the work being done by Bojrab *et al.*; however, in our emergency situation we had no idea of the complications that could arise from the surgery or even if the procedure had been proven effective. We hope this brief report of our experience will help other practitioners who might be faced with a need to perform similar surgery.

ACKNOWLEDGMENT

Special gratitude is expressed to Mr. Bill Castleberry for the excellent photographs.

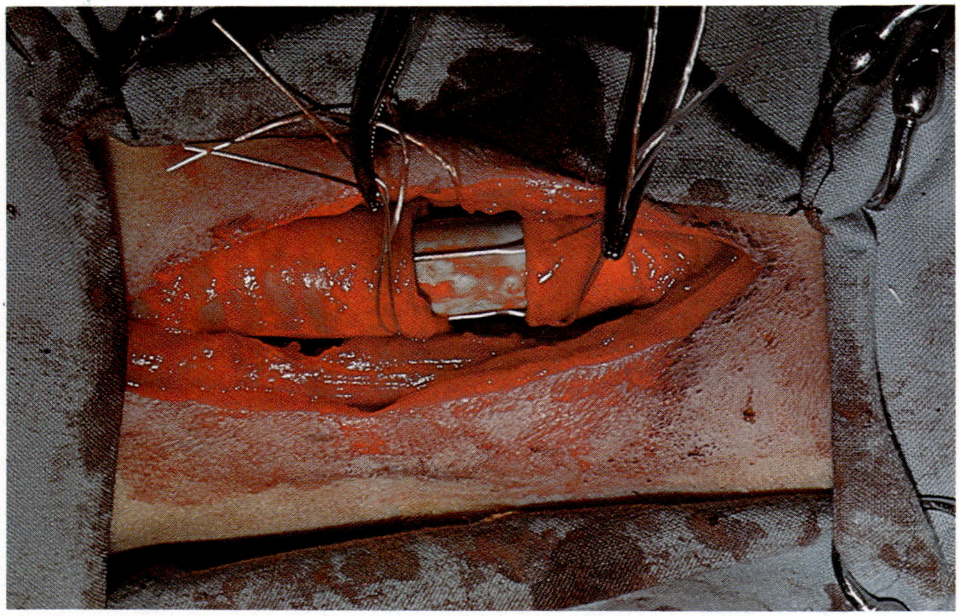

Figure 9
The second endotracheal tube has been removed and the original repositioned in the lumen of the distal segment of the trachea.

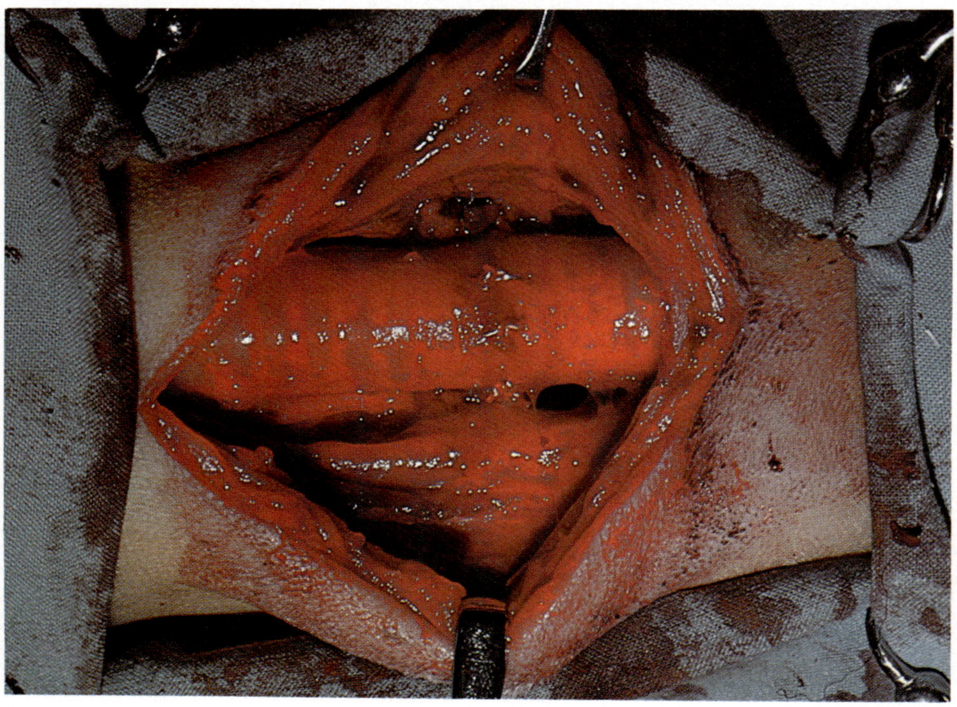

Figure 10
The ends of the anastomosis are apposed. Closure is routine.

GUNSHOT WOUND
in the head of a dog

Mark A. Zimmer, DVM*
Wayne E. Hoppe, DVM
Lakeside Animal Hospital, Ltd.
211 West Bender Road
Glendale, Wisconsin 53217

* Present address: 6904 Oakland Drive, Portage, Mishigan 49801.

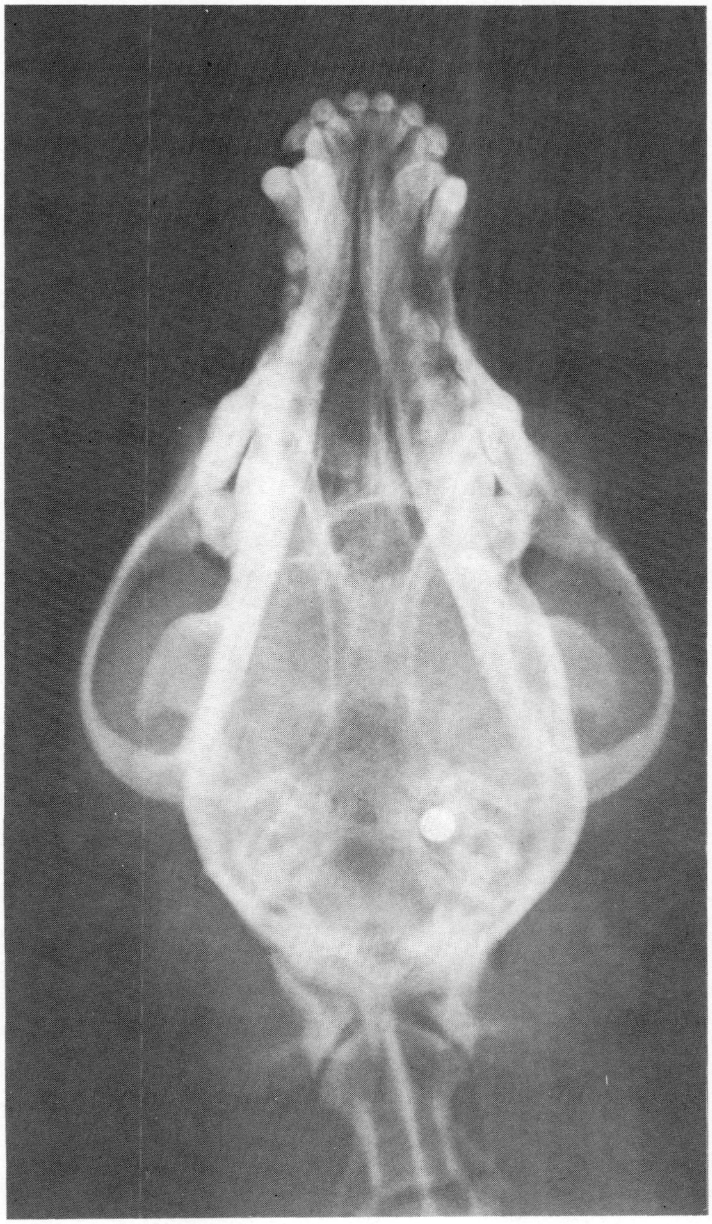

A 4-year-old dog was treated for a gunshot wound of the head which involved the brain. A year and a half after the injury a pellet remains in the animal's brain. Except for loss of vision in one eye, the dog is clinically normal and leading a normal life.

A 4-YEAR-OLD, male Poodle was presented for treatment of a gunshot wound of the head. The dog had been shot with a pellet rifle at close range 10 minutes before admission.

The dog was in shock, vomiting, and extremely ataxic. A puncture wound, where the pellet entered, was noted above the left eye. In addition, epistaxis from the left nostril was evident.

An intravenous catheter was positioned and treatment was begun with Multisol® -R (Abbott) in a dosage for shock. A bolus of 60 mg Solu-Delta-Cortef® (Upjohn) was given and 40 mg was added to the intravenous fluids. When the shock was under control, 0.15 ml Lasix® (National) was given intravenously; 0.5 ml of this was also added to the intravenous fluids. Also to help control cerebral edema, 5 ml dextran 75 (Travenol) was given as an intravenous bolus. A 25-mg dose of Gentocin® (Schering) was given by intramuscular injection.

After the animal's condition stabilized, radiographs of the head were taken. These showed the pellet lodged in the dog's brain (*Figures 1A & 1B*). During the next four days, dexamethasone (Med-Tech) and Gentocin were given by injection. The emesis gradually subsided, so medication by mouth was started with chloramphenicol (25 mg/lb) and

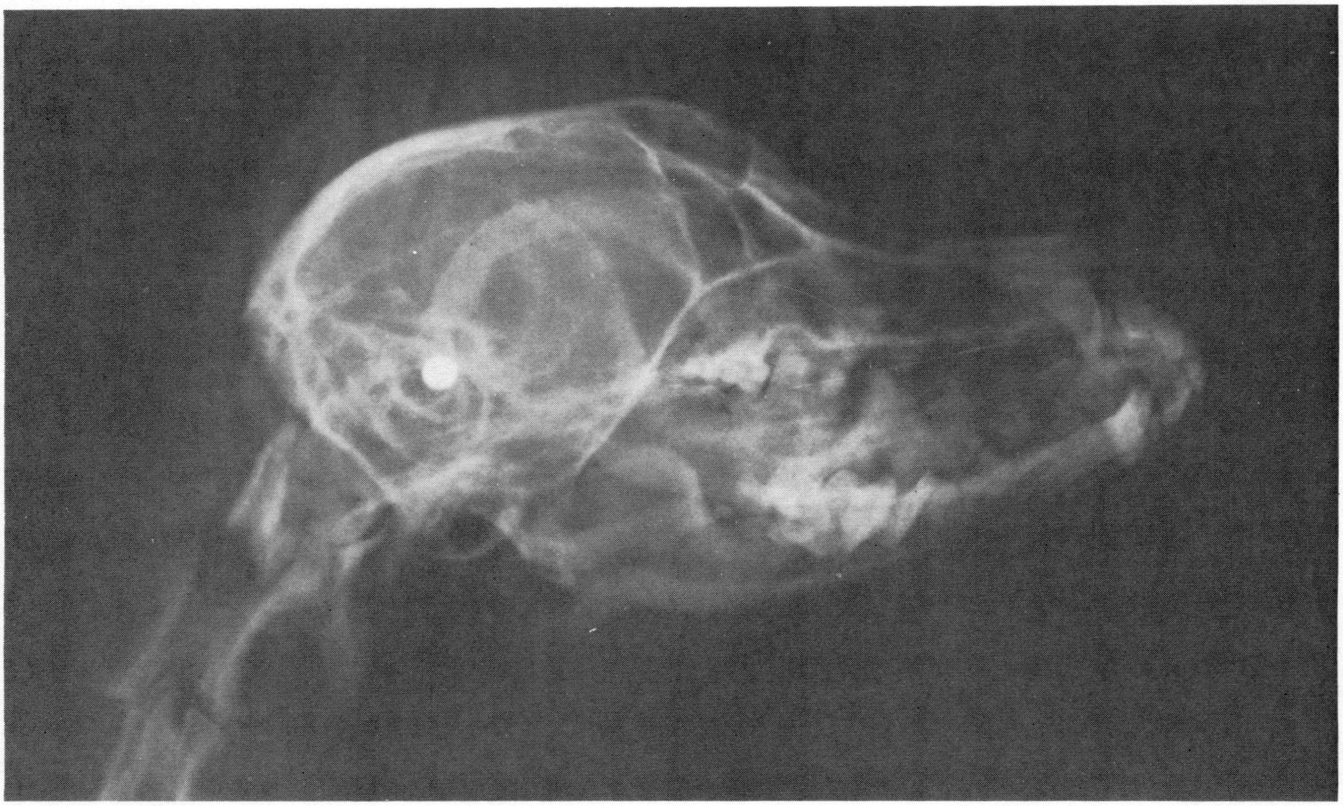

Figures 1A & 1B
Lateral and dorsoventral radiographic views of the head of a 4-year-old Poodle showing a shot pellet lodged in the brain.

decreasing doses of dexamethasone.

Over a period of several weeks, the dog began to function and behave almost normally. Eighteen months after the incident the dog can ambulate normally, shows no personality change, and is as alert and active as before the shooting. The Poodle has no vision in the left eye, but functional vision provided by the right eye is sufficient for the dog's usual activities.

Discussion

The entry of the pellet through the left frontal sinus caused the unilateral epistaxis. As inferred from the clinical signs, the pellet then entered the cranium and passed through the optic nerve; hence the lack of vision in the left eye. The pellet finally lodged in the ventral portion of the cranial vault. Because of the dog's relatively quick response to the initial treatment, we can assume that no major cerebral vascular supply was damaged.

The treatment for cerebral edema and possible infection was sufficiently successful to let us return a near normal pet to the owner. Radiographs taken one year after the incident indicate that the pellet has not migrated. This seems to presage a healthy and active life for this dog. ■

DERMOID SINUS in a Rhodesian Ridgeback

John T. Hathcock, DVM
Edwin G. Clampett, DVM
Richard V. Broadstone, DVM
University Blvd. Animal Hospital
5150 University Blvd., W.
Jacksonville, Florida 32216

THE DERMOID SINUS of the Rhodesian Ridgeback dog appears as an abnormal opening of the skin on the dorsal midline.[1] A tube-like sinus, which extends toward the spinal column, may end blindly at any level from just under the skin, down to the supraspinous ligament, or beyond to the dura mater.[2] Characteristically, tufts of hair protrude from the opening of the sinus in the skin. Modified skin that contains hair follicles and sebaceous

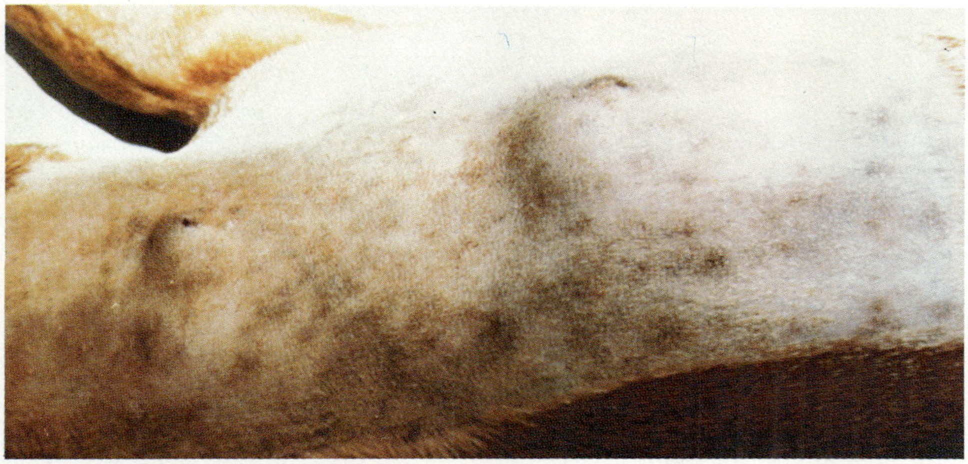

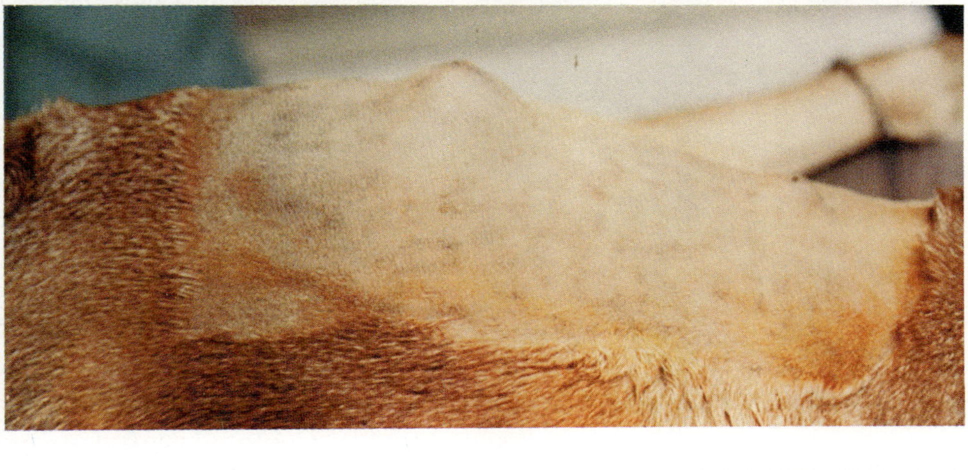

Figures 1 & 2
The dermoid cysts after the hair was clipped from around them.

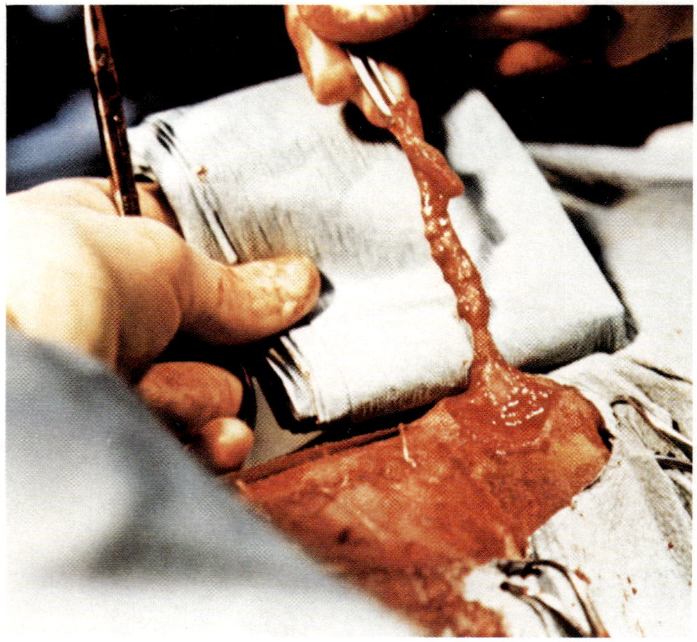

Figure 3—A tuft of hair protrudes from the smaller cyst.

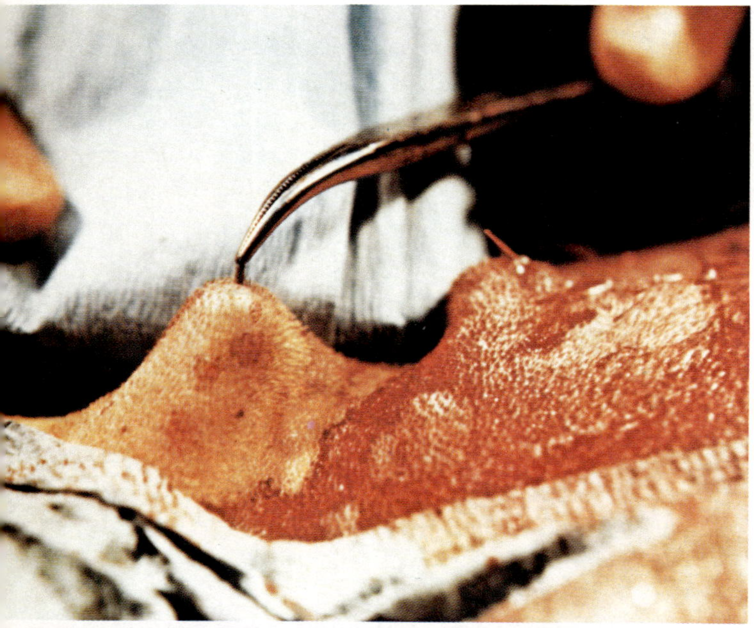

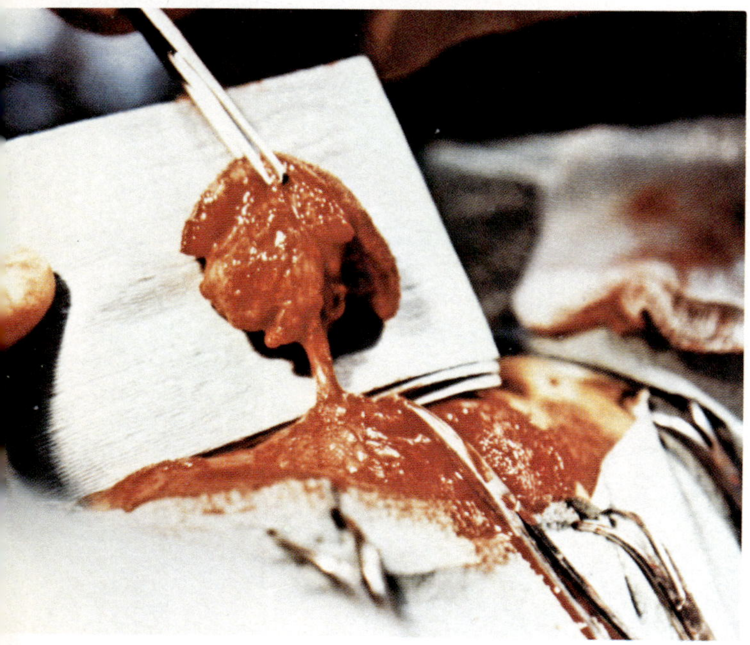

Figure 4—Dissection of the larger cyst and isolation of the sinus.

glands lines the sinus tract. Consequently, the lumen of the sinus may contain hair and sebum.[3]

The dermoid sinus is a congenital defect caused by incomplete separation of the spinal cord and the skin from the ectodermal layer during embryonic development. Data concerning the heritabilty of the defect suggest that it may be inherited as a simple recessive gene.[2]

Surgical excision is usually curative. However, because the attachments of the sinus are sometimes deep, complete surgical excision is not always possible.[2,3] Strict asepsis should be observed during surgery because the sinus is sometimes attached to the dura mater.[1]

Case Report

A 4-month-old female Rhodesian Ridgeback was presented because of two swellings on top of its neck. These swellings, first noticed when the dog was about 8 weeks old, had become larger and drained intermittently.

When the dog was examined closely, two draining cysts of different sizes were found on the dorsal cervical midline. The smaller cyst was situated at a site approximately dorsal to C3-4. The larger cyst was at about C6-7 (*Figures 1 & 2*). Although the cysts were in the

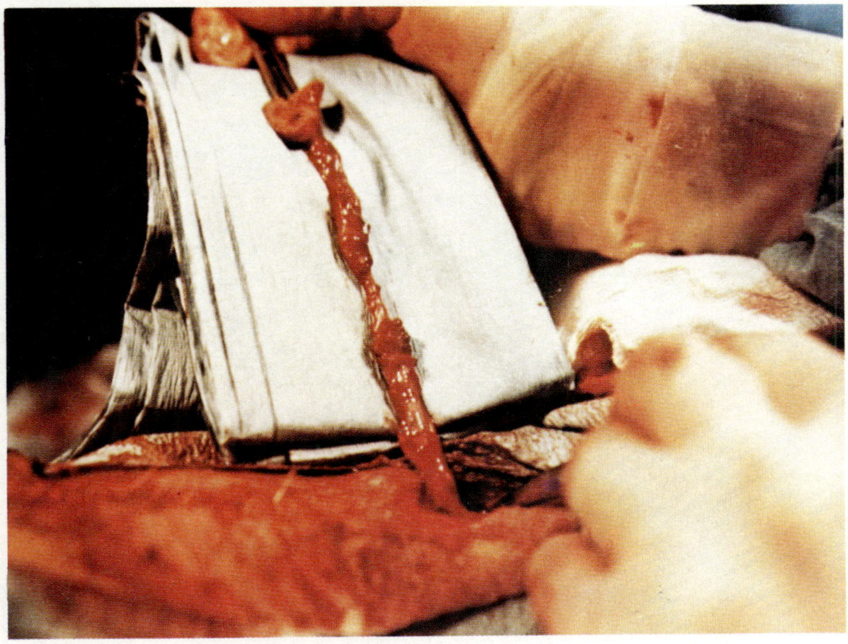

Figures 5-7
The smaller cyst and sinus at various stages of dissection. The length of the sinus tract can be seen.

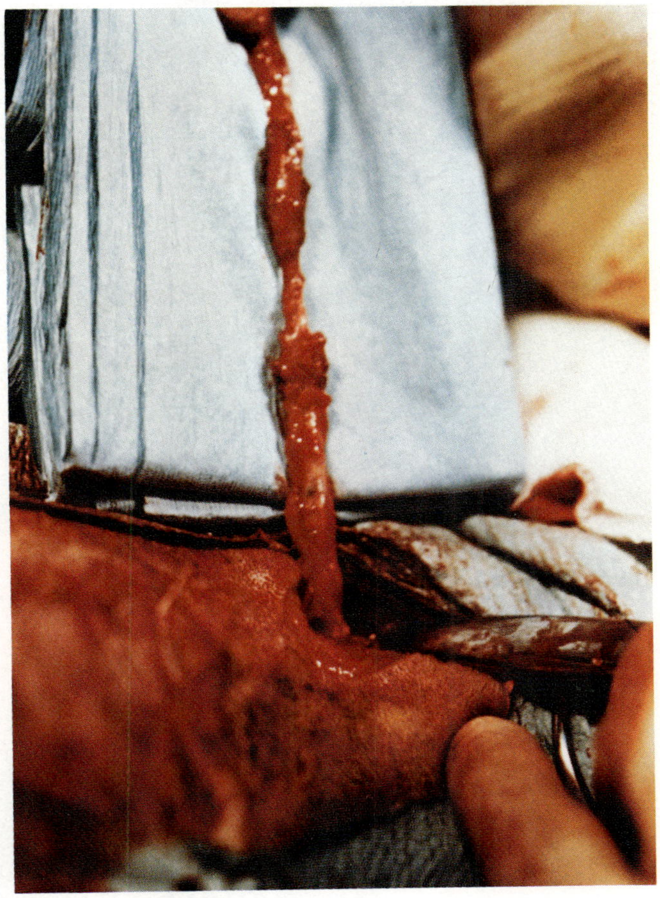

subcutaneous tissue, a tough, tube-like structure, which extended beneath the cysts into the cervical musculature, could be palpated. Small tufts of hair protruded from the openings of the cysts (*Figure 3*). A tentative diagnosis of dermoid sinus was made and surgical removal was recommended.

The hair was clipped and the area prepared routinely for aseptic surgery. An elliptical skin incision was made around the larger cyst. Blunt dissection around the cyst was begun and the sinus tract was isolated (*Figure 4*). Blunt dissection around the sinus continued through the cervical musculature, down to the supraspinous ligament, and the tract was removed. The smaller cyst and sinus were removed in the same way (*Figures 5-7*). Closure of the incisions was routine.

Postoperative care consisted of antibiotics, drainage of accumulated serum, and treatment of self-trauma caused by the dog scratching the surgical site with its rear legs. The surgical wound healed routinely.

When the cysts and sinus tracts were opened, hair and an oily greenish-yellow exudate were seen (*Figures 8-10*). Findings of histopathology were compatible with the tentative diagnosis of dermoid sinus. *(Continued)*

ACKNOWLEDGMENTS

The authors thank R.E. Thompson for his assistance with the photography, and E. Pritchard and T.L. Gandy for their assistance in preparing the manuscript.

REFERENCES

1. Muller, G.H.; Kirk, R.W.: Dermoid Sinus. *Small Animal Dermatology*, 2nd ed. W.B. Saunders Co., Philadelphia, Pa.. 1976; pp 482-483.
2. Mann, G.E.; Stratton, J.: Dermoid Sinus in the Rhodesian Ridgeback. *J. Sm. Anim. Prac.* 7:631-642; 1966.
3. Antin, I.P.: Dermoid Sinus in a Rhodesian Ridgeback Dog. *JAVMA 157*:961-962; 1970.

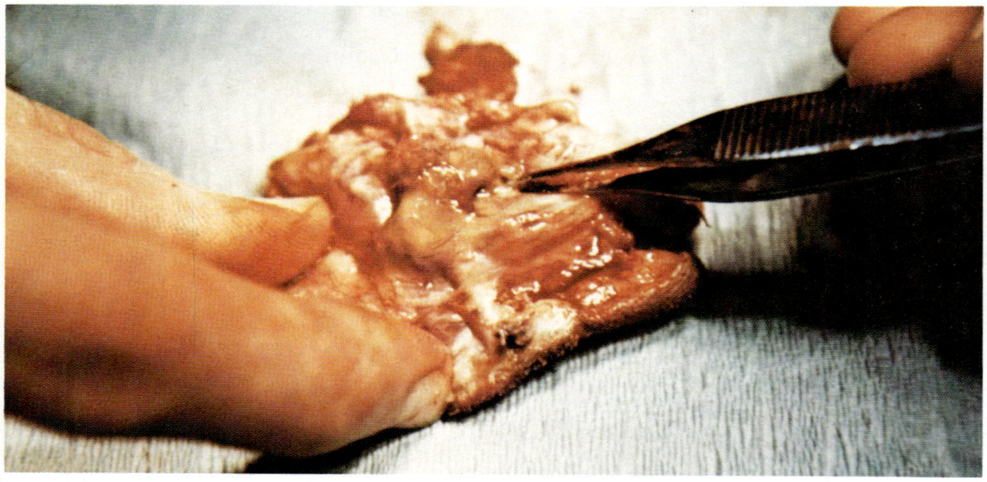

Figures 8-10
Opening the cyst and the sinus. Note the accumulation of hair and sebum.

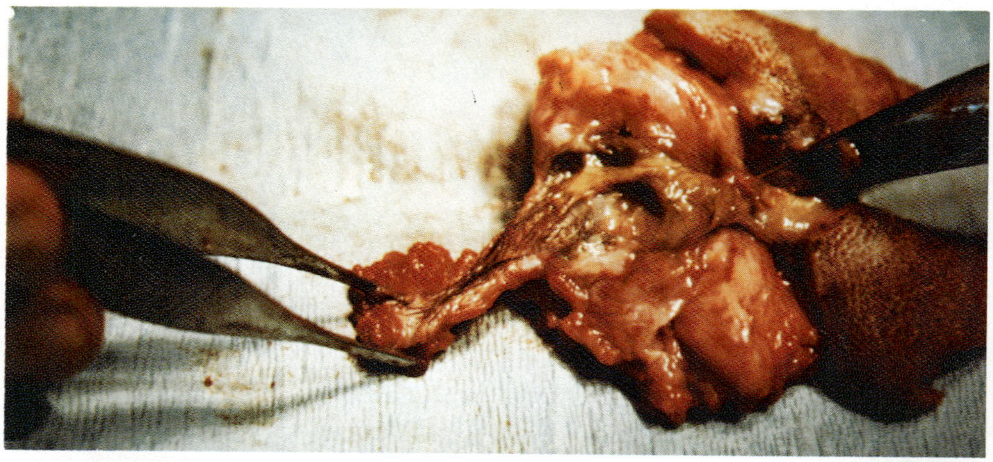

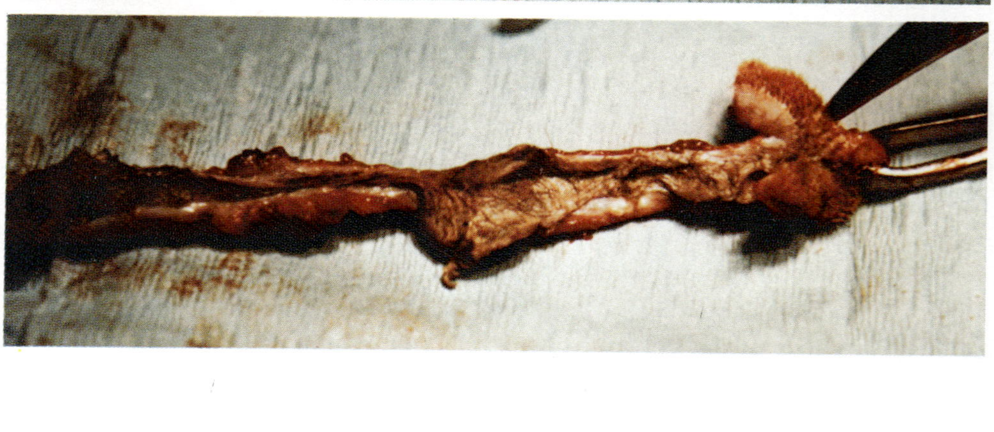

effects of postsurgical ligation of a

TRANSPOSED PAROTID DUCT

E.L. Kuhns, DVM, MS
2754 Burlingame, SW
Wyoming, Michigan 49509
W.F. Keller, DVM, MS
Professor and Chairman
Dept. of Small Animal Surgery and Medicine
Michigan State University
East Lansing, Michigan 48824

Ligation of a transposed parotid salivary duct at a point near its entrance into the cul-de-sac was accomplished without untoward effects on the parotid salivary gland. This procedure was indicated in 2 dogs in which excessive parotid secretion caused undesirable complications.

TRANSPOSITION of the parotid salivary duct and its use as an effective means of managing keratoconjunctivitis sicca has been described.[1-5] Various degrees of pathology may develop in the cornea as a result of excessive accumulation of mineral deposits from the transposed parotid duct. Concurrently, severe blepharospasm and matting of facial hair may also occur. In certain cases, stopping secretion from the parotid gland would be beneficial when persistent, uncontrollable complications occur. Several options that may be considered to accomplish this are as follows: 1) Retransposition of the salivary duct from the affected eye back into the buccal cavity. 2) Surgical removal of the involved parotid salivary gland. 3) Ligation of the parotid duct at a site before it enters the conjunctival sac.

Case No. 1

A 2-year-old male Yorkshire Terrier had a severe unilateral keratoconjunctivitis sicca of the right eye that had been present at least one year. For several months, artificial tears were instilled, topical antibiotic-steroid preparations were applied, and intermittent supportive therapy was given. Despite these measures, tear production continued to fluctuate between zero and 2 mm/minute as determined by Schirmer tear test strips.

Transposition of the parotid duct was successfully accomplished. Then, for 11 months, secretion by the parotid gland was so excessive that one of the three options described above became necessary. Accumulations of grayish-white mineral from the parotid secretion could be scraped from the eyelids and lifted from the cornea in small plaques measuring 3 to 5 mm in diameter. The secretions constantly soaked the patient from the eye to the right forefoot, causing an offensive odor. Pain was manifested by a persistent blepharospasm.

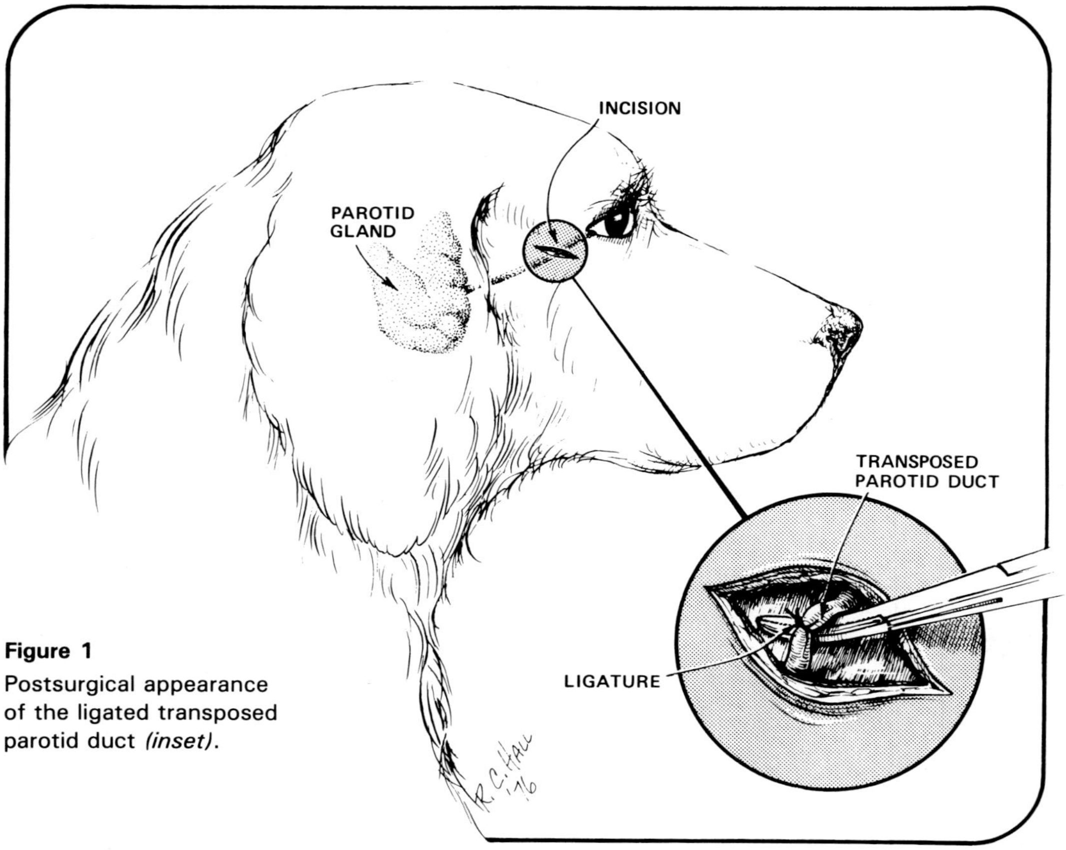

Figure 1
Postsurgical appearance of the ligated transposed parotid duct *(inset)*.

Eleven months after transposition of the parotid duct, the keratopathy, including edema, was so severe that the pupil and anterior chamber could not be seen under any type of illumination. A decision was made to stop the secretion from the parotid gland by ligating the parotid duct.

After the patient was given a preanesthetic agent and intubated, gas anesthesia was administered via a closed system. The hair ventral and adjacent to the lateral canthus was clipped and the operative site was scrubbed and draped.

A short strand of 4-0 Vetafil® (S. Jackson) was inserted into the parotid papilla within the cul-de-sac. This helped identify the duct by making it more rigid. A horizontal skin incision was made approximately 1.5 cm ventrolateral to the lateral canthus (*Figure 1*). By moving the strand of Vetafil, the duct could be easily found within the subcutaneous tissues.

The duct was isolated by blunt dissection, the tip of a mosquito forceps was introduced beneath it, and the duct was ligated with 4-0 Vetafil. Closure was completed with an interrupted suture pattern of 4-0 silk.

Immediately after the patient had recovered from the anesthetic, the excessive salivary flow had ceased and the cornea began to show signs of dryness. The next day the patient was discharged and artificial tears were dispensed to be administered several times daily.

When the patient was returned after one week for removal of the sutures, examination of the affected eye revealed a normal cornea. The edema was gone, the pupil and anterior chamber were easily viewed, and the facial hair ventral to the eye was dry. No signs of blepharospasm or discomfort were present.

Normal lacrimation had spontaneously recurred in this dog at some time after the parotid duct was transposed. This explains the rapid recovery of the cornea after ligation of the functional parotid duct. All medication, including the artificial tears, was discontinued and the eye remains normal after one year.

Case No. 2

Transposition of both parotid ducts was performed on a 6-year-old male Maltese suffering from chronic keratoconjunctivitis sicca. At the time of surgery, the animal was blind and had no normal corneal tissue. The surgery was performed in an effort to make the animal comfortable. From this standpoint, the surgery proved successful.

One year later the left eye was becoming phthisical and apparently painful. The decision was made to enucleate this eye. During this surgery the parotid duct was identified and ligated approximately 0.5 inch from its attachment to the conjunctiva. The ligation was completed using 4-0 surgical gut.

The postoperative period was without incident. During the two years of observation after surgery, neither swelling nor drainage occurred as a result of the parotid-duct ligation.

Conclusions

Three significant points may be inferred from these cases: 1) Normal lacrimation may recur spontaneously after prolonged absence. 2) Pathologic changes of the cornea may be rapidly reversed if physiologic factors such as lacrimation return to a normal state. 3) The transposed parotid duct may be ligated without undesirable consequences.

ACKNOWLEDGMENT

The authors thank medical artist, Rick Hall, for his contributions to this article.

REFERENCES

1. Baker, G.J.; Formston, C.: An Evaluation of Transplantation of the Parotid Duct in the Treatment of Keratoconjunctivitis Sicca in the Dog. *J. Small Anim. Prac.* 9:261-268; 1968.
2. Gelatt, K.N.: Treatment of Canine Keratoconjunctivitis Sicca by Parotid Duct Transposition. *JAAHA* 6:1-12; 1970.
3. Glen, J.B.; Lawson, D.D.: Modified Technique of Parotid Duct Transposition. *Vet. Rec.* 88(8):210-213; 1971.
4. Lavignette, A.M.: Keratoconjunctivitis Sicca Treated by Parotid Duct Transposition. *JAVMA 148*(7):778-786; 1966.
5. Magrane, E.G.: *Canine Ophthalmology*, 2nd Ed. Lea & Febiger, Philadelphia, Pa., 1971; pp 111-115.

Catheter Technique for Removing a Foreign Body from the Canine Esophagus

Richard S. Hawe, DVM
Alexandria Animal Hospital
2660 Duke Street
Alexandria, Virginia 22314

THE PREFERRED TREATMENT for removing a foreign body from the esophagus of the dog is a matter of opinion.[1-4] The choice of method should be based on the individual case, the type of foreign body to be removed, the available equipment, and the surgeon's skill. Current methods of management include conservative treatment, which involves esophagoscopy and removal of the foreign body with forceps, and surgery.[1-4]

Esophagoscopy and removal of the foreign body with forceps has been shown to be safe and effective.[2] The consensus is that this conservative approach should be attempted before surgical intervention.[1-4] However, the conservative treatment has disadvantages. In very small animals, esophagoscopy can be difficult. When the necessity of removing a foreign body is added, the procedure becomes even more challenging because of the limit on the size of the instruments that can be used. Smooth spherical objects may be difficult to grasp by endoscopic means because a suitable retrieving instrument is not available.[5,6] When conventional foreign-body forceps are used, the mucosa of the esophagus may be grasped inadvertently. If more than gentle traction is required to remove a foreign body, efforts employing the esophagoscope should be abandoned because perforation is probable.

Esophageal surgery can be trying due to lack of serosa, constant motility, segmental blood supply, and difficult exposure.[1] Potential postsurgical problems are formation of stricture and leakage through the incision.[7] Pneumonia, mediastinitis, pleuritis, and pyothorax can result from dehiscence.[2,4]

Foley urethral catheters have been used in man to extract esophageal foreign bodies.[5,6,8-11] This technique has also been mentioned in the veterinary literature.[2] Described here is the use of Foley urethral catheters as an alternative method for removing a foreign body from the canine esophagus.

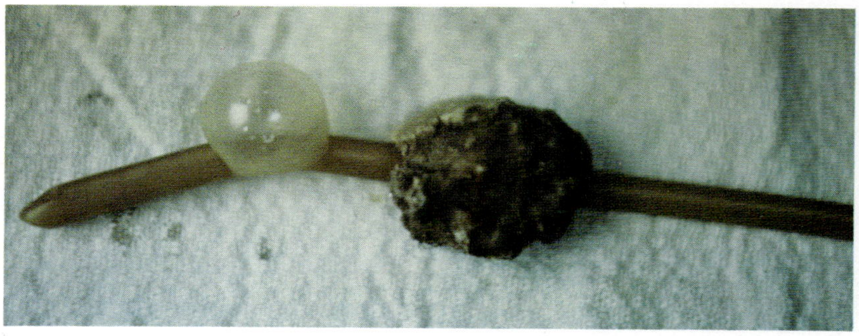

Figure 1—*In vitro* demonstration of the proper relationship of the catheter balloon to the foreign body. When traction is applied to the catheter, the balloon acts as a shelf on which the foreign body rests as it is lifted out of the esophagus.

Indications and procedures

Clinical signs of esophageal foreign bodies are ptyalism, progressive dysphagia, and persistent regurgitation of undigested food or quantities of alkaline mucus. Ptyalism in an animal with a recent history of anorexia and regurgitation should be considered highly suggestive of a foreign body in the esophagus. Rabies also must be considered in the differential diagnosis, since clinical signs may be similar.[1] A diagnosis of esophageal foreign body can be confirmed radiographically.

Whenever possible, esophagoscopy should be performed. This allows an evaluation of the position and shape of the foreign body and the condition of the esophageal mucosa. Such information can be invaluable in determining the choice of therapy. If a blunt esophageal foreign body is seen, especially a smooth one, extraction can be accomplished with a catheter.

A urethral catheter of appropriate size (No. 8 to No. 14 F Foley) is introduced through the mouth and into the esophagus until the balloon passes the obstruction. The balloon is then filled with water-soluble contrast medium, the amount depending on the size of the patient. A lateral radiograph is taken to verify the position of the catheter. Inflation of the balloon causes the esophagus to dilate and thereby release its grip on the foreign body.

The mobility of the foreign body should be tested with gentle traction on the catheter before extraction begins. If the object moves easily, the catheter is gently withdrawn and the foreign object rides up the esophagus on the balloon, which acts as a shelf (*Figure 1*). If the balloon slips past the foreign body, it is deflated and the procedure is repeated. Trial-and-error inflation of the balloon before passage of the catheter allows an estimation to be made of how much the balloon should be inflated and ensures symmetrical inflation of the balloon (*Figure 2*).

In some cases adequate dilation of the esophagus requires the passage of two catheters. In evaluating the procedure to be used for removing an esophageal foreign body, one must remember that these bodies tend to lodge at sites where the esophagus cannot fully dilate. These sites are the cricopharyngeal sphincter, the thoracic inlet, the base of the heart, and the esophageal hiatal region.[1-3]

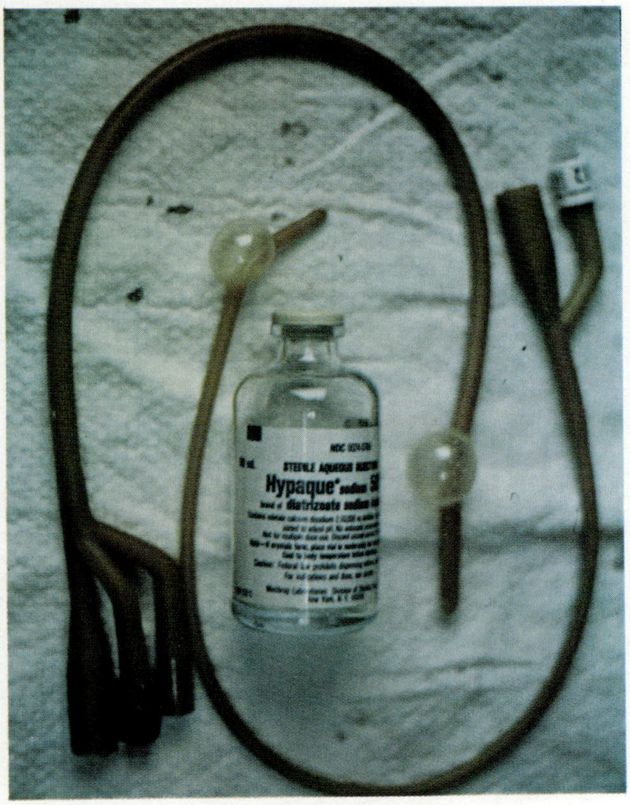

Figure 2—Catheter balloons inflated with water-soluble contrast medium. Symmetrically inflated balloons are more desirable.

Case report

A 10-year-old male Scottish Terrier was presented because of retching, sialorrhea, anorexia, and depression of four days' duration. The dog's attempts to eat were evidently painful and resulted in immediate regurgitation of undigested food and mucus. However, liquids were swallowed without difficulty.

Findings of the physical examination were unremarkable, but they confirmed the presence of the signs described in the history. A tentative diagnosis of esophageal obstruction was made and survey radiographs of the esophagus were taken.

Lateral and ventrodorsal radiographs showed a bone lying just cranial to the base of the heart in the area of the cranial mediastinal esophagus (*Figures 3 & 4*). The lungs appeared normal.

The dog was anesthetized, intubated, and laid in lateral recumbency. A lubricated endoscope was passed down the esophagus to the level of the obstruction. Esophagoscopy confirmed the pres-

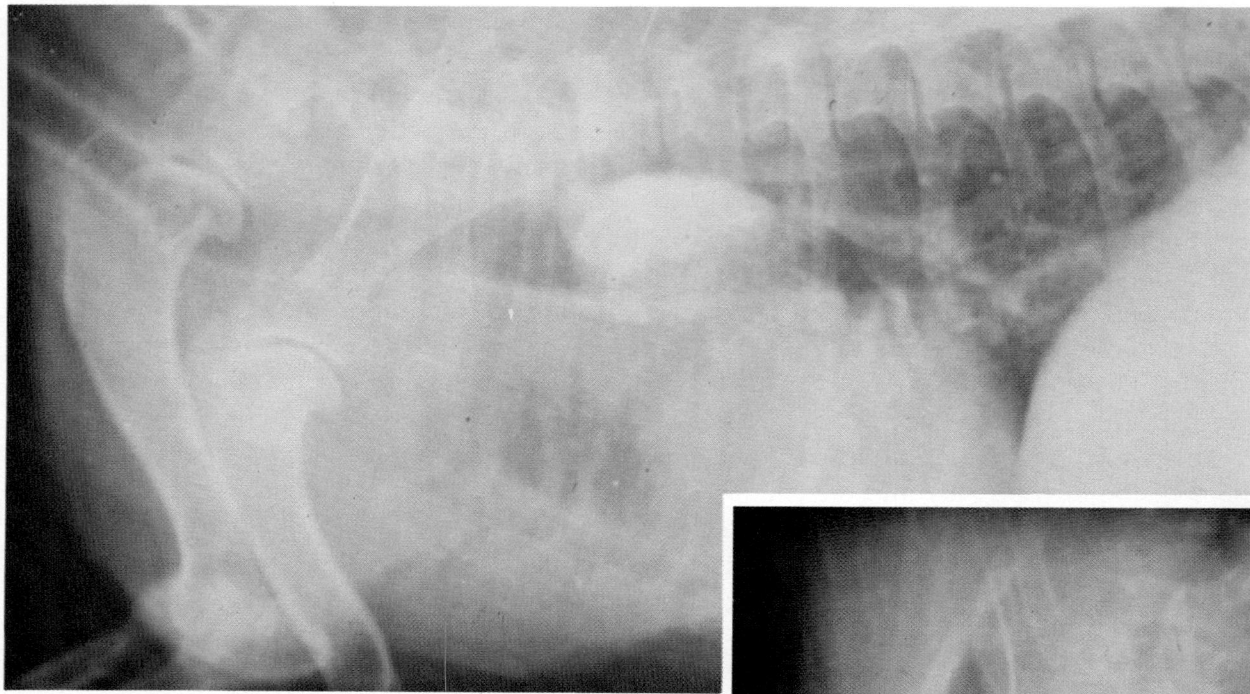

Figure 3—Lateral radiographic view of the thorax showing a bone lodged in the cranial mediastinal esophagus just cranial to the base of the heart.

ence of a bone with no visible sharp edges and disclosed minimal damage to the esophageal mucosa.

After the endoscope was withdrawn, a No. 12 Foley urethral catheter (Bard-Parker) was lubricated and passed down the esophagus to beyond the obstruction. The balloon of the catheter was gently inflated with 5 cc of contrast medium (Hypaque® 50%—Winthrop) and a lateral radiograph was taken to verify the position of the catheter (*Figure* 5). As the catheter was withdrawn, the balloon slipped past the bone. This was probably due to the asymmetrical inflation of the balloon.

A second attempt was made using two No. 12 Foley urethral catheters. The two catheters were passed, one on each side of the bone. The balloons were inflated with contrast medium and their positions were ascertained by radiography (*Figure 6*). The combined diameters of the inflated balloons expanded the esophagus, thereby relieving its hold on the bone. As gentle traction was applied, the Foley catheters were slowly withdrawn, pulling the bone with them.

Endoscopic examination revealed no lacerations, and mucosal damage at the site of the obstruction was minimal. The dog was hospitalized overnight

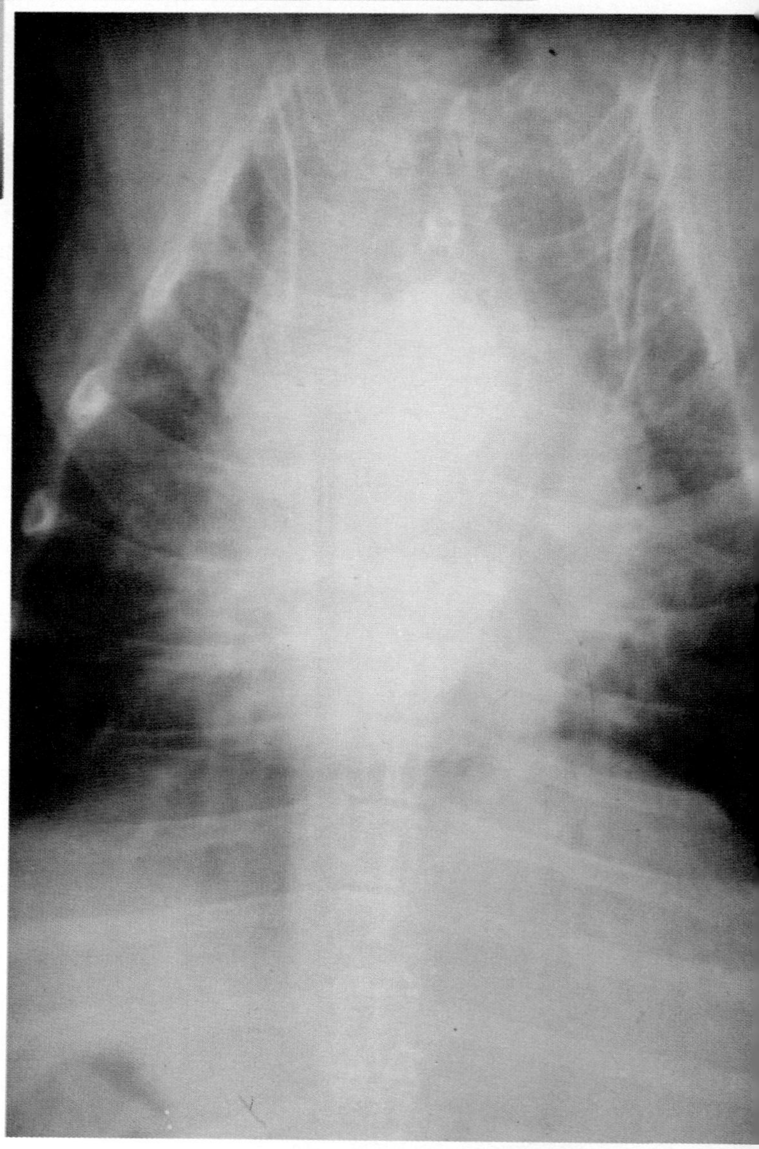

Figure 4—Ventrodorsal radiographic view of the thorax also showing the osseous foreign body at the base of the heart.

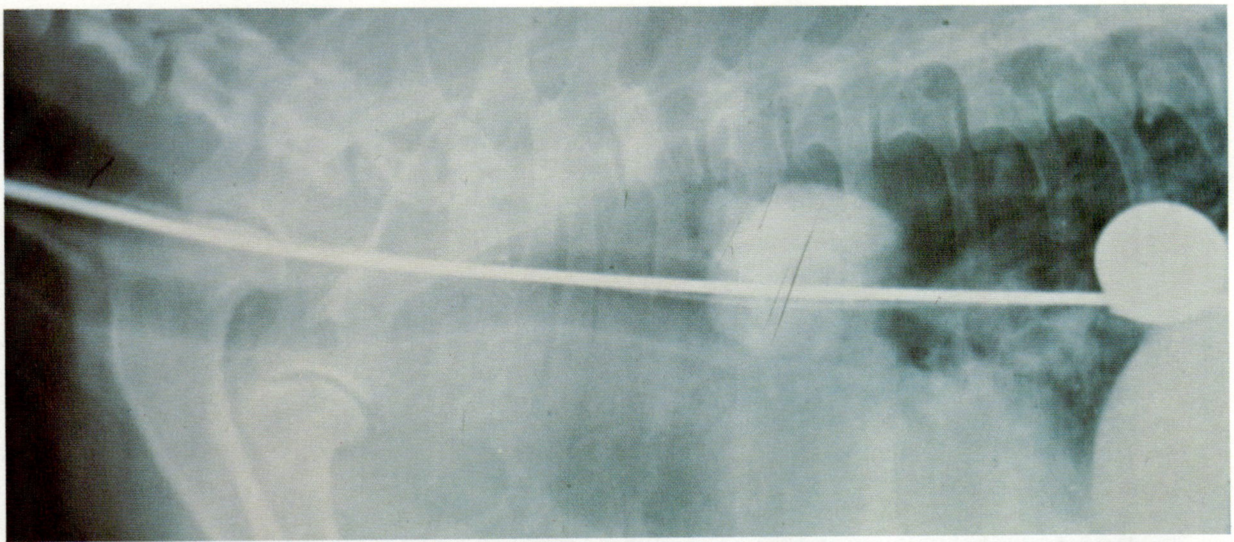

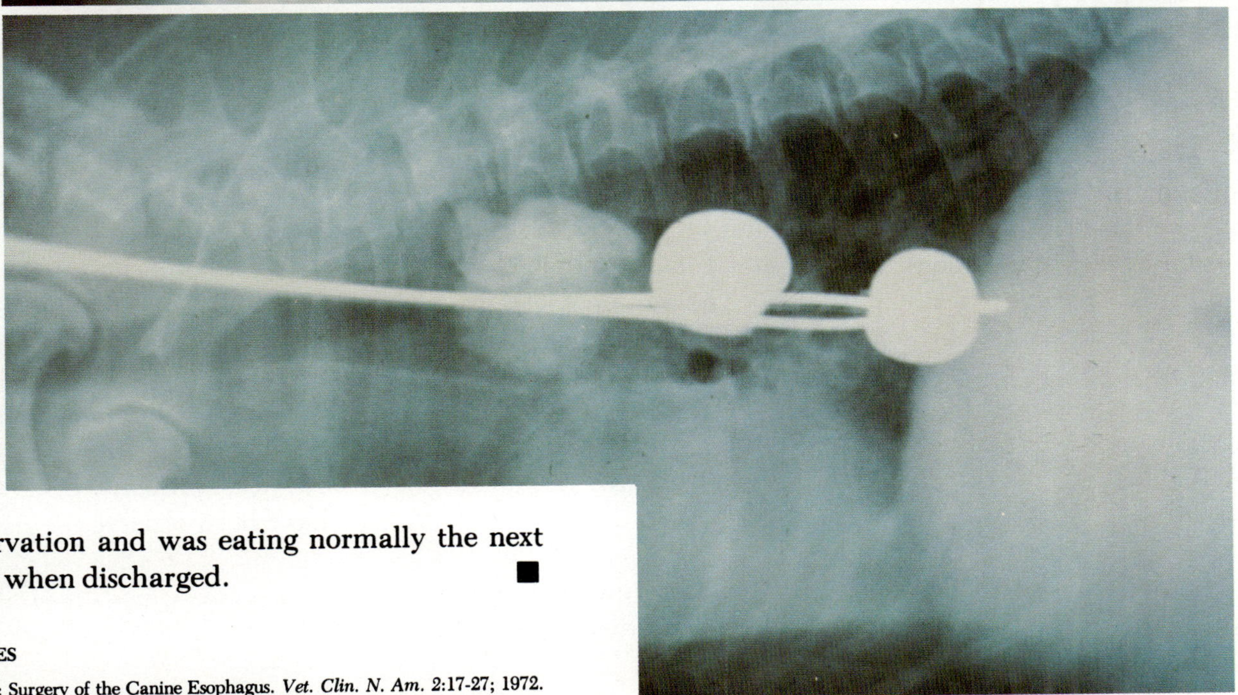

for observation and was eating normally the next morning when discharged. ■

REFERENCES

1. Rosin, E.: Surgery of the Canine Esophagus. *Vet. Clin. N. Am.* 2:17-27; 1972.
2. Ryan, W.W.; Greene, R.W.: The Conservative Management of Esophageal Foreign Bodies and Their Complications: A Review of 66 Cases in Dogs and Cats. *JAAHA 11*:243-249; 1975.
3. Hoffer, R.E.: Diseases of the Esophagus. In *Current Veterinary Therapy-VI* (R.W. Kirk, ed.). W.B. Saunders Co., Philadelphia, Pa., 1977.
4. Guffy, M.M.: Esophageal Disorders. In *Textbook of Veterinary Internal Medicine* (S.J. Ettinger, ed.). W.B. Saunders Co., Philadelphia, Pa., 1975.
5. Kretschmer, K.P.: Another Useful Application of the Balloon-Tipped Fogarty Catheter. *Am. J. Surg. 122*:417; 1971.
6. Stein, L.: Foreign Bodies of the Tracheobronchial Tree and Esophagus. *Ann. Thorac. Surg.* 9:382-383; 1970.
7. Faulkner, R.T. *et al*: A Case of Esophageal Foreign Body with Mediastinal Abscess Formation in a Dog. *JAAHA 12*:70-76; 1976.
8. Brown, L.P.: Blind Esophageal Coin Removal Using a Foley Catheter. *Arch. Surg. 96*:931-932; 1968.
9. Campbell, J.E.; Davis, W.S.: Catheter Technique for Extraction of Blunt Esophageal Foreign Bodies. *Radiology 108*:438-440; 1973.
10. Henry, L.N.; Chamberlain, J.W.: Removal of Foreign Bodies from the Esophagus and Nose with the Use of a Foley Catheter. *Surgery 71*:918-921; 1972.
11. Synbas, P.N.: Indirect Method of Extraction of Foreign Body from the Esophagus. *Ann. Surg. 167*:78-80; 1968.

Figure 5 *(top)*—This lateral radiograph of the thorax was taken to verify the position of the Foley catheter balloon. Note that the balloon was not inflated symmetrically.

Figure 6—This lateral radiograph of the thorax shows two Foley catheter balloons inflated caudal to the obstruction. The combined diameters of the two balloons prevented their slipping beyond the foreign body so that it rode on them out of the esophagus.

Lag-Screw Repair of FELINE MANDIBULAR SYMPHYSEAL FRACTURE

Christopher N. Garruba, Jr.
Veterinary Explorer Post President
200 Harrington C
University of Delaware
Newark, Delaware 19711

Richard D. Robertson, VMD
Veterinary Explorer Post Advisor
3975 Princeton Pike
Princeton, New Jersey 08540

PREVIOUSLY DESCRIBED techniques for repairing a mandibular symphyseal fracture in a cat lack the optimum efficiency required by busy small animal practitioners.

In one procedure, orthopedic wire or Kirschner stainless steel wire is looped in a figure-eight around the lower canine teeth or mandibles, or both. In the other method, a 1/8″ Steinmann pin is employed to connect the mandibles just posterior to the canine teeth. With either of these techniques the fracture segments are adequately aligned medially. However, the first method exerts pressure on the canine teeth, possibly resulting in malocclusion. The thinness of the bone itself limits the use of the Steinmann pin.

The application of a lag-screw technique appears ideal for repairing the mandibular symphyseal fracture in a cat.

Procedure

Anesthetization and preparation of the patient are routine.

After the fracture has been reduced and stabilized with towel forceps, a Steinmann pin (7/64″) is used to drill a hole through one mandible. This hole is started just caudal to the roots of the canine teeth and is directed into and through the corresponding site on the opposite mandible. A stainless steel, self-tapping lag screw* (5/8″ long) is then introduced (*Figure 1*) and adjusted to provide proper occlusion of the jaws and adequate compression of the fracture segments (*Figure 2*).

The screw is removed after four to six weeks.

The lag-screw causes no obstructive swelling or lesions, and the single hole heals without complications.

Discussion

The lag-screw technique offers numerous advantages:

1. The few supplies needed are mostly conventional and basic.
2. With threads in only one mandible, the two mandibles are easier to draw together, thus eliminating gaps and facilitating precise alignment.
3. Since only one hole is required, disruption of tissue is minimal and the risk of debris accumulating and causing infection is reduced.
4. Healing is rapid, and the patient may immediately resume a normal diet.
5. The minimal force required to remove the screw does not stress the fracture.

No significant disadvantages have been observed. ■

* Fixation screw, 15.8 mm long (Richards).

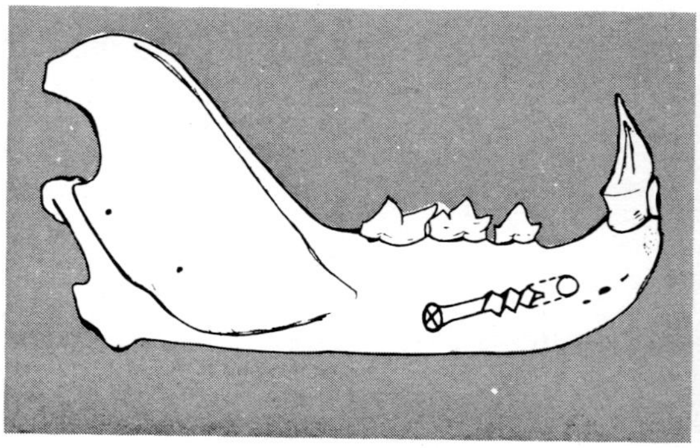

Figure 1— A 5/8″ self-tapping lag screw is inserted into the hole drilled with a Steinmann pin of 7/64″ diameter.

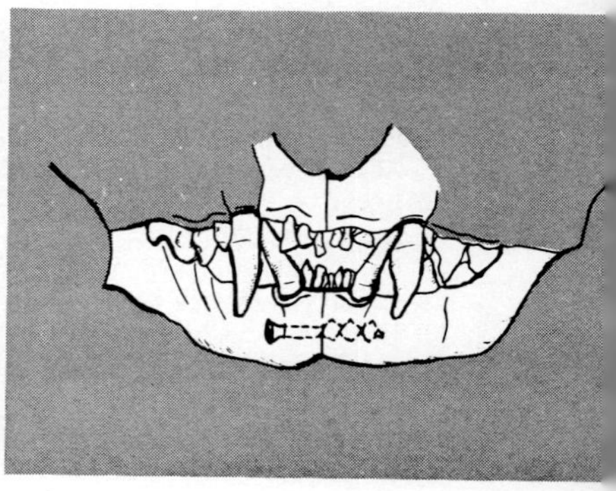

Figure 2—The completed lag-screw reduction of the fractured symphysis.

Ablation of the ear canal for treatment of chronic suppurative otitis externa in a cat

Mark E. Hitt, DVM
1200 S.W. 50th Avenue
Building 3, Apartment 207
Fort Lauderdale, Florida 33068

Ablation of the ear canal is an uncommon procedure that may be utilized in cases of nonresponsive otitis externa or diffuse neoplasia. The surgery described in this article was performed with cosmetic and therapeutically effective results. Suppurative granulation tissue, resembling a neoplastic mass, was the primary indication for use of this procedure.

A DOMESTIC long-hair cat was presented for examination because of a foul-smelling infection of the left ear. The cat had been found as a stray a few weeks previously. Findings from the physical examination were unremarkable except for the suppurative otitis externa.

When the ear was closely examined, a mass was found that blocked the entire vertical ear canal. The surface, ulcerated and bleeding, resembled a miniature cauliflower. Microscopic examination of debris from both ears was negative for ear mites.

Since the cat was a stray, the client decided to treat the ear topically until a decision could be reached regarding disposition of the animal. Liquichlor® (Evsco) was dispensed, with instructions to the client to clean the ear daily with peroxide.

Approximately three weeks later, the owner presented the cat for reexamination. The animal was depressed and the purulent discharge from the left ear was again apparent. The mass had enlarged and now protruded from the ear canal. A tentative diagnosis of neoplasia was made and surgical removal of the mass and attached tissue was recommended. The possibility of local invasion and metastasis was discussed. Our hope was to be able to remove very little tissue, utilizing resection of the lateral wall of the ear canal. Culturing and sensitivity testing of debris from the ears were not performed. Radiographic examination of the thorax for possible metastasis showed no discernible lesions. Also, a FeLV test (Leukassay*F® —Pitman-Moore) was negative.

Surgical technique

The cat was premedicated with atropine and Acepromazine (Fort Dodge). The anesthesia was induced and maintained with ketamine HCl. The surgical procedure required about 60 minutes.

Exposure of the vertical canal, and hence the origin of the mass, was achieved by a vertical incision overlying the vertical canal and extending ventrally to the level of the horizontal ear canal. A second incision of the skin was made, forming a T

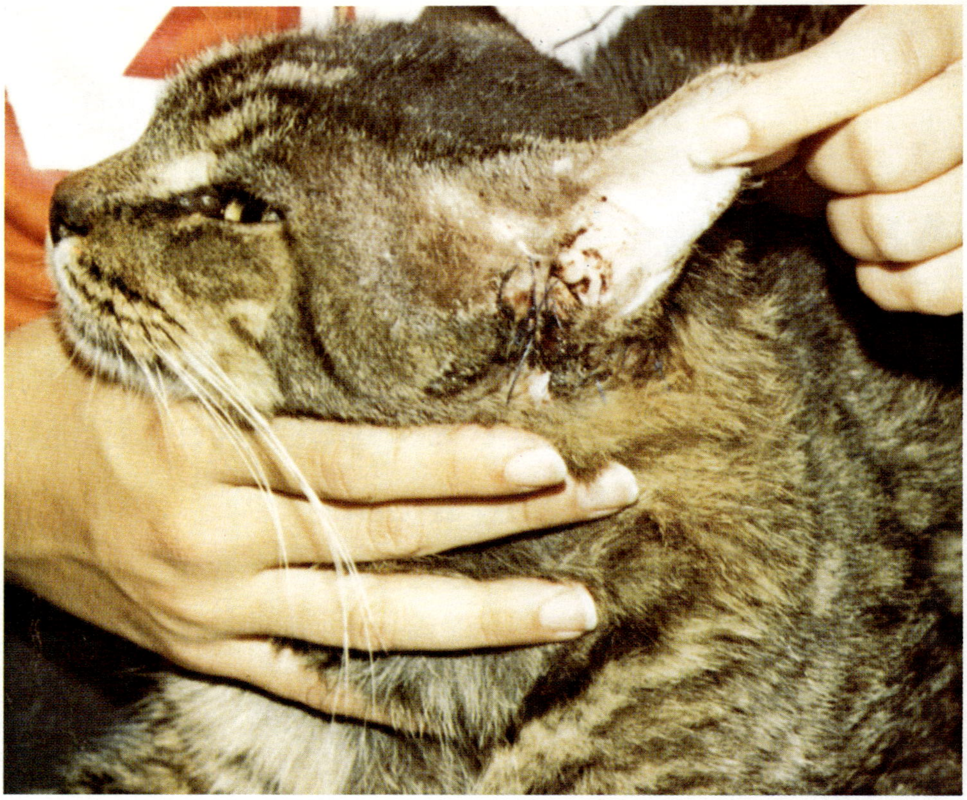

Figure 1
Appearance of the cat's ear three days postoperatively, after the drain had been removed.

with the first incision. The two flaps of skin were undermined bluntly and reflected. This exposed a portion of the cartilage of the vertical canal and the parotid salivary gland.

The parotid salivary gland was reflected caudally, giving more access to the area. A lateral incision was made in the cartilage of the canal in an attempt to find the origin of the mass. The mass was found to have four tentacle-like fingers that were diffusely attached near the tympanic membrane.

At this time removal of the entire ear canal (ablation of the ear canal) was deemed necessary in order to provide more assurance that the suspected neoplasm was completely excised.[1] By sharp and blunt dissection, the vertical and horizontal canals were isolated to a level approximately 2 mm lateral to the first osseous portion of the canal. Electrocautery was used to stop hemorrhage and destroy any remaining secretory lining cells.

The surgical area was flushed with saline solution and Betadine® (Purdue Frederick). A latex drain was positioned and the skin was closed with simple interrupted sutures of 2-0 Prolene. The suture line was T-shaped and composed of a vertical base 1 cm long and a horizontal top 3.5 cm long.

Postoperative medications consisted of atropine (for possible trauma to the parotid salivary gland), penicillin-streptomycin, and dexamethasone. The drain was removed on the third postoperative day (*Figure 1*), and the sutures on the tenth postoperative day (*Figure 2*).

The only postsurgical complications were a mild head tilt that lasted two days, and a small ulceration over an area of exposed cartilage. This lesion was treated with topical antibiotics and a single suture.

Three months after surgery, the ear is cosmetically acceptable. Absence of the vertical canal is hidden by the contour of the head and the cat's coat. Observation has been maintained for any draining tracts that might form from secretory products if any secretory cells remained after the incision was closed. No tracts have been seen.

Discussion

The mass measured 2 cm × 2.5 cm and resembled a miniature cauliflower (*Figure 3*). A diagnosis of neoplasia (basal cell tumor, ceruminous gland adenoma, etc.) was expected. A guarded prognosis was given both before and after the surgery due to the possibility of local invasion or metastasis.

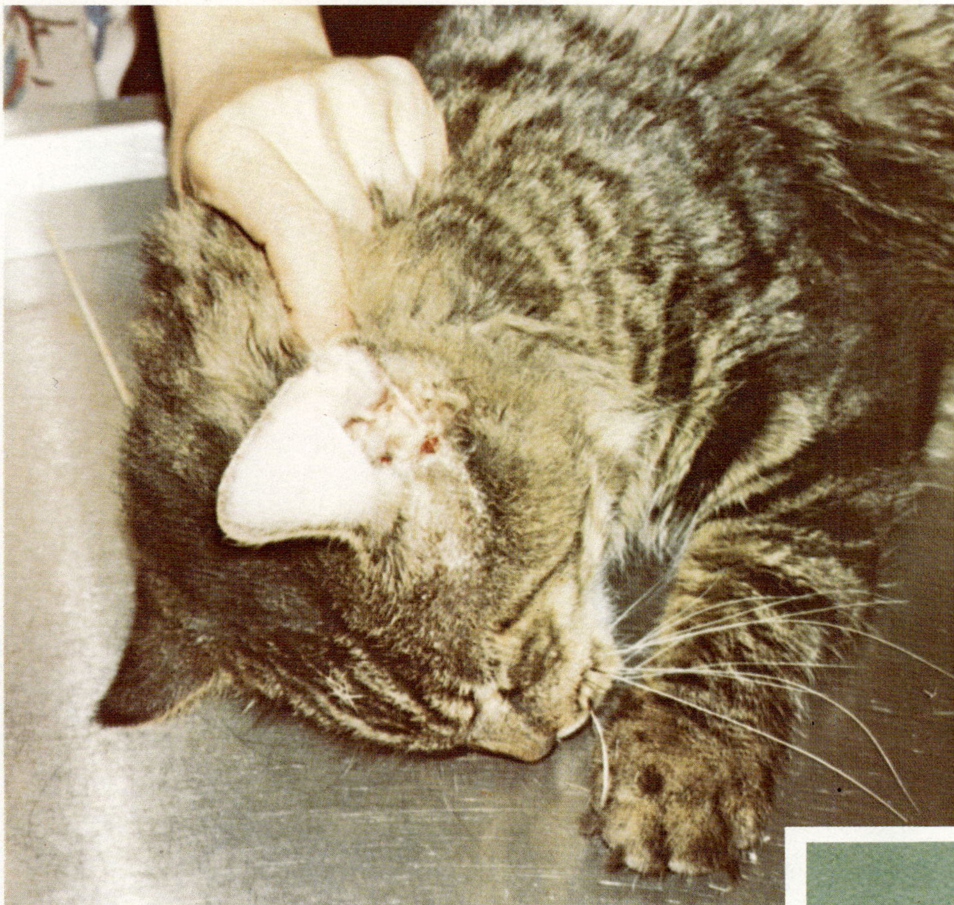

Figure 2
Appearance of the ear 10 days following the operation, after the sutures were removed.

Figure 3
The obstructing mass of granulation tissue shown next to a 5-inch hemostat. Note the tentacle-like fingers extending from the mass.

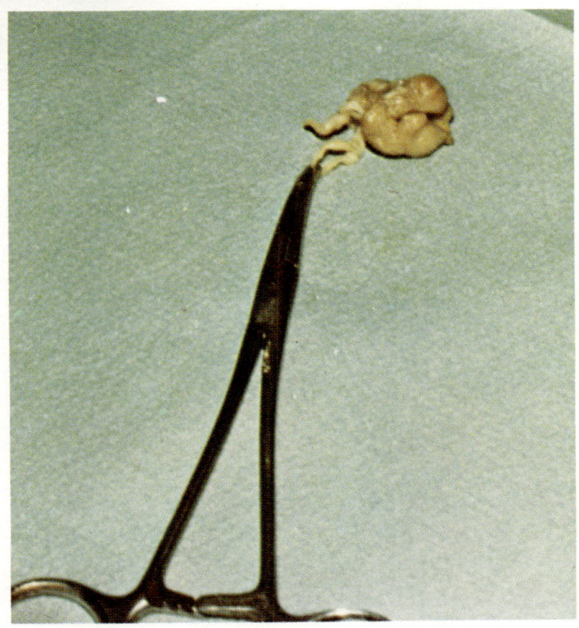

According to the histopathology report the ulcerated mass consisted of edematous granulation tissue that was heavily infiltrated with inflammatory cells, lymphocytes, plasma cells, neutrophils, and macrophages. The final diagnosis of chronic suppurative otitis externa improved the prognosis dramatically.

This unilateral occurrence of otitis externa with proliferative granulation tissue led me to think immediately of neoplasia of the ear canal. The clinical options considered by the owner and me after the initial topical treatment proved ineffective, included euthanasia as well as surgery. Without the owner's determination to do everything possible to help the cat, the animal probably would have been euthanatized because of a faulty diagnosis.

Perhaps this case illustrates the need to reevaluate the diagnosis arrived at too quickly because it seems so obvious. The cat is now a healthy and welcome addition to the client's household.

REFERENCE

1. Spreull, J.A.: Ablation of the Ear Canal; in *Current Techniques in Small Animal Surgery* (M.J. Bojrab, ed.). Lea & Febiger, Philadelphia, Pa., 1975; pp 68-70.

Small Animal Surgery

SKIN

a lay-open procedure for **anal sac resection** in the dog

Vincent W. Chaffee, DVM, MS, PhD*
School of Veterinary Medicine
Purdue University
West Lafayette, Indiana 47097

MANY METHODS have been used to resect the anal sacs of the dog. All methods are inodifications of two specific techniques, the open and the closed techniques.

The basic principle of the closed technique is filling the anal sacs with string, acrylic resins, plaster of Paris, Play-Doh®, wax, or silicone[1-5] and performing a closed dissection of the anal sac. In these cases, the skin incision is made directly over the anal sac just lateral to the circumference of the anus.

In the open technique, the anal sacs are left empty. A groove director is placed through the anal sac duct, and the entire anal sac is opened with an incision through the duct to the bottom of the sac.[6] The sacs are then resected. This makes the entire mucosal lining visible.

In both techniques the anal sacs are initially flushed with an appropriate antiseptic solution before surgery.

Pictured here is a modification of the open technique. Scissors are used to lay open the anal sacs. During the opening of the anal sacs, the scissors must be tipped up to prevent severing the external sphincter muscle.

*Diplomate, American College of Veterinary Surgeons and American College of Laboratory Animal Medicine

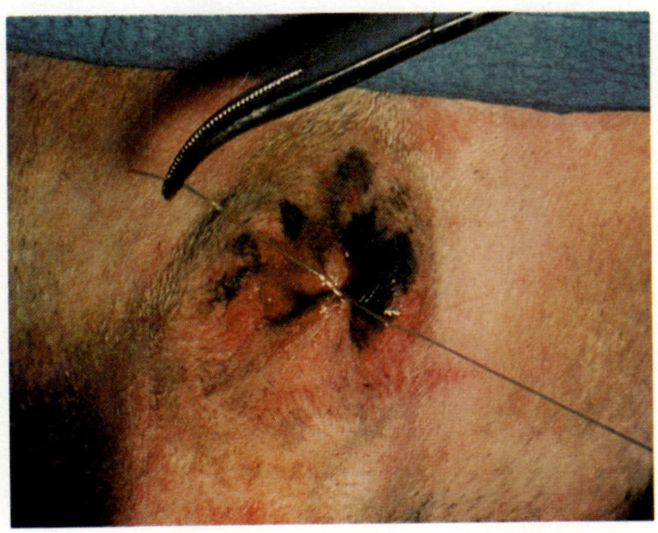

Figure 1
The anal canal is packed with a lubricated gauze sponge and a purse-string suture is placed to close the anus. The ducts of the anal sac are not included in this closure.

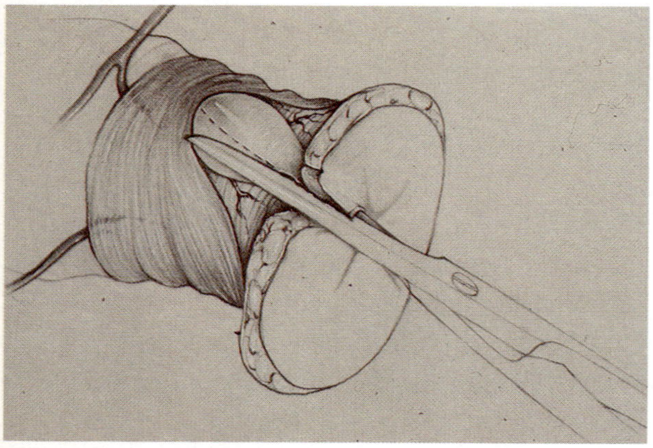

Figure 2—The anal sac is layed open by inserting the sharp-ended dissection scissors to the extreme depths of the sac. The scissors must be tipped up so that the external sphincter muscle rolls off the sac.

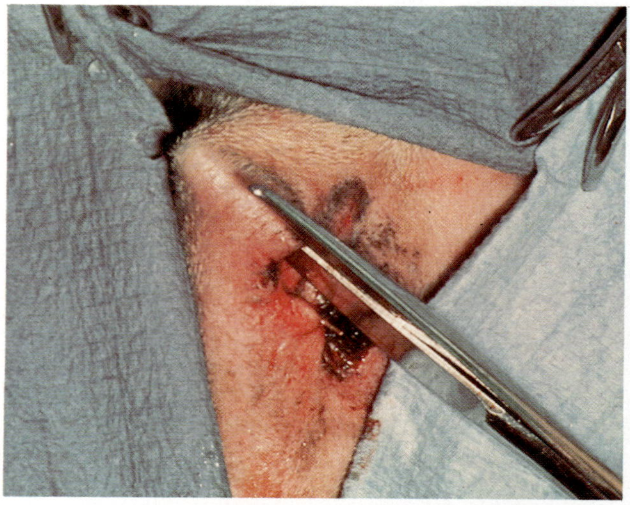

Figure 3—The blade of the scissor is placed through the duct of the anal sac to the bottom of the anal sac and tipped up.

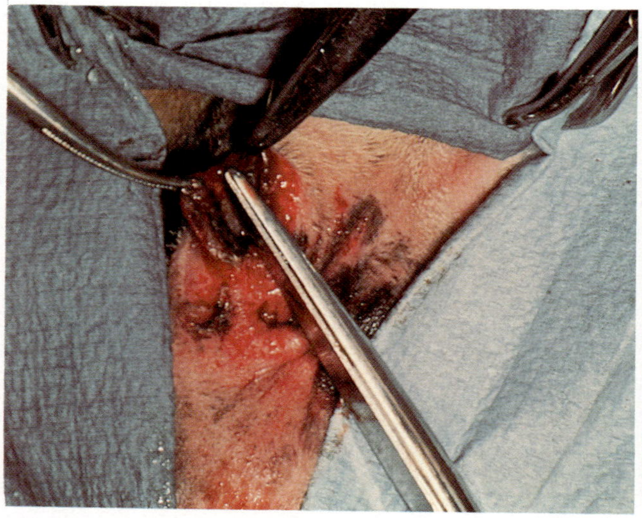

Figure 4—The anal sac is layed open to expose the mucosal lining.

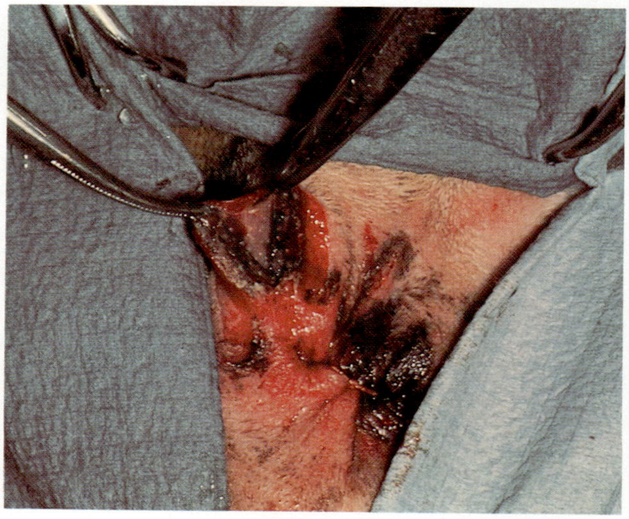

Figure 5—The entire anal sac and the duct are exposed and ready to be dissected.

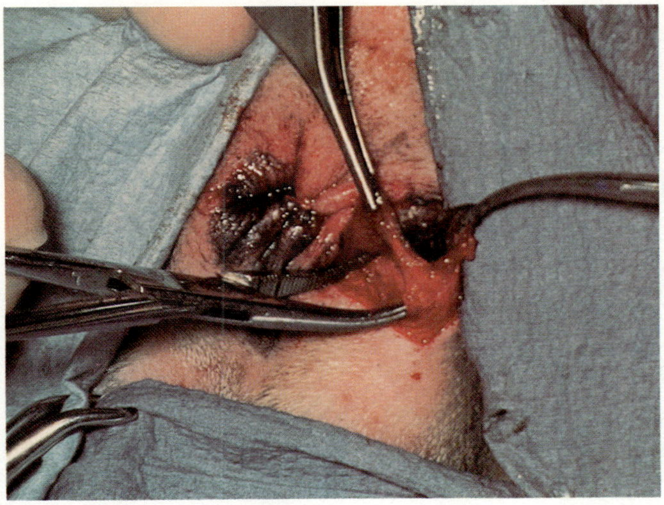

Figure 6—A small hemostat is used to dissect around the anal sac and duct. Dissection is performed close to the sac without tearing the mucosal lining.

Figure 7—The dissected anal sac and duct.

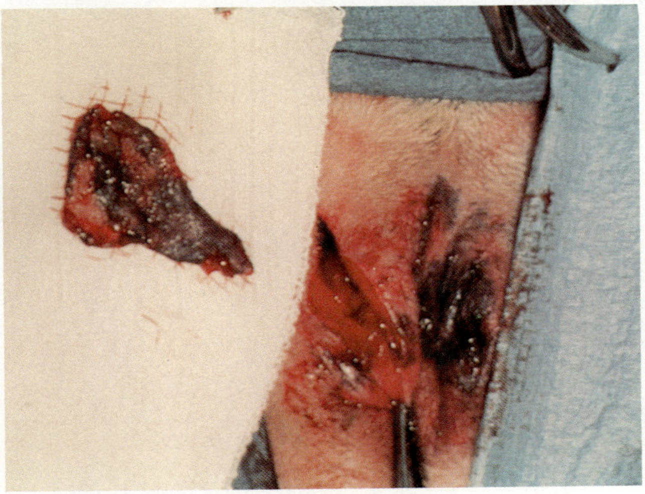

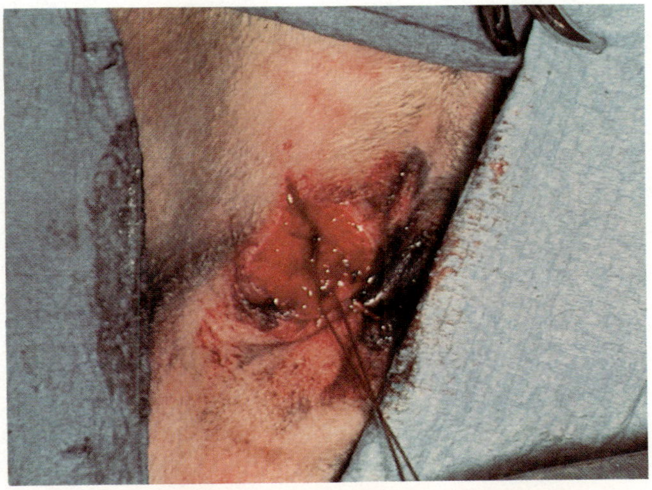

Figure 8—The dead space is obliterated with one or two subcutaneous sutures in an interrupted pattern. If the caudal rectal artery was torn, it is ligated at this time.

Figure 9—The skin is routinely closed and the purse-string suture is removed from the anus.

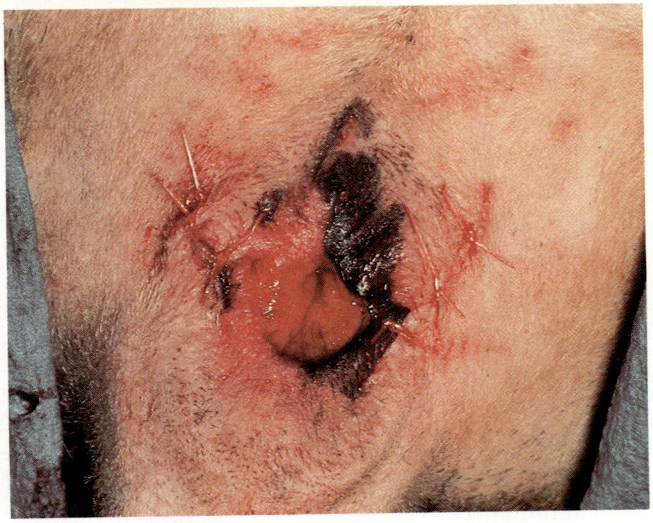

REFERENCES

1. Theobald, A.R.: Surgery of the Anal Sacs. *N. Am. Vet. 23*:44-47; 1942.
2. Taylor, D.C.; Chesworth, A.T.: Acrylic Resins in Anal Gland Resection. *Vet. Rec. 74*:843; 1962.
3. Young, M.: Extirpation of the Anal Sacs of the Dog. *Vet. Rec. 72*:369-370; 1960.
4. Vice, T.E.: A New Approach to Anal Gland Surgery. *Small Animal Clin. 2*:250-253; May 1962.
5. Frye, F.L. *et al:* Silicone Sealant for Preoperative Packing of Canine Anal Sacs. *JAVMA 156*:1030; April 15, 1970.
6. Archibald, J.; Horney, F.D.: Colon, Rectum, and Anus. In *Canine Surgery II,* J. Archibald, ed. American Veterinary Publications, Inc., Santa Barbara, Calif., 1975; p 626.

Shifting local tissues to repair surgical wounds

R.P. Barrett, DVM*
Canyon Veterinary Hospital
20897 Redwood Road
Castro Valley, California 94546

Case No. 1

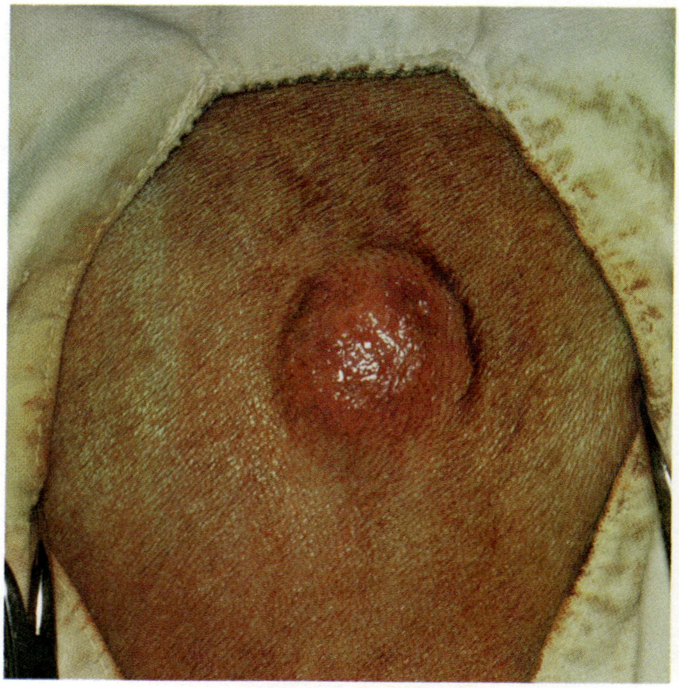

Figure 1—A mast-cell tumor on the shoulder of a dog.

SHIFTING OF LOCAL TISSUES is a simple way to repair defects created by excision of tissue masses. The procedure has several advantages over conventional elliptical excision and repair. These are:

1. Often a surgical wound on an extremity cannot be closed with an elliptical excision, whereas shifting local tissues provides complete closure and thus more rapid healing.
2. The tension on suture lines when local tissue is shifted is frequently minimal, thus reducing inflammatory response. The reduction of inflammation also reduces the amount of itching that occurs during healing, and consequently the amount of self-mutilation.
3. Repairs using shifted local tissue are cosmetic.
4. Surgical time required for these techniques is usually only slightly longer than for conventional elliptical excision and repair.

Two basic techniques of shifting local tissues are described and illustrated here. The first technique involves circumferential excision of a mass. A pedicle is then created which is undermined, rotated into the excision bed, and sutured in place. When a flap of tissue is prepared, a wide base to the flap must be maintained so that there is a generous supply of blood to the graft. As a guideline, the length of the flap should be no greater

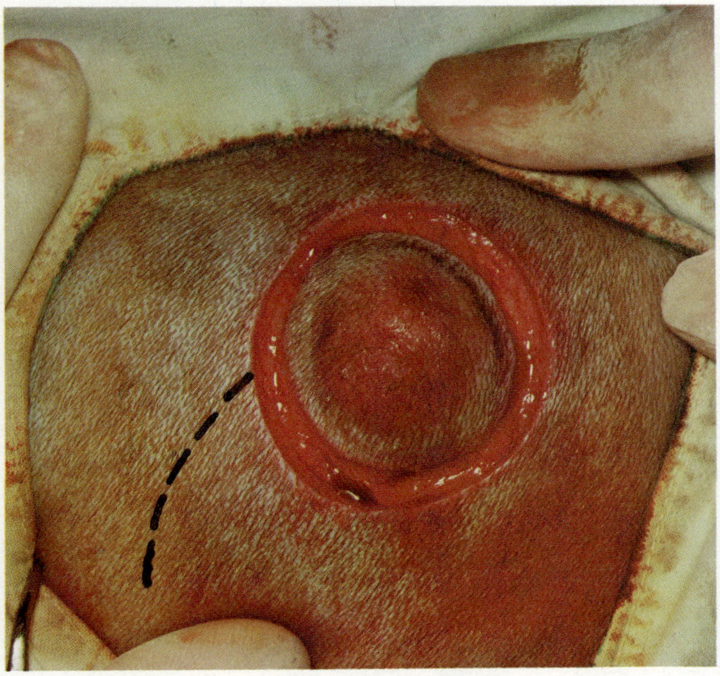

Figure 2—A circumferential incision is made, and the tumor is undermined and excised. The dotted line indicates the line of incision used to create the flap.

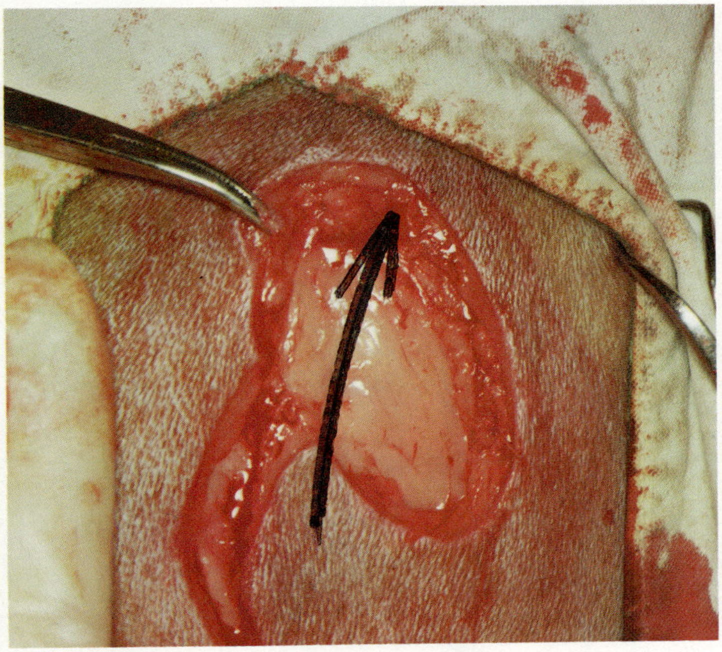

Figure 3—The flap is undermined to include the subcutaneous tissue. The arrow indicates the direction in which the flap is rotated.

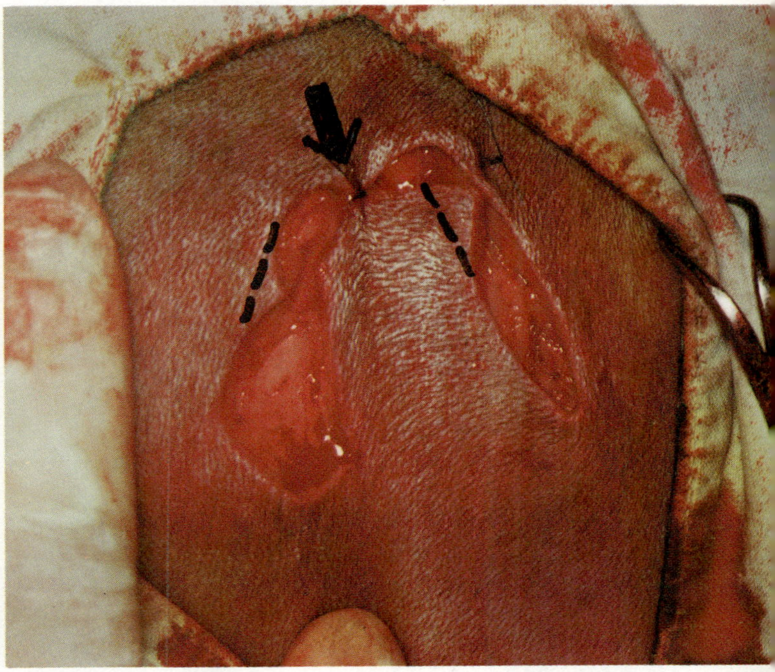

Figure 4—A suture is placed at the apex of the graft to hold it in place *(arrow)*. The dotted lines indicate the excess tissue to be removed to contour the graft to the graft bed.

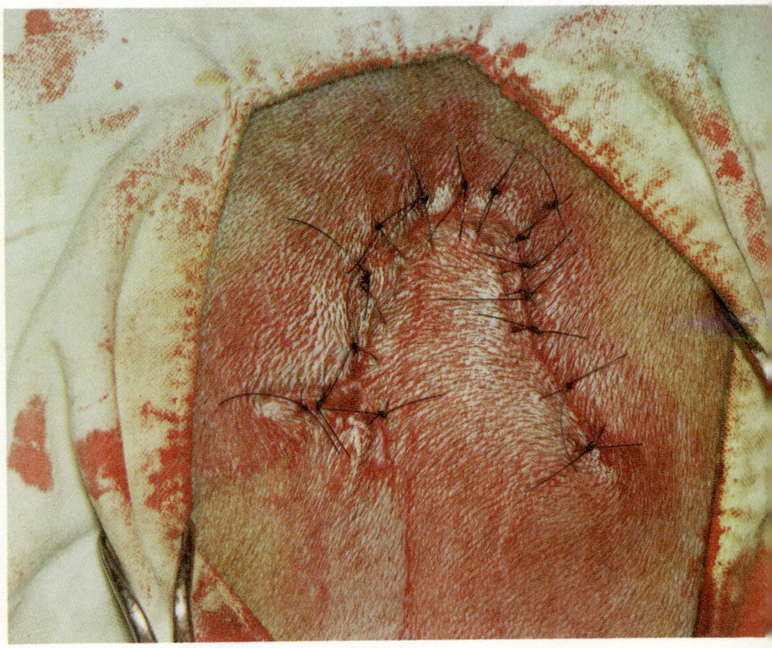

Figure 5—The graft is completed by closing with simple interrupted sutures. Neither a wound dressing nor antibiotics are used after surgery.

Case No. 2

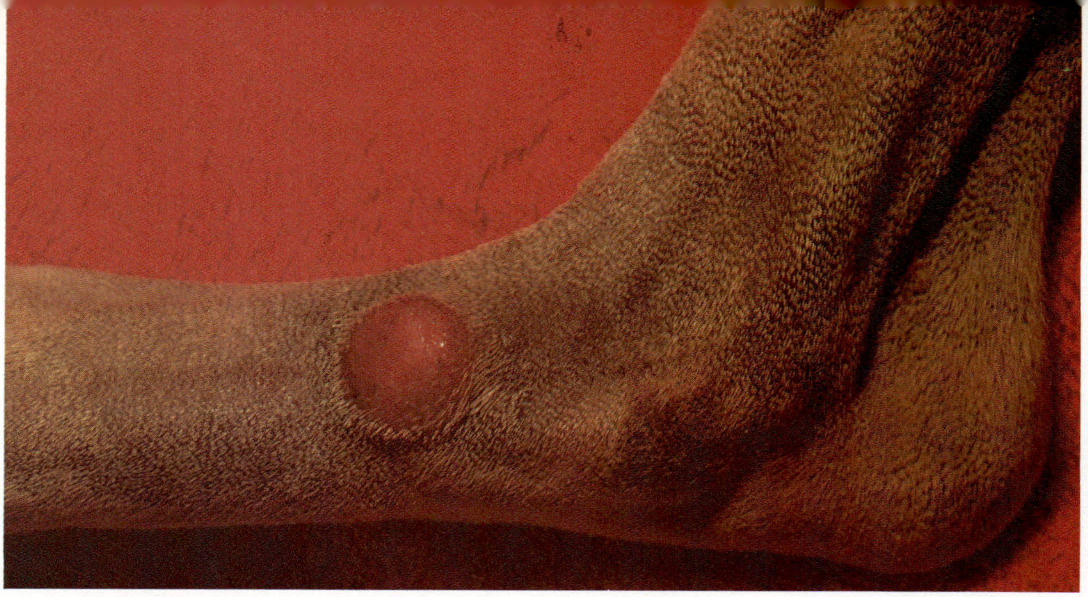

Figure 6
Histiocytoma on the lateral tarsus of a dog.

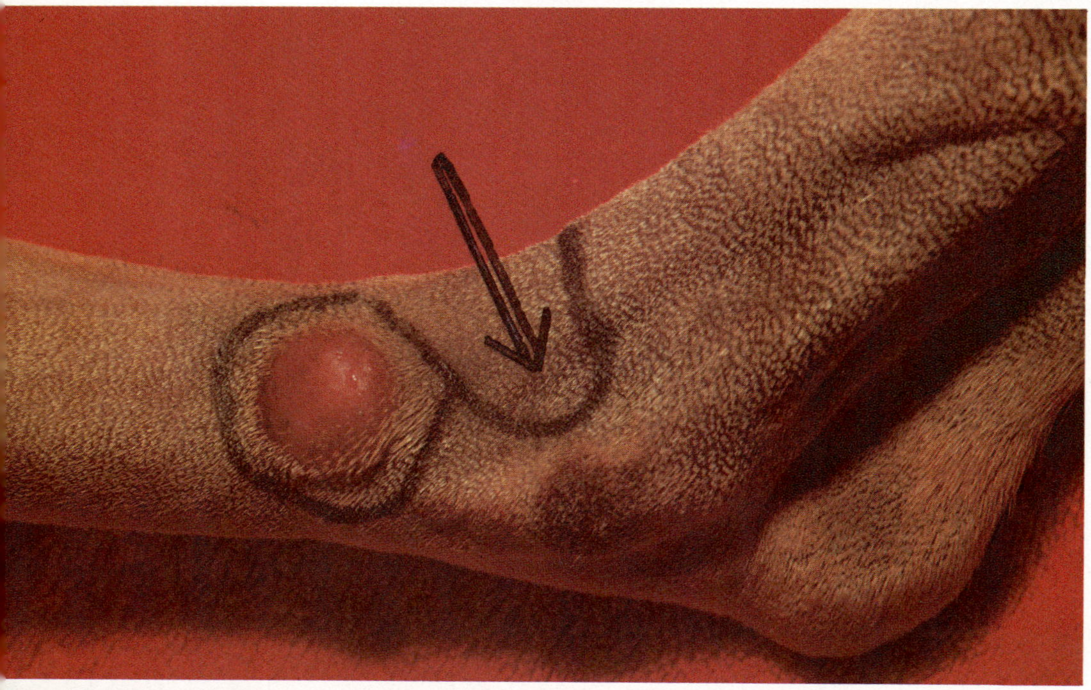

Figure 7
The line indicates the circumferential incision and incision used to create the flap *(arrow).*

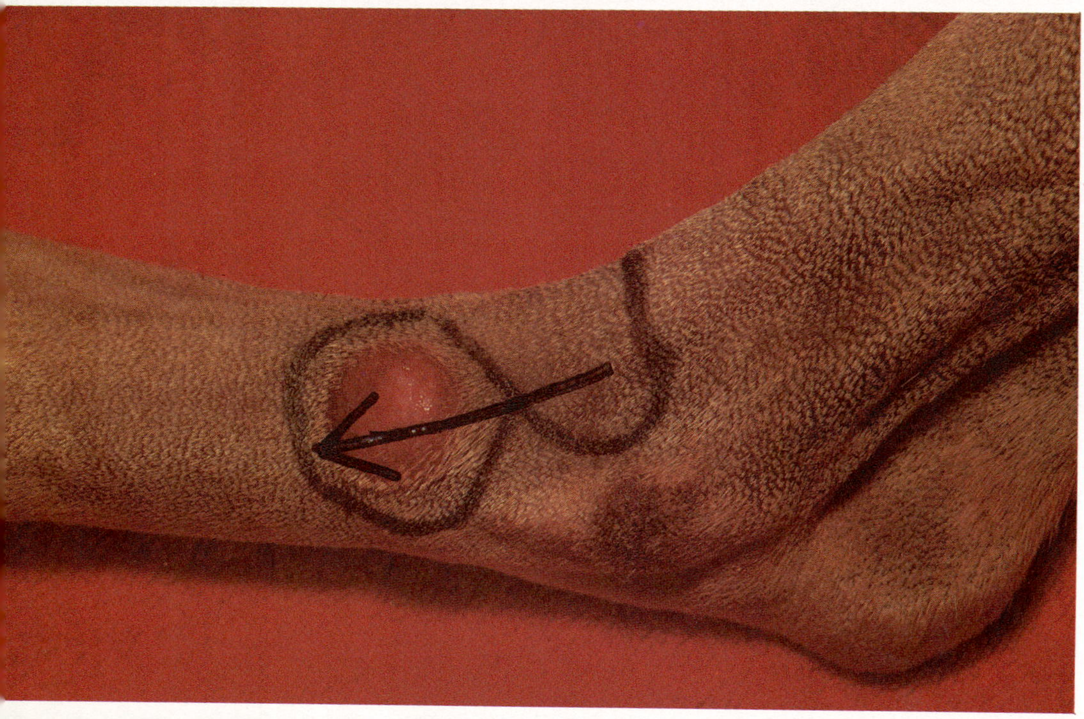

Figure 8
The tumor is undermined and removed. The arrow indicates the direction in which the flap is rotated.

than twice the width of its base. If it is possible for the length to equal the width, viability of the flap is almost certain. Careful aseptic technique must be used to preclude postoperative infection. Two variations of the rotating-pedicle-flap technique are illustrated in Cases 1 and 2 *(Figures 1 through 8)*.

The second technique involves advancing the pedicle in a linear direction rather than rotating it. This technique is ideal for lesions on the extremities where tissue is inadequate to rotate a flap and where a conventional elliptical excision would provide no means for closure. Case 3 *(Figures 9 & 10)* illustrates this technique.

The two techniques described in this article are illustrated diagramatically in the references listed below.[1,2]

REFERENCES

1. Bojrab, M.: *Current Techniques in Small Animal Surgery*, Vol. I. Lea & Febiger, Philadelphia, Pa., 1975; pp 284-286.
2. Stashak, T.S.: Reconstructive Surgery in the Horse. *JAVMA 170*(2):143-149; Jan. 15, 1977.

Case No. 3

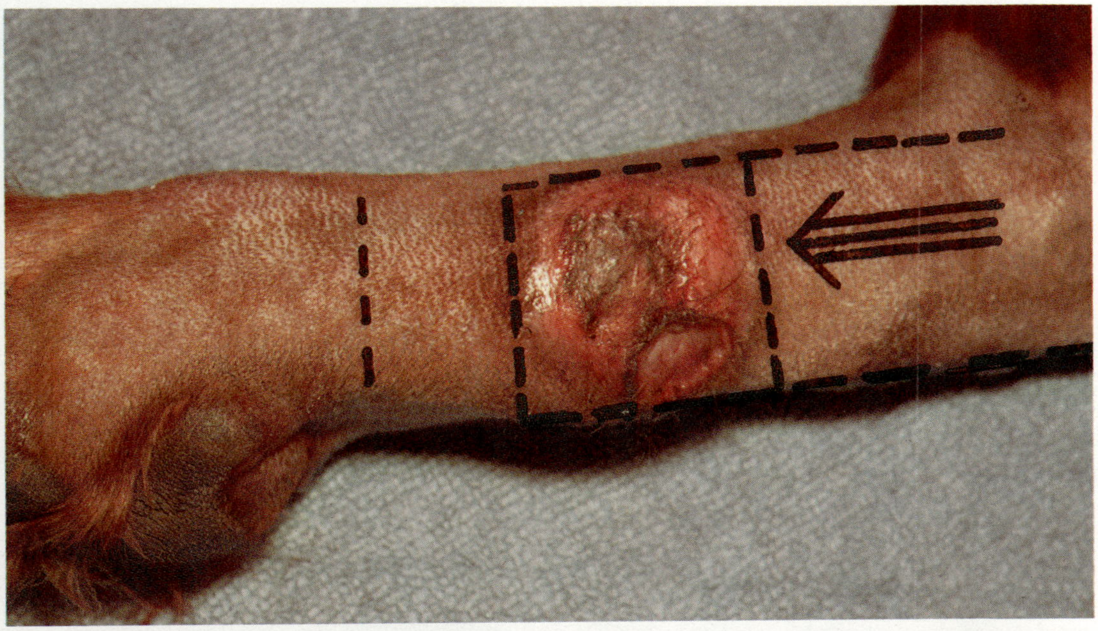

Figure 9
An acral lick granuloma on the medial tarsus of a dog. The dotted lines indicate the incision used to minimize tension on the suture line of the graft. The arrow overlies the advancement flap, which is undermined and advanced in the direction of the arrow.

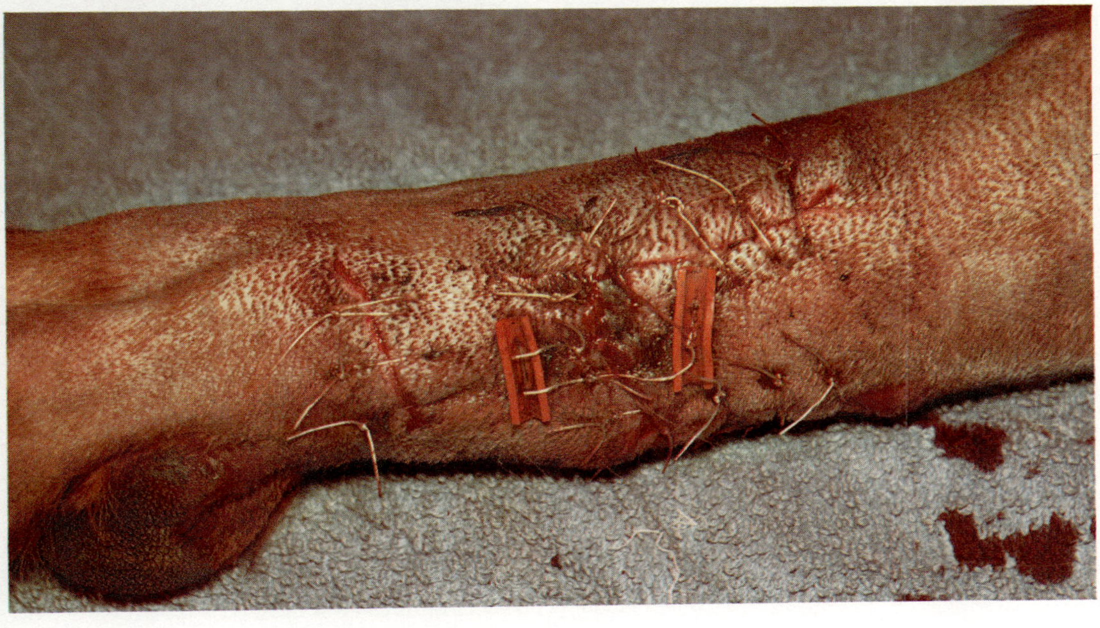

Figure 10
Completed repair. Two tension tubes secured by horizontal mattress sutures have been placed to reduce further tension on the suture line.

emergency care of

SKIN TRAUMA:

case report and discussion

Stephanie J. Sherman, RN, MS, DVM*
R.L. Bradley, DVM**
Veterinary Teaching Hospital
Colorado State Hospital
Fort Collins, Colorado 80523

SKIN is an organ of remarkable versatility. Wounds of the skin have a high potential for complete functional recovery after trauma. Three main factors that affect this full recovery are epithelialization, synthesis of connective tissue, and wound contraction.[1,2] In acute traumatic injuries, this potential for recovery can be greatly influenced by the treatment the tissue receives.

In this article we describe an approach to treating acute, extensive skin wounds. The significance of prompt treatment, methods of cleaning and debridement, approximation of the wound edges, and care after debridement are discussed.

Case Report

A 9-year-old male Schipperke-Poodle cross was admitted to the emergency room of the Colorado State University Veterinary Teaching Hospital 30 minutes after being struck by a car. The patient was in stable condition. An intravenous catheter was inserted for administration of fluids.

The dog's main injury was an extensive full-thickness laceration of the skin on the left foreleg, 5 cm proximal to the elbow and extending to the level of the carpus. The skin had been undermined and torn free 360 degrees both proximally and distally. The skin flap had curled upon itself. Its viability was questionable due to the extensive undermining of subcutaneous tissue and the subsequent potential for loss of blood supply. Other minor skin abrasions and lacerations elsewhere on the dog's body required minimal treatment.

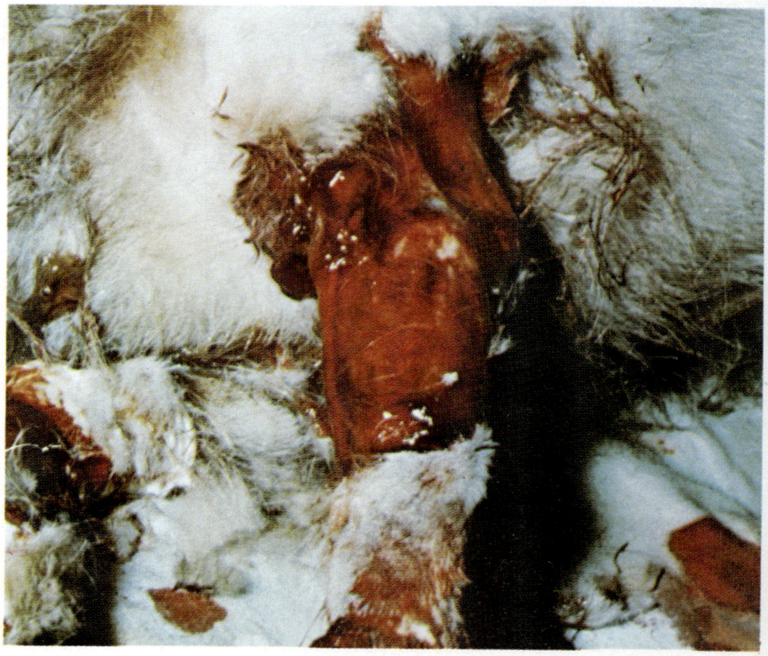

Figure 1—Lateral view of the wound.

* Dr. Sherman graduated from CSU in May, 1979.
** Direct reprint requests to Dr. Bradley at CSU.

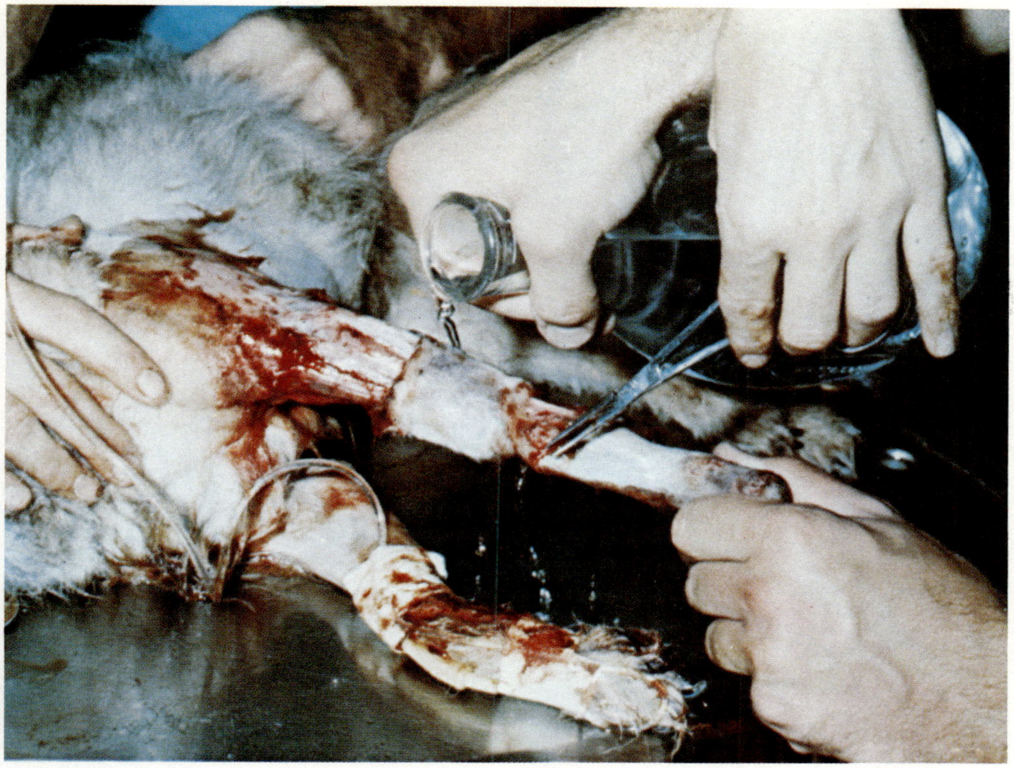

Figures 2 & 3
Flushing and debridement of the wound. Sterile gloves should be worn by all persons involved and the affected area should be draped.

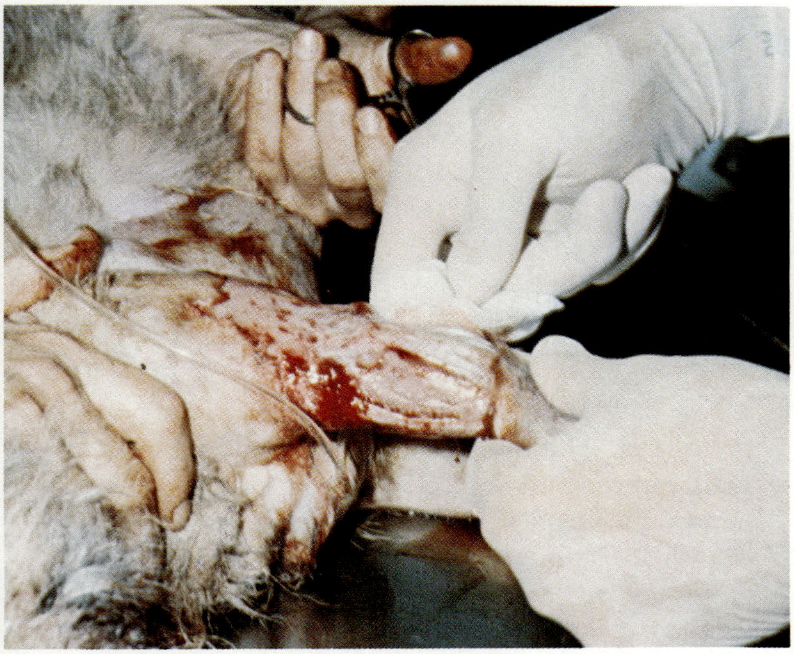

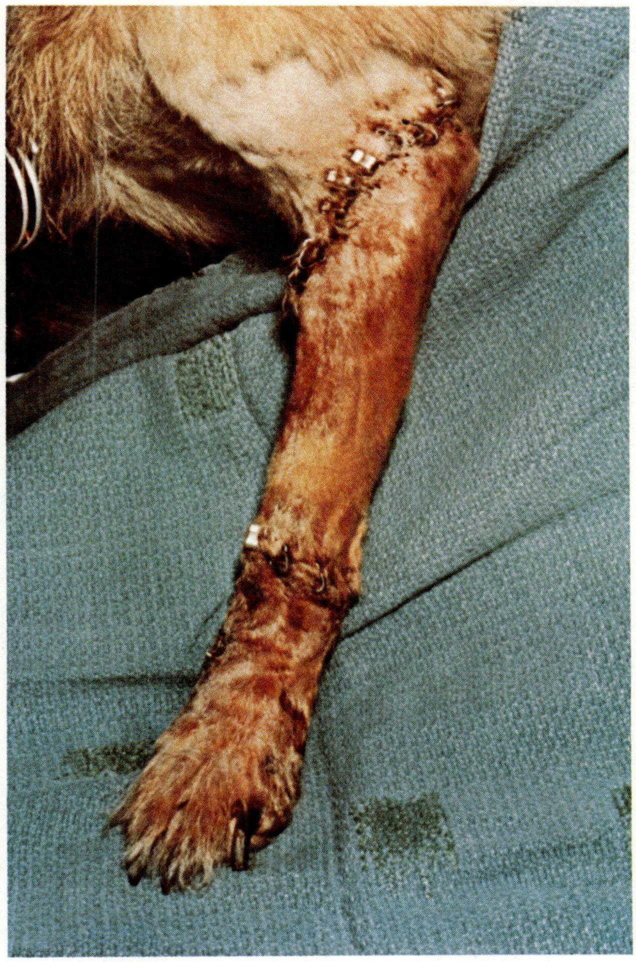

Figure 4
The edges of the wound were approximated with Michel clips.

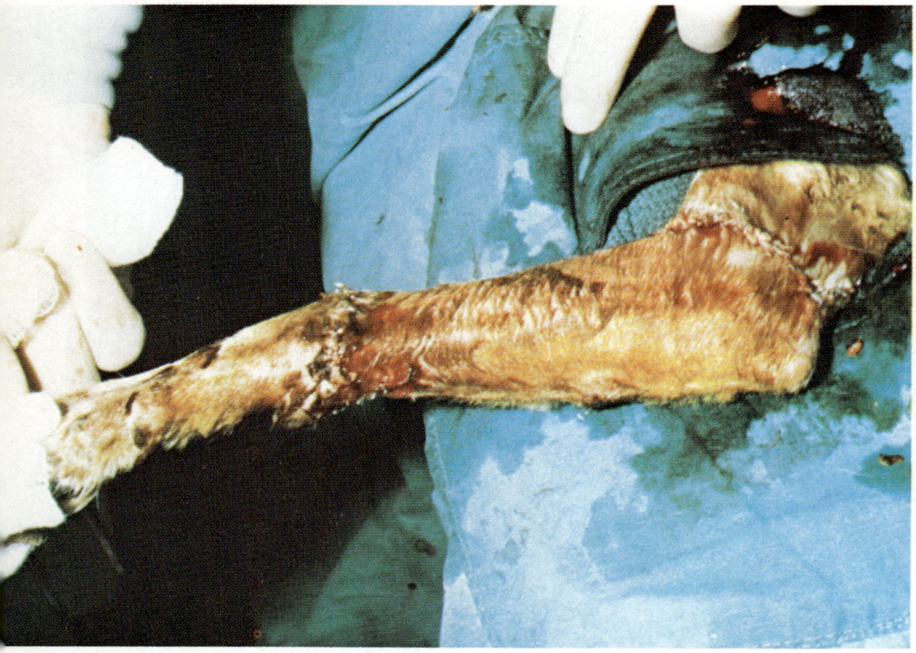

Figure 5
Delayed primary closure, accomplished six days after the injury was sustained.

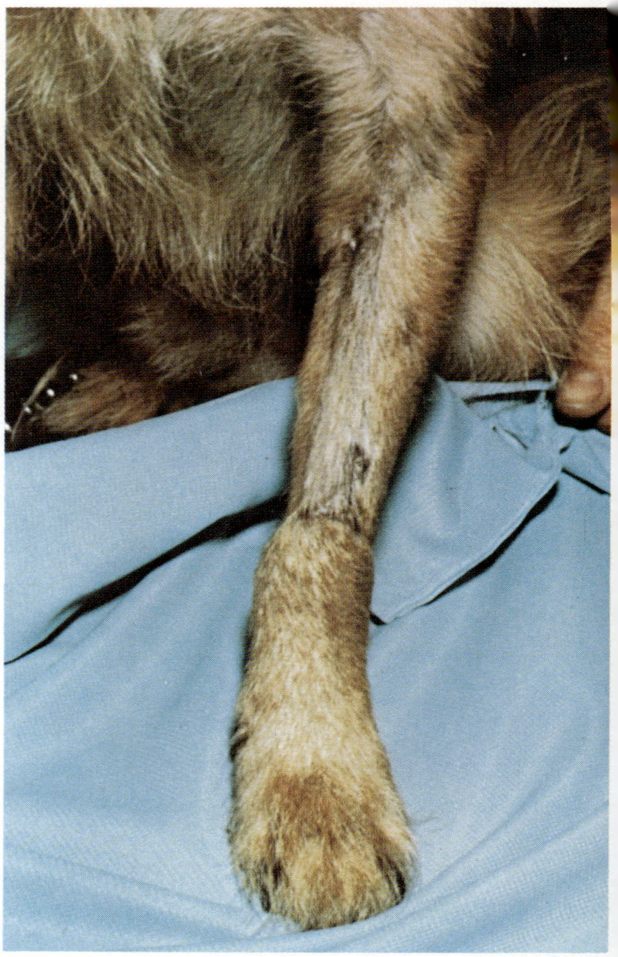

Figure 6
The wound 48 days after injury.

Treatment

The patient was sedated with oxymorphone, and the skin wound was packed with sterile K-Y® Jelly (Johnson & Johnson) to prevent introduction of hair particles into the wound (*Figure 1*). After the long hair was scissored from the wound, the site was clipped for surgery. The wound was flushed with 2 liters of warm sterile physiological saline solution, followed by another liter to which povidone iodine solution was added (*Figure 2*).

Manual debridement with sterile instruments and gauze was performed (*Figure 3*). The skin edges were approximated with Michel wound clips and the wound was packed with nitrofurazone ointment (*Figure 4*). A well-padded sterile bandage was applied. The bandage was changed daily.

Six days later, surgical debridement was again performed. The freshened skin edges were closed with sutures of 5-0 monofilament stainless steel (*Figure 5*). Good approximation of the edges was achieved. Capillary bleeding and the color of the skin edges indicated that the tissue was viable. The leg was dressed with nonadherent pads, elastic gauze, and elastic wrap.

One day after surgery the patient was discharged with a light dressing on the wound. The patient's progress was evaluated every third day until the sutures were removed.

Figure 6 shows the wound 48 days after the injury. The patient had full use of the leg, and functional recovery of the skin wound appeared to be complete.

Discussion

This case report illustrates four basic principles of treating acute skin trauma:

1. *Time*

Traumatic skin injuries should be treated as soon as possible, preferably within six hours. With prompt attention and proper care, even a heavily contaminated wound can be cleaned sufficiently for primary closure.[3]

Contaminated wounds must be differentiated from infected wounds. The difference is often a factor of time and environment. Fresh traumatic wounds like the one in the case described are considered contaminated. Traumatic wounds with retained devitalized tissue or fecal contamination should be considered infected, as should wounds treated more than six hours after injury.

Delaying treatment of traumatic wounds jeopardizes the amount of tissue that can be saved. Loss of tissue is usually caused by infection and retraction of the wound margin. Primary closure promotes rapid healing, but this advantage must be weighed against the devastation sepsis can cause if the wound is still contaminated when closed.[3]

2. *Asepsis*

Iatrogenic sources of pathogenic contamination can pose the greatest threat of wound infection. Thus, all treatment should be rendered as aseptically as possible. Gloves, cap, mask, instruments, and cleansing solutions should all be sterile.

3. *Debridement and Closure*

The skin wound should be thoroughly cleansed and debrided, with a minimum of additional trauma being imposed. Only tissue that is obviously contaminated and devitalized should be removed.[3,4] Devitalized tissue can act as a culture medium, promoting bacterial growth and inhibiting the host's defense mechanism.[4] All foreign material must also be removed. Sharp dissection and flushing with sterile solutions accomplish much of the necessary debridement. Flushing solutions should be isotonic and should be applied aseptically.

After debridement and cleansing, approximation of tissue edges should be considered. Approximation is essentially equivalent to primary closure.[1,3] Michel clips are useful for this purpose because they can be quickly applied and removed, and they allow drainage if infection occurs.

Primary or secondary closure can be delayed until a contaminated wound has been converted to a clean wound.[1,3] Delaying definitive closure a minimum of four to five days is recommended when the full extent of injury to the tissue is in doubt. This delay allows more-accurate evaluation of viable tissue.[4] With secondary closure of a wound, development of healthy granulation tissue within 10 to 14 days is anticipated. Primary skin closure may then be feasible.[1,3]

4. *Wound Coverage*

Covering an extensive leg wound with a thick, cotton-padded bandage provides four advantages:

- Uniform but minimal pressure is applied to the skin, allowing adherence to underlying tissue.
- Motion is limited.
- The patient cannot further traumatize the wound.
- Contamination is prevented.

In bandaging the wound, care should always be taken not to compromise available blood supply.

In consequence of delay, sepsis and degree of debridement must be considered to achieve best results in managing a skin wound. Early closure of a leg laceration is especially desirable to avoid difficulties due to contraction of the wound.

REFERENCES

1. Peacock, E.E., Jr.: Van Winkle, W.: *Surgery and Biology of Wound Repair.* W.B. Saunders Co., Philadelphia, Pa., 1970.
2. Johnston, D.E.: The Processes in Wound Healing. *JAAHA 13*:186-196; 1977.
3. Burke, J.F.: Fundamentals of Wound Management in Surgery "Infection". Chirurgecom, Inc., S. Plainfield, N.J., 1977; p 49.
4. Haury, B. *et al*: Debridement: An Essential Component of Traumatic Wound Care. *Am. J. Surgery 135*:238-242; 1978.

surgical correction of

TAIL-FOLD DERMATITIS

in the English bulldog

L.D. Rubin, VMD
Rhawnhurst Animal Hospital
7905 Bustleton Avenue
Philadelphia, Pennsylvania 19152

IN ENGLISH BULLDOGS, ankylosis of the coccygeal vertebrae, coupled with a tightly curled tail, can cause severe intertriginous dermatitis. As the dog matures and gains weight, a skin fold develops that encircles the base of the tail (*Figure 1*). A moist and malodorous dermatitis usually ensues. Frequently the skin comprising the fold deteriorates, and sometimes a granulomatous lesion develops.

Topical treatment of tail-fold dermatitis is not satisfactory because the pathologic anatomy will certainly cause a recurrence. Surgical removal of the skin fold is the only permanent cure. This operation is complicated by the need to remove the entire tailbone in order to expose the skin fold to its full depth.

Figure 1
The base of the tail is encircled by a fold of skin.

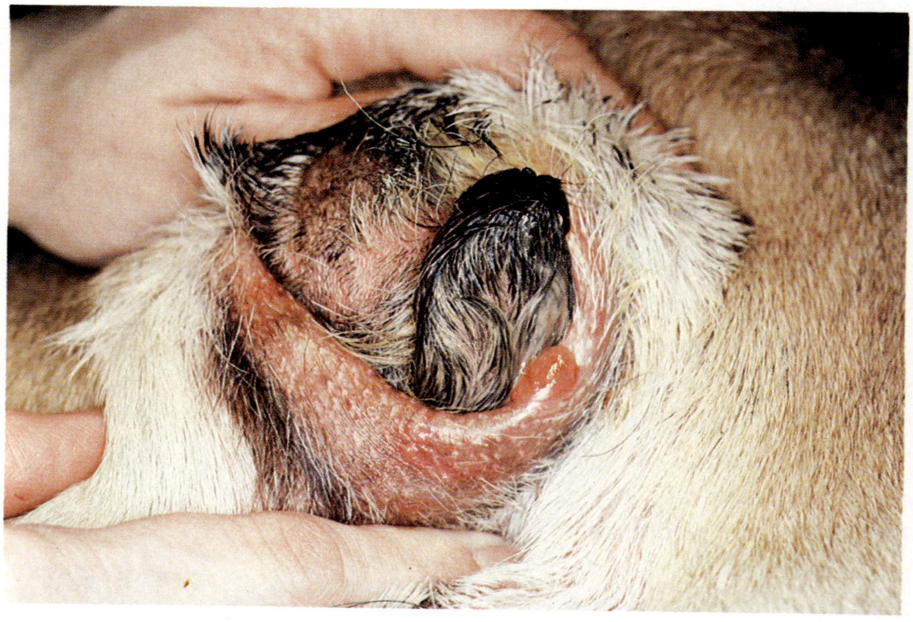

Surgical Procedure

The dog is put in dorsal recumbency and the incision site is prepared routinely, except for the obviously impossible task of shaving the tail into the full depth of the fold. A deep incision is made through the dorsal skin fold, beginning 3 cm anterior to the sacrococcygeal articulation and extending posteriorly over the mid-dorsal line of the base of the tail. The sacrococcygeal articulation is palpated, and the bone is then exposed by sharp and blunt dissection.

The index finger of one hand is inserted into the ventral skin fold to the depth of the sacrum. With the other hand, a small Liston bone cutter is applied over the articulation (*Figure 2*). As the sacrococcyx is separated, the finger inserted into the skin fold is used to ensure that the points of the bone cutter penetrate no deeper than through the bone and accompanying coccygeal muscles.

When the separation is complete, the entire tail is retracted caudally. This everts the skin folds. At this time the remainder of the tail can be shaved and prepared for surgery. The area is redraped and new gloves are donned.

The freed base of the tail is exposed and the midline dorsal incision is extended caudally to the tip of the tail (*Figure 3*). The entire coccyx is then

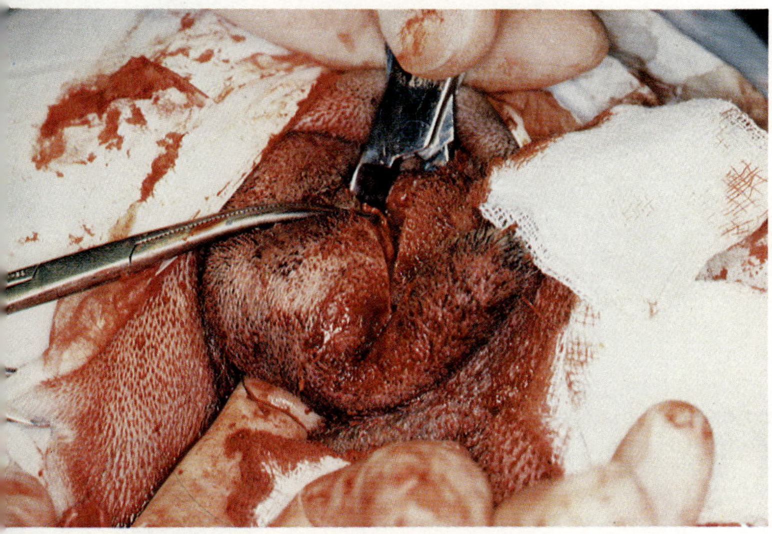

Figure 2
A Liston bone cutter is used to cut through the bone and coccygeal muscles at the articulation of the sacrococcyx joint.

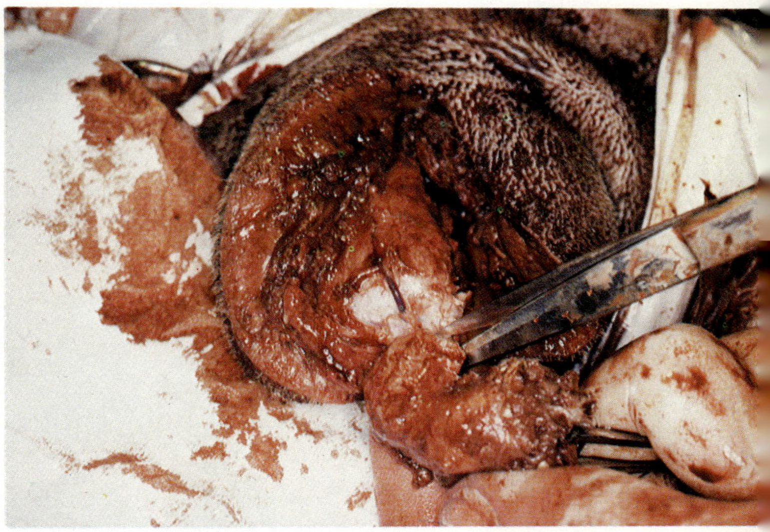

Figure 3
The dorsal midline incision is extended from the base of the tail to the tip of the tail.

dissected and removed (*Figure 4*). Care must be taken to leave as much subcutis as possible attached to the remaining skin.

The boneless tail hangs straight down. It is rather long, actually resembling a turtle's tail.

The dorsal incision is closed with stainless steel sutures in a simple interrupted pattern starting from the base of the tail and progressing toward the tip of the tail (*Figure 5*). A cosmetically pleasing length is determined and the tip of the tail is amputated. Skin closure is then completed (*Figure 6*).

When healing is complete, the tail wags as vigorously as the tail on any other Bulldog. ■

Figure 6

The tip of the tail has been amputated to give a cosmetically pleasing appearance, and closure of the skin incision has been completed.

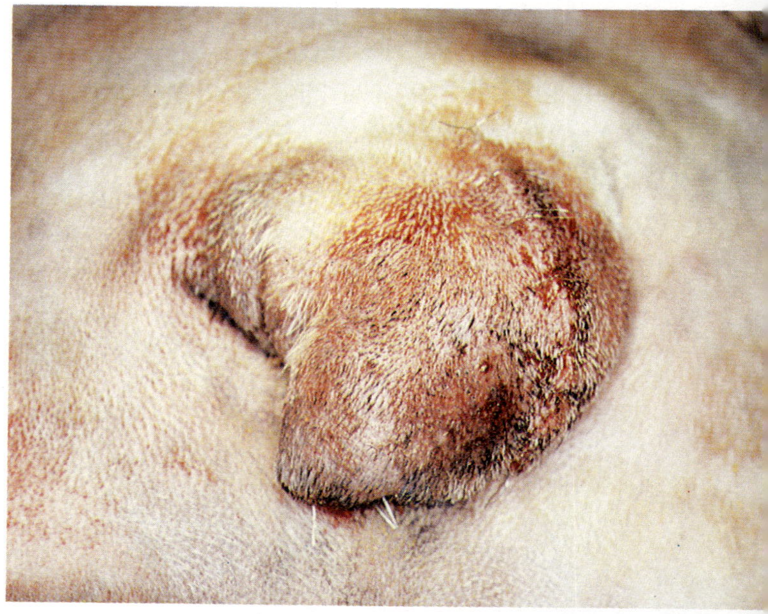

Figure 4

Appearance of the coccyx after dissection and removal.

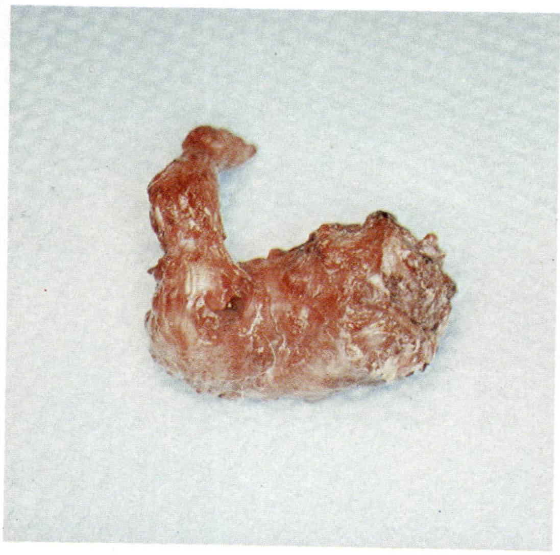

Figure 5

The incision is sutured from the base of the tail to the tip using stainless steel in a simple interrupted pattern.

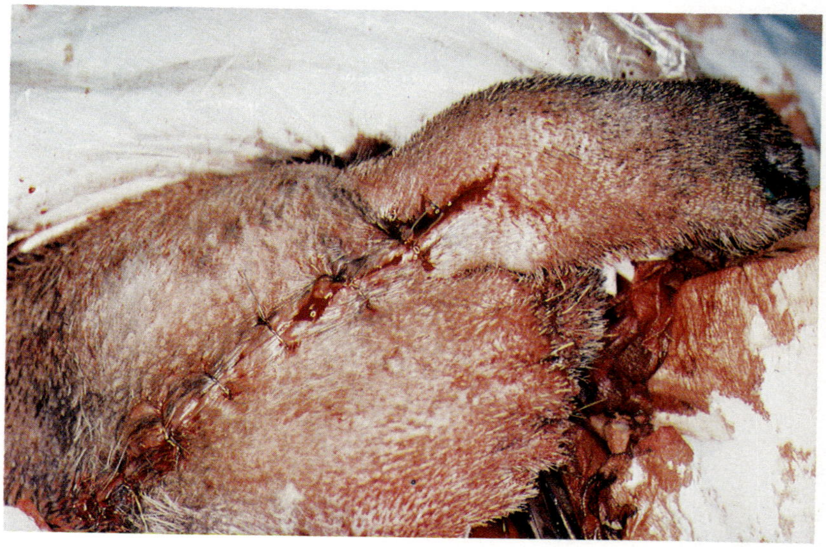

reconstructive surgery for a BITE-WOUND ABSCESS

Michael B. Auslander, DVM
Auslander Animal Hospital
501 South First Street
LaGrange, Kentucky 40031

Veterinarians frequently treat cats suffering infected bite wounds, or animals with large areas of the body from which the skin has been lost. Skin loss from an extensive area is usually associated with traumatic injuries such as burns, automobile accidents, and fights with other animals. This report concerns a cat which sustained loss of a large area of skin as a sequela to a probable bite wound. The cat was treated successfully with antibiotics and an autogenous skin graft.

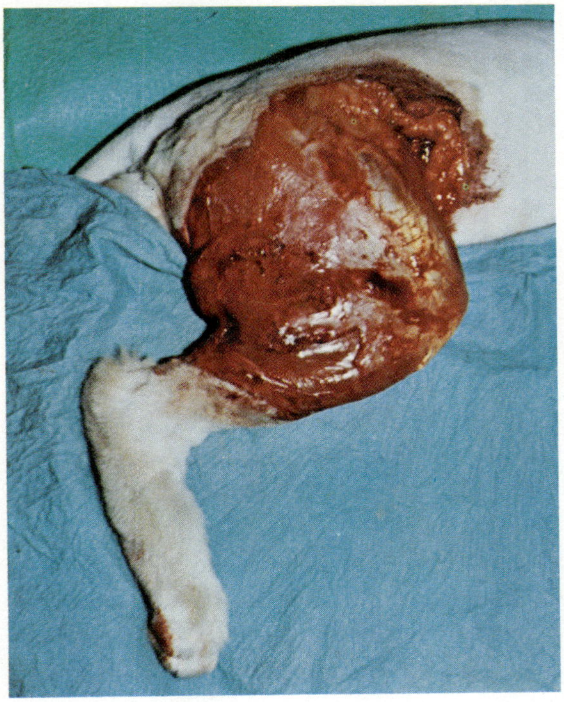

Figure 1—Appearance of the lesion after surgical debridement.

Case report

An 18-month-old, male cat was presented because of anorexia, depression, and a draining lesion on the upper right side of the rear leg. The cat's temperature was 104 F (40 C). Purulent material could be expressed from an opening 1 cm in diameter in the leg. The diagnosis was bite-wound abscess.

When an effort was made to clip the affected site so that it could be scrubbed and the lesion flushed, the hair did not cut normally. Instead, the clippers pulled the hair and large patches of necrotic skin from the leg. The animal was anesthetized and the leg was debrided of all necrotic tissue. Adjacent areas of healthy skin were clipped, and the entire upper leg was cleaned with a surgical scrub.

The resulting lesion was a full-thickness loss of skin encompassing an area from the coxofemoral joint distally to just above the hock and extending over the complete dorsal surface and part of the ventral surface of the leg (*Figure 1*). A skin graft seemed to be the treatment of choice.

Figure 2—The skin flap prepared for transposition.

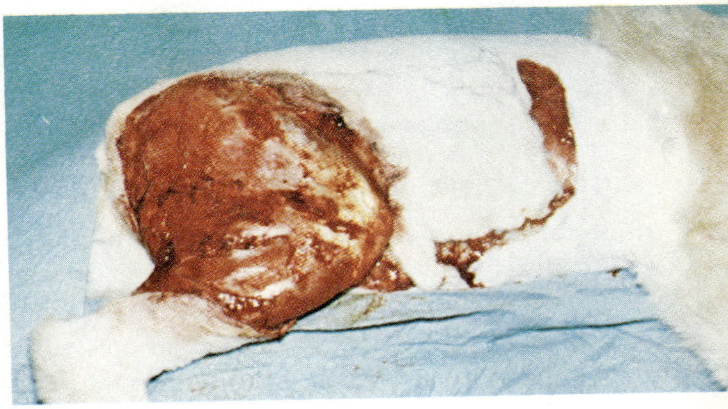

Surgical procedure

The length and width of the affected area were measured and a rectangle of these dimensions was drawn on the skin immediately cranial to the lesion. The ventral and cranial sides of the rectangle

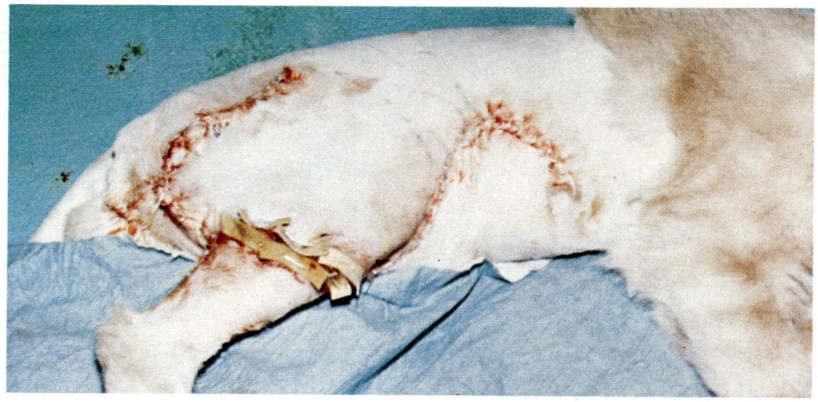

Figure 3—Appearance of wound after suturing. Pieces of rubber band were incorporated in the mattress sutures to help prevent necrosis.

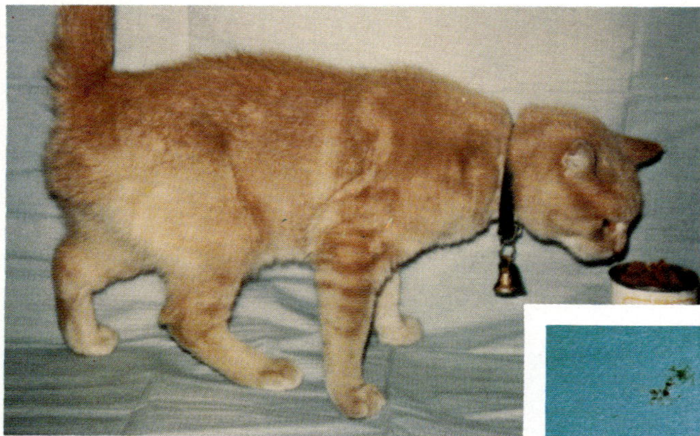

Figure 4—One year after the operation the cat appears almost normal.

were cut. The caudal edge was a free margin; the dorsal margin was not cut. The skin within the margins was undermined from the subcutis to form a flap attached dorsally (*Figure 2*).

All skin margins were undermined 1 cm to 3 cm back from the free edge. The flap thus formed for grafting was pulled over the leg and sutured at the margins. A combination of interrupted simple and continuous interlocking sutures was used at the cranial and caudal suture lines. Interrupted horizontal mattress sutures were used at the junction of the graft and the mid-tibial area. There was moderate tension on the distal suture line. Pieces of a rubber band (8-mm wide) were incorporated in the mattress sutures to help prevent necrosis (*Figure 3*).

The defect created at the donor site was closed by undermining the skin margins, apposing the edges, and suturing with a continuous interlocking pattern. All sutures used were of 00 nylon.

Postsurgical care

An attempt was made to place the leg in a sling to keep it flexed after the surgery. However, the cat would not tolerate the sling. The cat did not lick the sutures excessively. Lincomycin was prescribed at a dosage of 100 mg b.i.d. The day after the operation the cat was sent home and the owner was instructed to confine it to the house.

When the cat was returned 10 days later for removal of the sutures, the graft seemed attached to the subcutis in most places. An area of necrosis was noted at both corners of the distal margin of the graft. These sites composed less than 10% of the total graft area and were exuding a small amount of purulent discharge. Also, an area of wound dehiscence measuring 1 cm was situated at the junction of the leg and the flank. Chloramphenicol at a dosage of 100 mg t.i.d. was prescribed. The animal was sent home and the owner was instructed to keep it confined.

The cat was rechecked seven days later. The necrotic areas were healing well by granulation and wound contraction. The area of dehiscence on the flank showed no change. With no further treatment this small area required approximately four months to close by wound contraction.

Postoperative care was minimal and consisted of confining the cat and giving it antibiotics. The skin healed rapidly except for the small area previously mentioned. The cat regained normal mobility within a month after the procedure. After one year, the cat appeared almost normal (*Figure 4*). ■

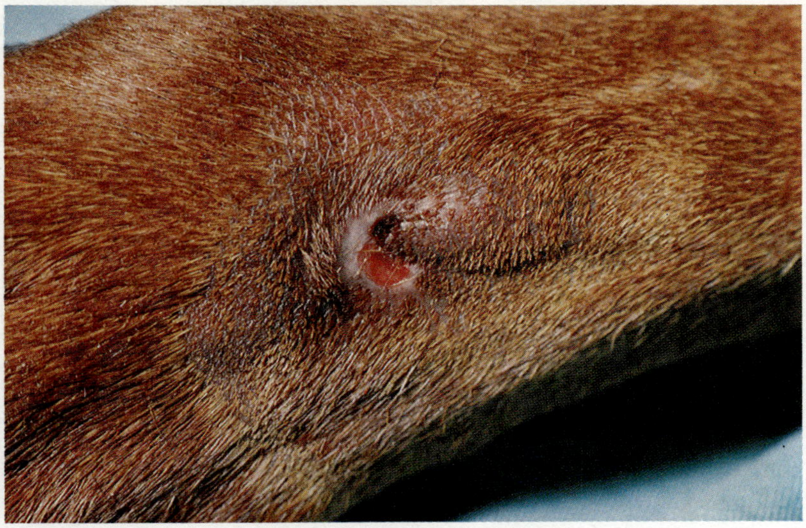

Figure 1
The opening of the fistulous tract is seen on the dorsal surface of the paw just proximal to the digits.

A FISTULOUS TRACT induced by a foreign body in a dog

Stephen J. Birchard, DVM
Russ L. Stickle, DVM
Jerry A. Thornhill, DVM
Dept. of Small Animal Clinics
School of Veterinary Medicine
Purdue University
West Lafayette, Indiana 47907

Cutaneous fistulous tracts that chronically drain pus are common in veterinary medicine.[1] Perianal fistulas have been well described,[2] but cutaneous fistulas in other sites have not been as well documented. They are assumed to be caused by irritants or foreign bodies that act as a constant source of inflammation. Classically, these fistulas begin as localized abscesses that do not respond to routine therapy; *i.e.*, drainage and antibiotics.

Surgical exploration of cutaneous fistulous tracts is, at best, difficult and time-consuming. Frequently, the source of the tract cannot be identified by surgical exploration. The tract or tracts may dissect near such vital structures as large arteries and nerves, hindering the surgeon's attempt to follow them.

The use of positive contrast fistulography has become an important preoperative tool for defining the extent and shape of the tracts. The fistulogram technique is practical, easily performed, and can give valuable information about the site of the tracts. The contrast material may even outline a foreign body.

In this paper we report a case of a chronic, draining, cutaneous fistulous tract caused by a

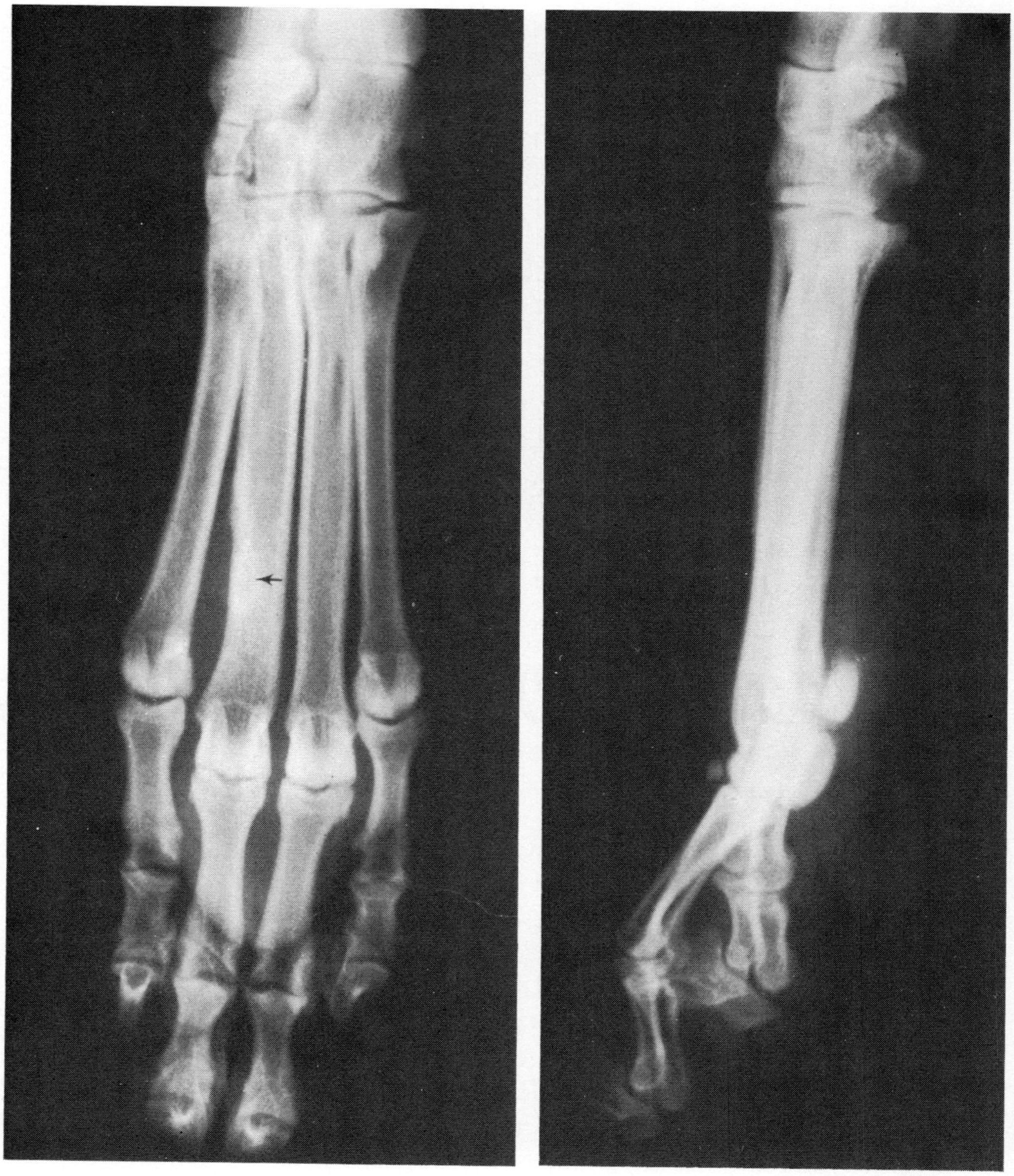

Figures 2A & B
Anteroposterior (*right*) and lateral (*far right*) radiographs showing tissue-swelling, separation of the distal portions of the second and third metatarsal, and sclerosis of the medial cortex of the third metatarsal (*small arrow*).

wooden foreign body in a dog's metatarsal region. The case is presented to illustrate the value of a preoperative fistulogram and to describe the surgical technique used to trace the tract to the foreign body. Postoperative management of the surgical wound is also described.

Case report

Signalment and history

A 1½-year-old, male, intact, Redbone Hound weighing 70 lb (31.5 kg) was presented to the Purdue University Small Animal Clinic with the primary complaint of a chronic draining fistulous tract on the dorsal surface of the left metatarsus (*Figure 1*). The tract had been apparent for approximately four months. No history of trauma to the paw was evident before the onset of the draining tract. Previous treatment for the condition included antibiotics, corticosteroids, and surgical probing of the tract. When exercised, the dog became noticeably lame on the affected leg.

Physical examination

When the dog was examined, a purulent fluid was draining from the lesion. A healed scar was

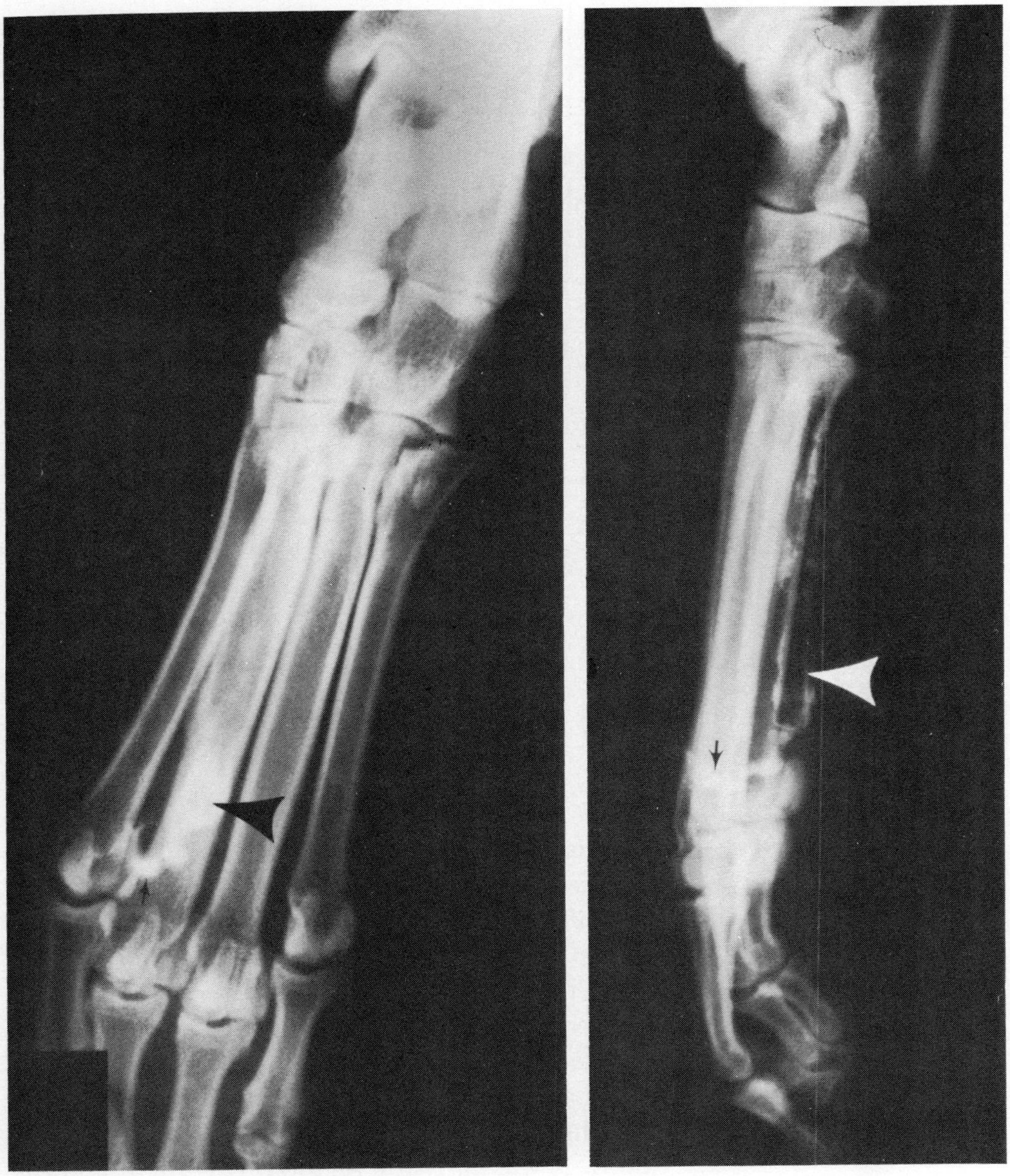

Figures 3A & B
Anteroposterior (*far left*) and lateral (*left*) radiographs taken after injection of positive contrast medium in the fistulous tract (*small arrows*). The foreign body is seen on the plantar aspect of the paw (*large arrows*).

seen on the plantar surface of the same paw. This scar corresponded to the wound made when the tract was previously probed by the referring veterinarian. No lameness of the leg was noticed.

The dog otherwise was in good physical condition and was not febrile.

Radiology

Survey radiographs (*Figure 2*) showed soft-tissue swelling, with separation of the distal ends of the second and third metatarsal bones. The cortex of the third metatarsal bone was sclerotic at the site of the fistulous tract.

A Sovereign® Tom Cat catheter (Sherwood) was inserted as far as possible into the tract. Thus, while pressure was applied with a surgical sponge to the opening into the tract, 2 cc of a water-soluble radiopaque contrast agent (Conray® —Mallinckrodt) was injected. On the resulting fistulogram a long, cone-shaped radiolucent foreign body in the metatarsal region could be seen as a filling defect in the positive contrast medium (*Figure 3*). Although the tract-opening was on the dorsal surface of the paw, the foreign body was in a plantar relationship to the third metatarsal bone.

Figure 4
The foreign body is seen with the blunted end facing distally. Notice the polyethylene catheter coming through from the dorsal side of the paw.

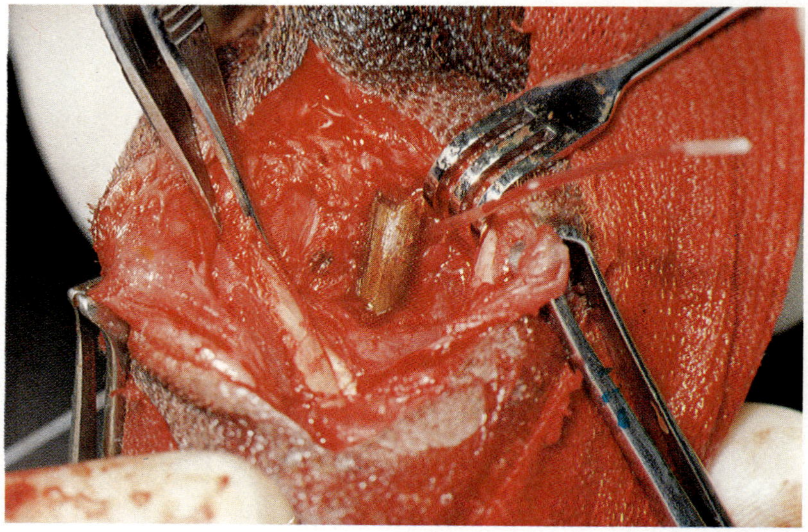

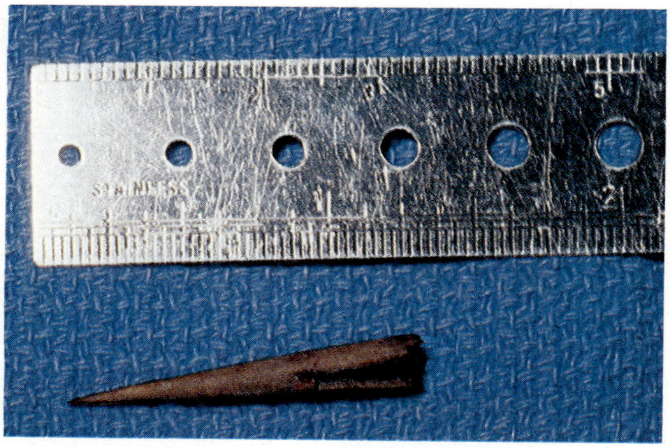

Figure 5—The wooden foreign body after its removal.

Surgical procedure

The dog was preanesthetized with 1.4 mg of atropine sulfate given subcutaneously. Anesthesia was induced with 8 cc of 5% thiopental and maintained with halothane and nitrous oxide delivered in a semi-closed rebreathing system via a cuffed endotracheal tube. During the surgery, lactated Ringer's solution was given intravenously at a dosage of 4 ml/lb/hour.

The entire left hind paw and tarsus were clipped and prepared for aseptic surgery.

An incision 8 cm long was made over the plantar surface of the third metatarsal bone. The deep soft tissues were carefully dissected and the tendons of the superficial and deep flexor muscles were identified as described[3] and retracted. A Sovereign® Tom Cat catheter was passed through the fistulous tract to help lead to the foreign body. Dissection was continued along the catheter until a wooden, pointed foreign body was found (*Figure 4*). The foreign body was situated on the plantar surface of the third metatarsal bone, deep to the flexor tendons. It was carefully removed (*Figure 5*) and the area was flushed with sterile saline solution to remove any residual debris.

A section of fenestrated Silastic® tubing (Intramedic® polyethylene tubing—Clay-Adams, Inc.) was passed through the deeper tissues of the wound, employing entry and exit holes separate from the incision. This tube facilitated postoperative flushing of the wound with sterile saline solution. A soft-rubber drainage tube (Penrose tube—Davol®) was inserted in the distal aspect of the wound to accommodate drainage of serum and the flushing solution (*Figure 6*).

Subcutaneous tissue was closed with sutures of 2-0 polyglycolic acid (Dexon® —American Cyanamid). This material was used instead of catgut in

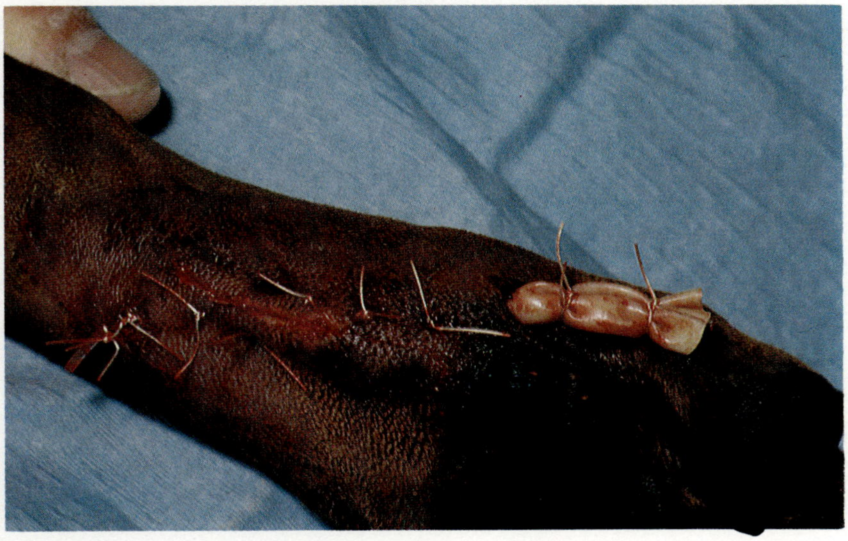

Figure 6
The plantar surface of the paw as seen postoperatively. Note the Silastic® tubing at the proximal end of the incision. The rubber drain is visible distally.

an attempt to reduce the inflammatory response around the wound. The skin was closed with 2-0 Vetafil® (S. Jackson) in a vertical mattress pattern. The incision then was covered with an antibiotic ointment (Biozide® wound dressing—Performance Products, Inc.) and the paw was bandaged.

Specimens were taken for culturing and sensitivity testing, but no significant growth was obtained. Postoperatively, the dog was given lincomycin (10 mg/lb) orally every 12 hours. The wound was flushed once a day and the bandage was changed daily. The dog was bearing weight on the leg within 24 hours after the operation.

The drain and tubing were left in place for three days.

Ten days postoperatively the skin sutures were removed by the referring veterinarian. The wound and fistulous tract were healing well at that time. No recurrence of the tract has been reported.

Discussion

This case is a good example of how integration of radiology and surgery can hasten diagnosis and therapy of a chronic disease. Without preoperative radiology, surgery on this patient would have been more difficult—possibly fruitless. The surgeon, not knowing the foreign body was on the plantar surface, could conceivably have made the incision and exploration on the dorsum of the paw.

The feeding of a polyethylene catheter through the tract during surgery is another helpful means of finding the source of the infection, in this case, the wooden foreign body. Without this advantage, it is possible to lose sight of the tract in the deeper tissues.

Immediately after the foreign body is removed, the tissue must be flushed with copious amounts of sterile saline solution. Postoperative flushing of the wound for two to three days is not mandatory, but is helpful in preventing delayed healing of the wound as a result of sepsis.

ACKNOWLEDGMENTS

The authors thank Dr. Terry Woolwine for referring this case to the Purdue Small Animal Clinic, and Mr. Tom Huffman for the photos.

REFERENCES

1. Thordal-Christensen, A.: In *Canine Surgery*, 1st ed. (J. Archibald, ed.). American Veterinary Publications, Inc., Wheaton, Ill., 1965; p 346.
2. Lowry, E.C.: In *Current Techniques in Small Animal Surgery* (M.J. Bojrab, ed.). Lea & Febiger, Philadelphia, Pa., 1975; pp 159-161.
3. Miller, M.E. *et al: Anatomy of the Dog*. W.B. Saunders Co., Philadelphia, Pa., 1964; pp 260-261.

Small Animal Surgery

CHEST

Pacemaker and sutureless lead implantation in a dog with third-degree heart block

Greg P. Sykes, VMD
Guilford Veterinary Hospital
81 Saw Mill Road
Guilford, Connecticut 06437

EIGHTEEN YEARS HAVE PASSED since the introduction of means to pace the heart by surgically implanting electronic devices in the patient's body.[1] Implantation of a self-contained pulse generator and cardiac electrodes quickly became the therapy of choice for certain rhythm disorders of the heart. Direct ventricular stimulation allows cardiac output to be maintained despite interrupted atrioventricular (AV) conduction.

Normal cardiac conduction begins in the sinoatrial (SA) node, passes through the atrial musculature, and excites the AV node. From the AV node, current continues through the Bundle of His and Purkinje fibers to discharge both the left and right ventricular myocardia.

Complete (third degree) heart block occurs when conduction along the Bundle of His has been totally interrupted. In these cases, for initiation of systole, the ventricles rely on their own cells or on the automaticity of the His-Purkinje cells. A variety of lesions of the AV node or Bundle of His may disturb conduction.[2]

The following case of idiopathic third-degree

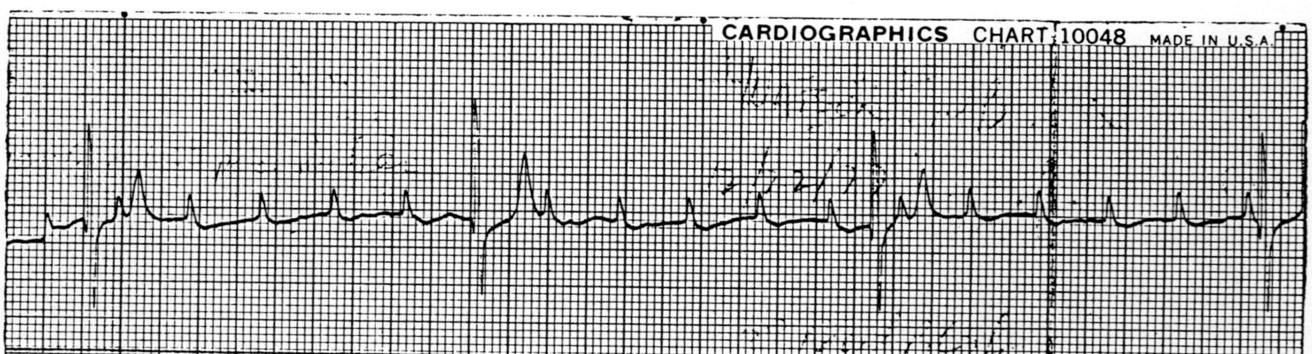

Figure 1
Lead II of the electrocardiogram taken the day after the onset of clinical signs. The shape of the QRS complex is normal but completely dissociated from the p-waves. The atrial rate is 175 beats/minute; the ventricular rate is 35 beats/minute.

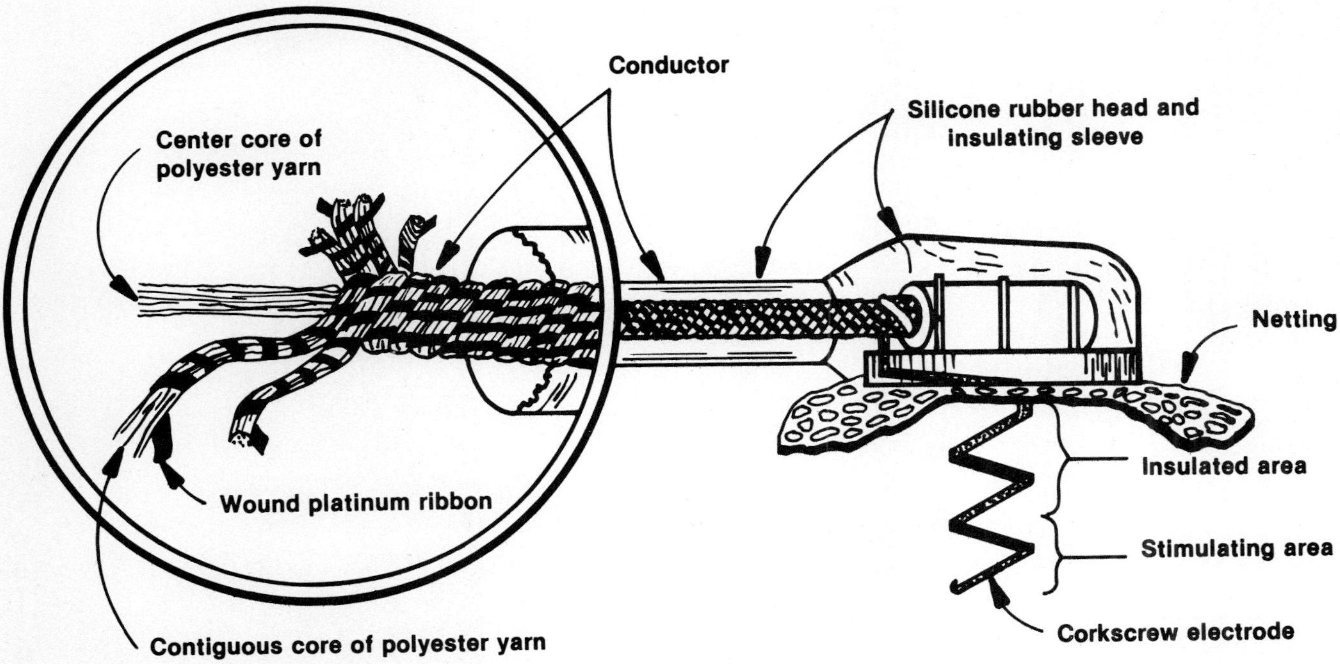

Figure 2—Diagram of the sutureless corkscrew electrode and conductor.

heart block was successfully treated by surgically implanting a pulse generator and unipolar sutureless electrode.

Case history

A 9-year-old male Basset Hound weighing 52.8 lb (24 kg) was presented with clinical signs of vomiting and lethargy of one day's duration. The heart rate, measured by auscultation and palpation of the femoral pulse, was 30 to 40 beats/minute. Complete blood count (CBC), blood urea nitrogen (BUN), and serum creatinine values were normal, as were sodium, potassium, calcium, and chloride. Serum liver enzymes were elevated (*Table 1*).

An ECG was performed. Results supported a diagnosis of third-degree heart block with an atrial rate of 175 beats/minute (*Figure 1*). Radiographs showed mild enlargement of the heart. The lung field was clear. The dog was maintained with cage rest for one week while a pacemaker and electrode were being obtained.

A unipolar, demand pacemaker was used (Xytron Pulse Generator, Model 5951—Medtronic, Inc., Minneapolis, Minn. 55418). This type of pacemaker delivers impulses through the conductor lead and electrode when the intrinsic heart rate falls below the designated setting of the pacemaker (in this case 80 beats/minute). The pacemaker is

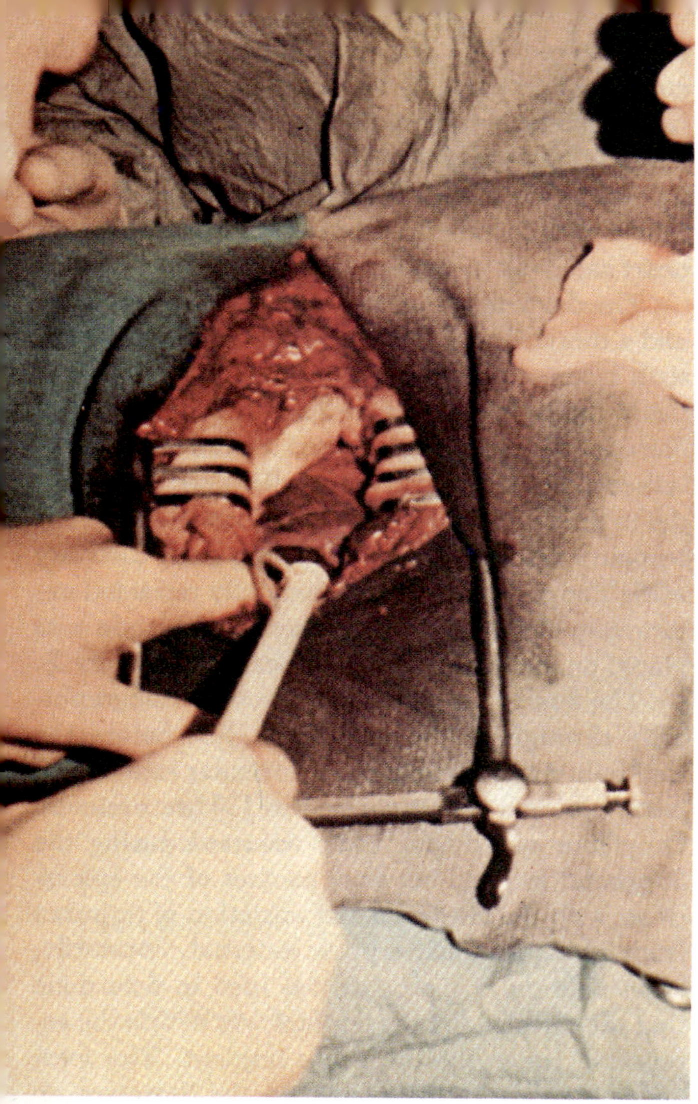

Figure 3—The electrode and lead are held in their handle and twisted into the left ventricular wall.

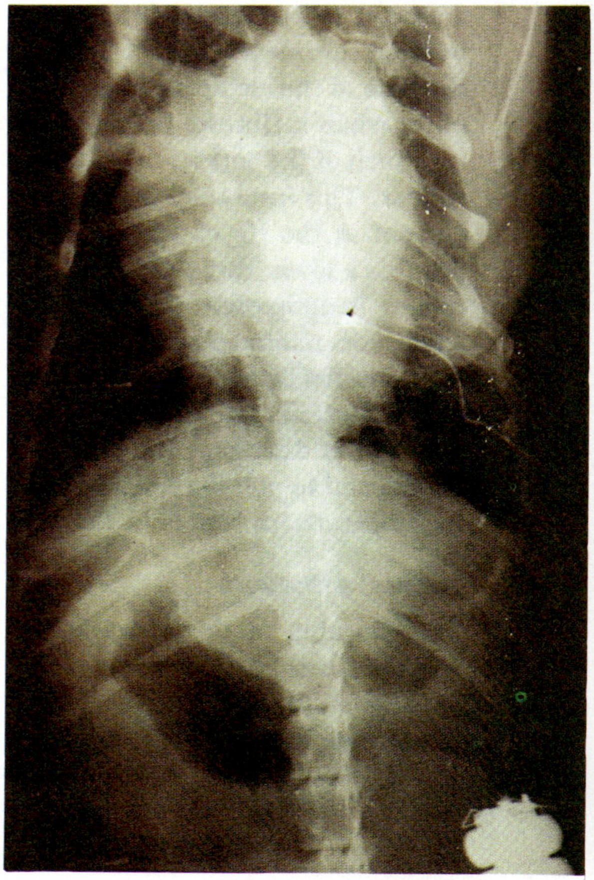

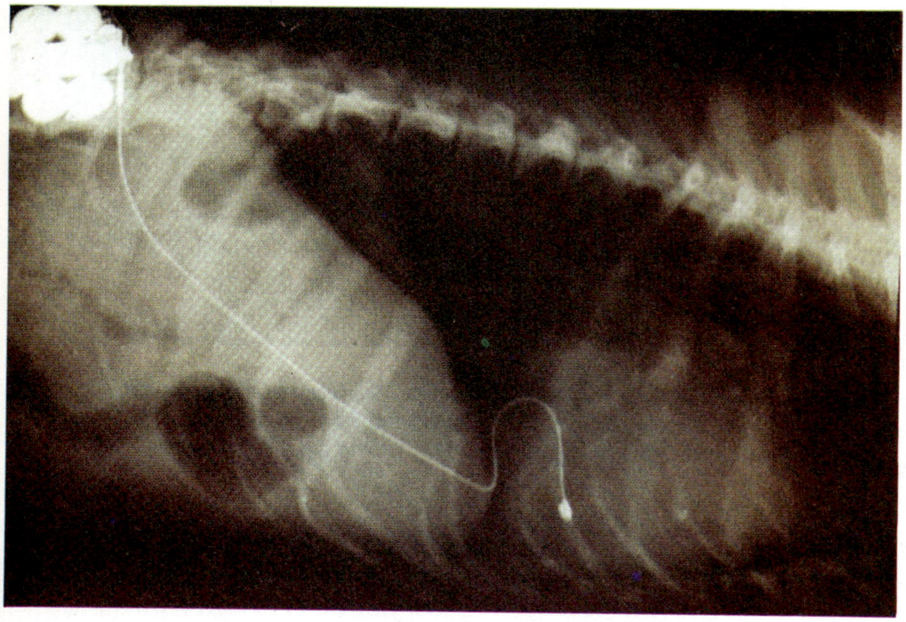

Figures 4A & B

Appearance of the corkscrew electrode and pulse generator as seen on the postoperative radiographs.

administered. The dog was clipped to reduce the amount of preparation necessary under anesthesia. Immediately before induction of anesthesia, the animal's heart rate was 18 beats/minute. Anesthesia was induced with 200 mg thiamylal and maintained with halothane. Under anesthesia, the dog's heart rate was 25 beats/minute.

The dog was placed in right lateral recumbency and a thoracotomy was performed through the left sixth intercostal space. An incision 7 cm long was made through the pericardium in a dorsoventral direction. This incision exposed a relatively avascular section of left ventricular wall immediately caudal to the ventral interventricular branch of the left coronary artery and accompanying great coronary vein. The pericardium was manually retracted anteroventrally while the corkscrew electrode was placed on the selected area of epicardium (*Figure 3*).

The heart was monitored electrocardiographically throughout the procedure. Just before the electrode was attached, the ventricular rate was 10 beats/min. and the atrial rate was 130 beats/minute. Only four ventricular beats occurred during the 30-second interval between contact of the epicardium with the electrode and initiation of impulses from an external battery. An external, nonsterile, adjustable pulse generator was used to determine that the threshold of the implant was within the acceptable range for the acute implant. The term *acute implant* has been used in the literature on powered by four mercury-zinc cells that offer a minimum projected service life of four years.

A single myocardial pacing lead with a corkscrew-shaped electrode (Medtronic Sutureless Myocardial Pacing Lead, Model 6917) was selected for implantation. The electrode's spiral design allows it to be affixed firmly to the myocardium without sutures (*Figure 2*). Dacron mesh netting at the base of the electrode head provides further stability when it fibroses to the epicardium.

Much of the corkscrew is insulated with silicone rubber. This insulation concentrates density of the current at the tip of the corkscrew, thus making possible a lower threshold of stimulation. The conductor is composed of six intertwined platinum conductors reinforced with polyester. The electrode-lead unit fits into a handle that facilitates screwing of the electrode into the myocardium. A tunneler is supplied to disengage the electrode head from the handle and to pull the distal end of the lead through its subcutaneous tunnel to the pulse generator.

Surgical procedure

The morning of the operation, eight days after onset of heart block, the dog was extremely lethargic and could hardly walk. One hour before anesthesia was induced, 1.5 mg atropine sulfate was

Figure 5—Lead II electrocardiogram taken one hour after implantation. The bizarre QRS complex reflects the new path of ventricular depolarization. Still dissociated from all p-waves, the QRS complexes occur at 90 beats/min., the designated setting of the pacemaker.

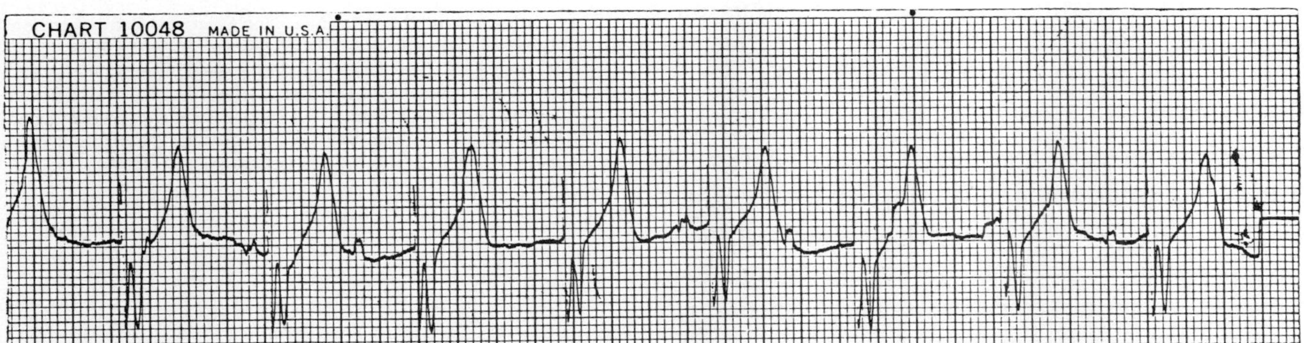

TABLE 1—Serum Hepatic Enzyme Values (IU/Liter) Before and After Implantation of the Pacemaker

	Before	One Month After
SGPT	323	70
LDH	183	81
Alk Phos	153	44

human medicine to refer to threshold values immediately after implantation. These values change with time, especially after scar formation.

A subcutaneous pouch to receive the battery was created in the left paralumbar fossa. The tunneler was passed backwards subcutaneously from the pouch, through the seventh intercostal space. The free end of the lead was attached to the implanted pacemaker. Two sutures of 00 monofilament nylon (Ethilon® —Ethicon, Inc.) were used to secure the lead to the pacemaker and the pacemaker to the lumbar musculature.

A chest tube was inserted and both incisions were closed routinely. Postoperative radiographs were taken (*Figures 4A&B*). Antibiotics were administered to prevent infection.

An ECG reading was taken one hour postoperatively while the dog was still under anesthesia (*Figure 5*). Additional ECG readings were taken one week, one month, and six months postoperatively. The ventricular rate consistently has been 80 beats/min., but the atrial rate has varied from 120 to 187 beats/minute. Shapes of the various complexes remain essentially unchanged with only minor, probably inconsequential, alterations in amplitude. Two months after the implantation, a blood profile was obtained and all values were within normal limits (*Table 1*). Nine months postoperatively, the dog remained vigorous. No abnormal signs have appeared.

Discussion

The development of a sutureless myocardial pacing lead is an important step in simplifying the procedure for implanting a pacemaker. Results of previous studies have indicated that the screwing action of the corkscrew electrode causes much less damage than the lancing action of other myocardial electrodes. Further, the corkscrew configuration of the electrode creates at least 10 times the force-bearing surface of a lead attached by sutures.[3]

In the human medical field many surgeons advocate implanting the sutureless electrode by means of a subxiphoid surgical approach under local anesthesia.[4] However, such an approach would surely not be applicable to the dog. The thickness of the canine right ventricular wall that would be exposed by such an approach would usually be less than the 6-mm depth of the corkscrew, and only the last three-quarter turn is not insulated. These circumstances seem to necessitate the use of a thoracic approach in dogs, with the animal under general anesthesia.

In the case presented here, the extremely low ventricular rate recorded during the operation, particularly after mechanical contact was made with the electrode, is worth noting. Apparently the patient was close to cardiac arrest and probably would have benefited from pharmacologic support. Isoproterenol has been used to stimulate ventricular contraction[5] but was unavailable at the time of implantation. A transvenous electrode also could have been used to maintain the heart during surgery[6] if one had been available.

An important point to remember is that even an attached unipolar pulse generator will not depolarize the heart until the metal face of the unit touches the patient's tissues. A patient could easily die while the surgeon held the connected pacemaker and waited for it to function.

REFERENCES

1. Chardack, W.M. *et al*: A Transistorized Self-Contained, Implantable Pacemaker for the Long-Term Correction of Complete Heart Block. *Surgery 48*: 643-654; 1960.
2. Webb, T.J. *et al*: Artificial Cardiac Pacemakers and Some Clinical Indications for Pacemaking. *Southwest. Vet. 28*:91-99; 1975.
3. Hunter, S.W. *et al*: A New Myocardial Pacemaker Lead (Sutureless). *Chest 63*:430-433; 1973.
4. Stewart, S.: Placement of the Sutureless Epicardial Pacemaker Lead by the Subxiphoid Approach. *Ann. Thorac. Surg. 18*:308-313; 1974.
5. Buchanan, J.W. *et al*: Medical and Pacemaker Therapy of Complete Heart Block and Congestive Heart Failure in a Dog. *JAVMA 152*:1099-1109; 1968.
6. Lombard, V.C.; Buchanan, J.W.: Implantation eines Elektronischen Herzschrittmachers bei einem Fall von AV-block III. Grad. Beim Hund. Berl. *Munch. tierarztl. Wchnschr. 89*:362-364, 371-373; 1976.

Paratracheal Mediastinotomy in the Dog and Cat*

Raymond F. Hinkle, DVM
Hilltop Animal Hospital
135 East Lake Cook Road
Palatine, Illinois 60007

AN APPROACH to dealing with pathologic processes that affect the mediastinal space in dogs and cats would be aided by a safe and simple technique used for direct inspection, biopsy, or treatment of this space. Because of its close relationship to vital anatomic and protective musculoskeletal structures, the mediastinal space is a difficult and often risky area in which to work.[1,2] With a good history and physical examination, and by using conventional diagnostic and therapeutic techniques, diagnosis of mediastinal disease can often be made. In cases where this is not possible, thoracotomy, empirical treatment, or euthanasia may be the alternative.

Presently a variety of diagnostic aids are being used by veterinarians to diagnose and treat mediastinal disease.[3–14] Once suspected, the presence of mediastinal disease is often confirmed using flat-film radiography. Additional applications might incorporate contrast, image intensification, and tomography. Nuclear medicine and ultrasound are considerations as well. Common questions concerning disease processes in the mediastinum include neoplasia *versus* infection *versus* inflammation? malignant *versus* benign *versus* hyperplasia?

Differentiation may require additional diagnostic procedures. Hematology and serology can help, but a more direct approach may be needed, such as tracheal sampling or needle aspiration in conjunction with cytology and culturing. Techniques using thin-needle aspiration and ultrasound may have application as well.[15] Immuno-testing, such as for leukemia virus, has also been supportive. Despite the many approaches to the diagnosis of mediastinal disease, a more direct diagnostic technique may be needed to make the definitive diagnosis.

In man, mediastinoscopy has been used as a direct yet simple approach to the mediastinum. Its use has been primarily as a diagnostic and prognostic indicator for neoplastic processes, most notably when thoracotomy is contemplated.[16–25] A variety of other diagnostic and therapeutic applications have been reported. For example, the techniques have been used to diagnose cases of bacterial and fungal infections, benign and cystic processes, and vascular and eosophageal abnormalities.[16,20,22,24–26] Techniques for radiographic contrast studies, pacemaker installations, and mediastinal drainage have also been reported.[10,26–29]

Since the concept of mediastinoscopy was first introduced, a variety of approaches to the mediastinal space in man have been discussed.[18,20,24,26,30–33] The most widely used technique is one initially described in 1959, in which the mediastinal space was approached through the thoracic inlet.[31] A small suprasternal and paratracheal incision was made. The same investigator developed the first mediastinoscope. Other approaches through the thoracic inlet are more paramedian. A subxiphoid approach

*This work was done while Dr. Hinkle was serving an internship program at Washington State University (1978-1979).

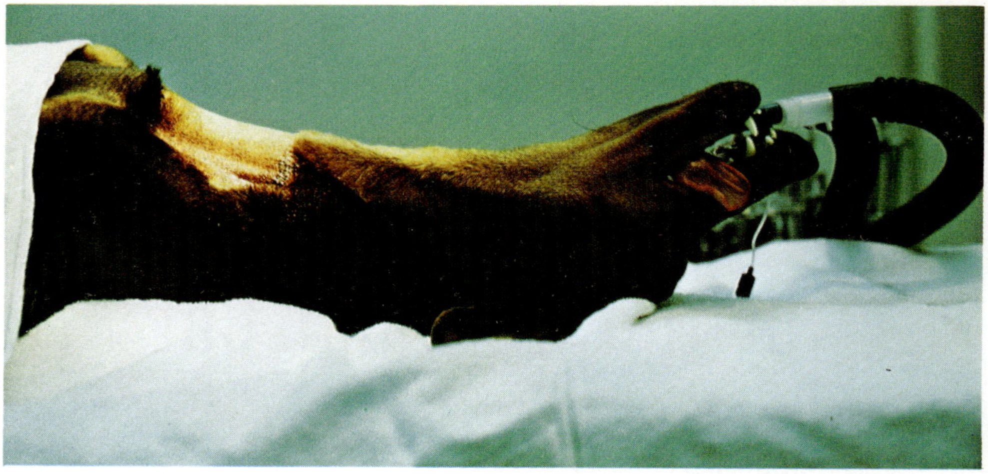

Figure 1—Positioning for paratracheal mediastinotomy requires that the animal be in dorsal recumbency with the neck extended and the forelegs extended posteriorly along the wall of the thorax.

has also been described.[30] General anesthesia, and local anesthesia alone have been used.[31,33,34]

Although controversy exists regarding specific indications for mediastinoscopy, it has been used extensively and is now generally accepted worldwide.[1,16,17,19-21,24-26,30,31,35-40] Studies indicate low morbidity and mortality.[1,2,17,24,26,33,35,36] The list of potential side effects is lengthy, but the reported frequencies are low, and the side effects were resolved with little difficulty.

In order of the highest reported frequency, the side effects include hemorrhage, pneumothorax, laryngeal paralysis, and infection.[16,18-20,24,26,31,33,35,36,39] Hemorrhage was controlled in all but a few cases by positive intermittent pressure. Major thoracic surgery was performed in very few cases, and hemostasis was achieved. The usual causes of hemorrhage have been aggressive biopsy and careless dissection.[35,37] In addition, fine-needle aspiration of any suspected hypervascular tissue to be sectioned could prevent most post-biopsy hemorrhage.

Pneumothorax was most frequent in cases where actual pulmonary biopsy was performed. These cases were managed by aspiration of the affected hemithorax after the biopsy specimen was taken. Several reports have cited the development of laryngeal paralysis, generally resulting from aggressive biopsy along the recurrent nerves. The majority of these cases involved only temporary pareses, but permanent paralyses have occurred. Postoperative infection was reported in few cases, and all of these infections were resolved using antibiotic therapy. Many of the affected patients were undergoing chemo or radiation therapy before mediastinoscopy was performed.

Considering the number and complexity of the structures in the mediastinal space, many other side effects are possible during mediastinoscopy. Infrequently reported side effects have included mediastinitis, minor postoperative discomfort, tumor seeding, impairment of the phrenic nerve, injury of the esophagus, chylothorax, air embolism, and hemiparesis of extremities secondary to arterial compression by instrumentation.[1,16,17,20,24,26,30,31,33,35,36,38] Complications are uncommon.

Generally, patients tolerate mediastinoscopy quite well, even when local anesthesia alone is used.[35,36,38] Very few pain receptors are believed present in the mediastinal space. Patients can be treated on an out-patient basis. Aspirin given for a few days postoperatively controls most discomfort caused by the incision.

Direct access to the mediastinal space is greatly simplified by the use of mediastinoscopy; however, when the procedure is attempted by poorly trained or unprepared individuals, the incidence of complication increases.[1,2,33,37,40] The technique warrants serious consideration before it is attempted. Also, anticipation of possible complications can forestall a fatal result. Preparation for positive-pressure ventilation, proper instrumentation, sterile technique, and preparations for performing thoracotomy (if necessary) all have contributed to survival of patients and widespread acceptance of the technique.

Veterinarians occasionally are confronted with a mediastinal problem that is difficult to diagnose. A definitive diagnosis is usually obtained using conventional approaches discussed previously. The use of a paratracheal mediastinotomy for diagnosis, prognosis, and treatment has not been reported in the veterinary literature. Nevertheless, for reasons of safety, economics, and diagnostic potential, paratracheal mediastinotomy has real application in select cases seen in veterinary practice.

Several approaches to the mediastinum for mediastinoscopy in man have been reported.[18,20,21,26,31–33] A medial approach, paratracheal in direction, was introduced in 1959.[31] Because of the simplicity, popularity, and diverse application of this method, a similar approach was believed to be of possible value in small animal medicine.

Mediastinoscopy in man has routinely been carried out with the patient under local or general anesthesia. Due to lack of cooperation from animal patients, general anesthesia is believed to be necessary for exploration of the medial space in the dog or cat. Also, preparations should be made for positive-pressure ventilation and thoracotomy, in the event that a serious respiratory or vascular insult should make such a procedure necessary.

Instrumentation is routine—usually requiring only a small laceration pack. Additional instruments may be needed, depending on the procedures being attempted in the mediastinal space. Catheters, endoscopes, and surgical drains have all been used experimentally in the mediastinal space.

Once anesthetized, the patient is positioned in dorsal recumbency with the forelegs held along the thoracic wall and the mandible extended as far anterior as possible. This allows for better exposure of the operative site (*Figure 1*). Also, less difficulty is met in passing linear instruments parallel to the trachea and into the mediastinal space. Routine surgical preparation and draping are carried out in the ventral cervical area over the bifurcation of the sternomastoideus muscle.

A small skin incision, 2 to 4 cm long, is made on the midline over the bifurcation of the sternomastoideus. Usually this incision is large enough to accommodate most instruments and the insertion of fingers (*Figure 2*). Making of the incision is followed by blunt dissection, dorsally, to the trachea, which is easily palpated. Only a separation of the sternomastoideus and sternohyoideus muscles, with minimal displacement of fascia, is necessary (*Figure 3*). Little vasculature is encountered. As the dissection nears the trachea, the accessory

Figure 2—The initial incision for paratracheal mediastinotomy exposes the sternomastoideus and sternohyoideus muscles.

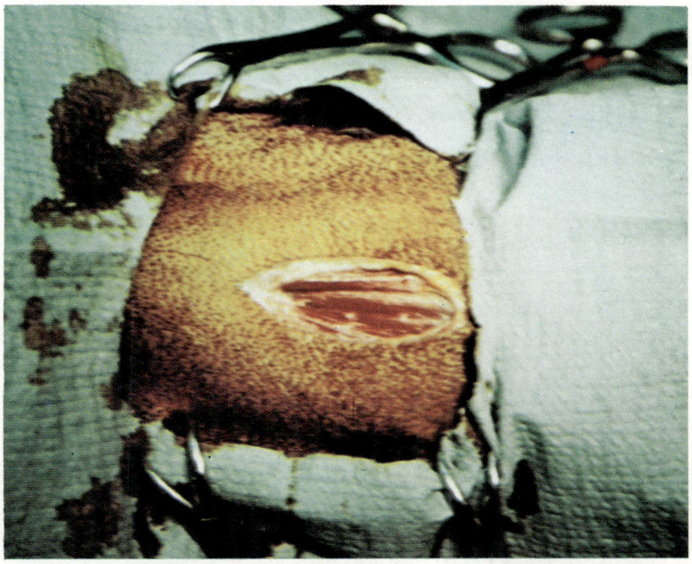

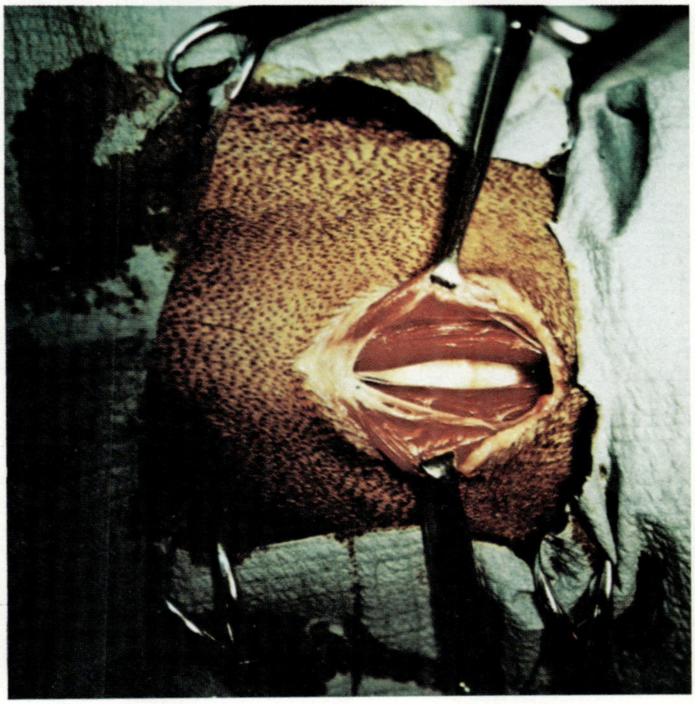

Figure 3—Blunt dissection and midline separation of the sternomastoideus and sternohyoideus muscles exposes the trachea.

thyroid (thyroidea ima) vein can be retracted laterally if necessary. Hemorrhage is minimal.

When the trachea has been identified, blunt dissection continues caudally and along the ventral paratracheal fascia until a finger or linear instrument can be passed through the thoracic inlet and into the mediastinal space. In animals weighing 12 kg or more, digital dissection is especially useful.

Depending on the animal's size and the length of the surgeon's fingers, the mediastinal space may be invaded as far caudally as the heart base. Major anterior mediastinal vasculature is easily palpated and presents little difficulty when a finger or instrument is inserted. In man, the gloved index finger is commonly used for blunt dissection before an endoscope is placed. The distance from the incision to the heart base is surprisingly short in man as well as the dog and cat.

When the mediastinal space has been entered, a number of procedures can be performed. One of the simple techniques is a mediastinal wash for harvesting cells for cytology or culturing, or both. This procedure can be carried out by inserting a large-bore catheter along the trachea and using it for blunt dissection as it is advanced caudally. However, results are more consistent when a sterile, stainless steel, female urinary catheter is used (*Figures 4 & 5*). Being very rigid, this type of catheter can be well controlled when used for blunt dissection and during its caudal advancement along the trachea. Proper placement of the catheter is easy to confirm using image intensification or plain-film radiography (*Figures 8 & 9*). Dissection is minimal and the catheter falls almost unaided into the mediastinal space.

To prevent pneumomediastinum, a small, sterile, rubber adaptor hose is attached to the external opening in the feline catheter; a syringe in series with a three-way valve is attached to the free end of the adaptor (*Figures 5 & 6*). Adaptors can be obtained from the ends of used intravenous-fluid ad-

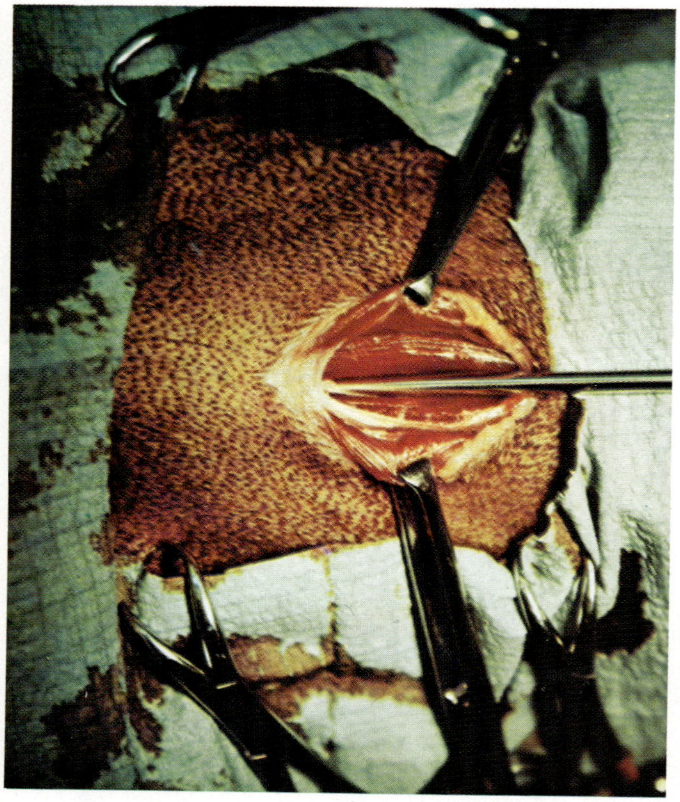

Figure 4—Blunt dissection and catheterization along the paratracheal fascia can be done using a stainless steel female urinary catheter.

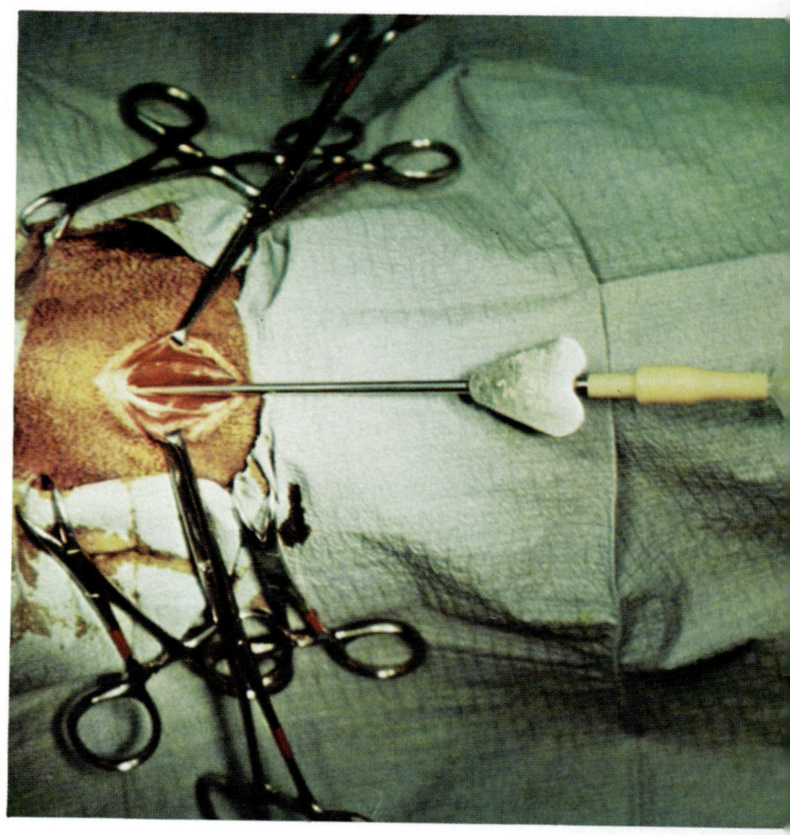

Figure 5—Mediastinal aspiration for cytology and culture samples can be done using a female urinary catheter, rubber adaptor, and syringe.

ministration sets. Although intentional pneumomediastinum has created no problems experimentally, a pneumothorax could easily occur subsequent to mediastinal insult or disease.

In trials with normal dogs and cats, no problems have been encountered in placing instruments and maintaining mediastinal integrity. Female catheters have been advanced as far as the carina and heart base. Ventrally, the mediastinum is thinner, and this is a consideration. Contrast studies of normal dogs and cats have shown that the mediastinum is an effective barrier to rapid movement of aqueous fluid or gas[41,42] (*Figures 10 & 11*). In man, the mediastinum is more rigid, and during mediastinoscopy it can even be incised to obtain lung parenchyma for biopsy.[16] Any pneumothorax that occurs is easily controlled with positive-pressure ventilation.

A female catheter can be placed anywhere within the cranial mediastinal space or anterior thoracic space, if desired. Once the catheter is positioned, aspiration, cytologic washing, drainage, or injection of contrast medium can be accomplished. As much as 30 cc of fluid or gas has been injected, without adverse effect, into the mediastinal space of a cat weighing 3 kg.[3] Generally, 5 to 10 cc can be retrieved from a 30-cc fluid wash if aspiration immediately follows the infusion.

If visual inspection of mediastinal structure is required, as during excisional biopsy, pacemaker implantation, or tissue inspections, a more extensive dissection is required. This is most easily accomplished by digital technique. Use of conventional endoscopes permits viewing of the connective tissues, major vessels, and enlarged lymphoid tissues (*Figures 12 & 13*). Intentional injection of gas into the mediastinal space at this time improves the visibility of mediastinal structures.

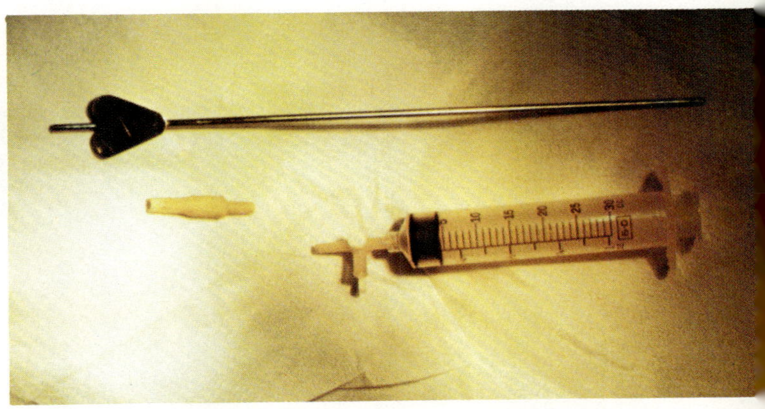

Figure 6—A female urinary catheter, rubber adapter hose, three-way valve, and syringe can be used for either mediastinal aspiration or injection.

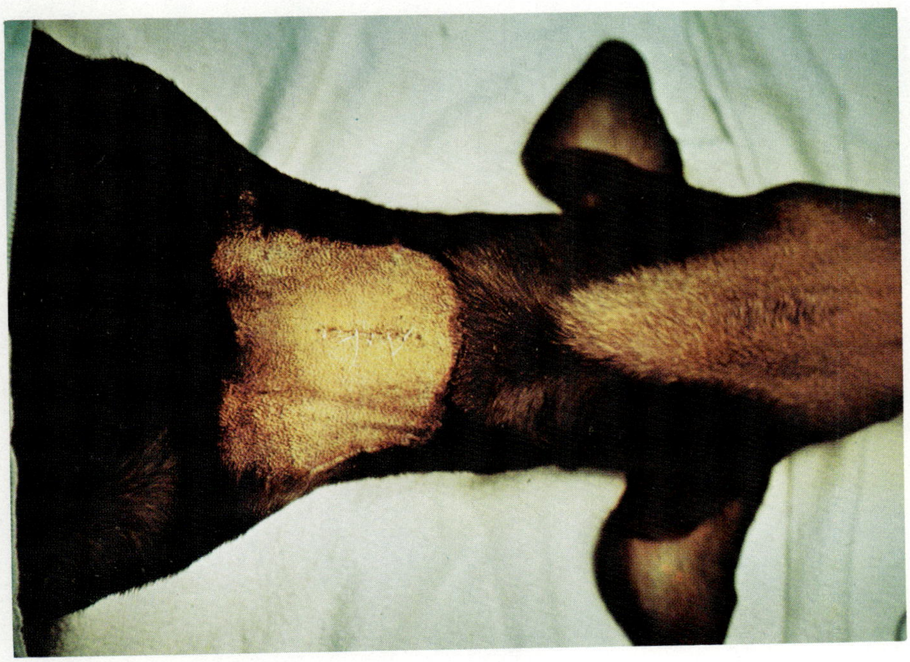

Figure 7—A simple interrupted suture pattern is used to close the skin incision.

When the procedure is terminated a reasonably good pneumatic seal is attained just by removing the instruments. Before any catheters are removed, aspiration may be performed to reduce attainable unnecessary gas or fluid. A simple interrupted subcutaneous suture pattern and standard skin closure are required to close the incision (*Figure 7*).

Discussion

Postoperative edema and hemorrhage have not been a problem. In man, little postoperative discomfort is reported. Aspirin or a similar analgesic generally is all that is needed to relieve the discomfort.[35,36,38] If no breach of sterile technique occurred, antibiotics are not used.[35,38]

Specific contraindications to paratracheal mediastinotomy would be the same as those applicable to general anesthesia and surgical procedures. In particular, a large thymus gland in a young animal inhibits easy passage of instruments into the mediastinal space. In the case of aggressive neoplasms or in the presence of sepsis, invasion of the mediastinal space may advance the process. Physicians have been cautioned that paratracheal mediastinotomy is no substitute for an indicated major thoracotomy.

The types of mediastinal disease are diverse (*Table 1*) and not unusual in small animal veterinary medicine.[43] Conventional diagnostic approaches can lead to a definitive diagnosis. In cases where a more direct approach to the mediastinal space is indicated—whether for diagnosis, therapy, or a prognosis—the option of thoracotomy may be refused

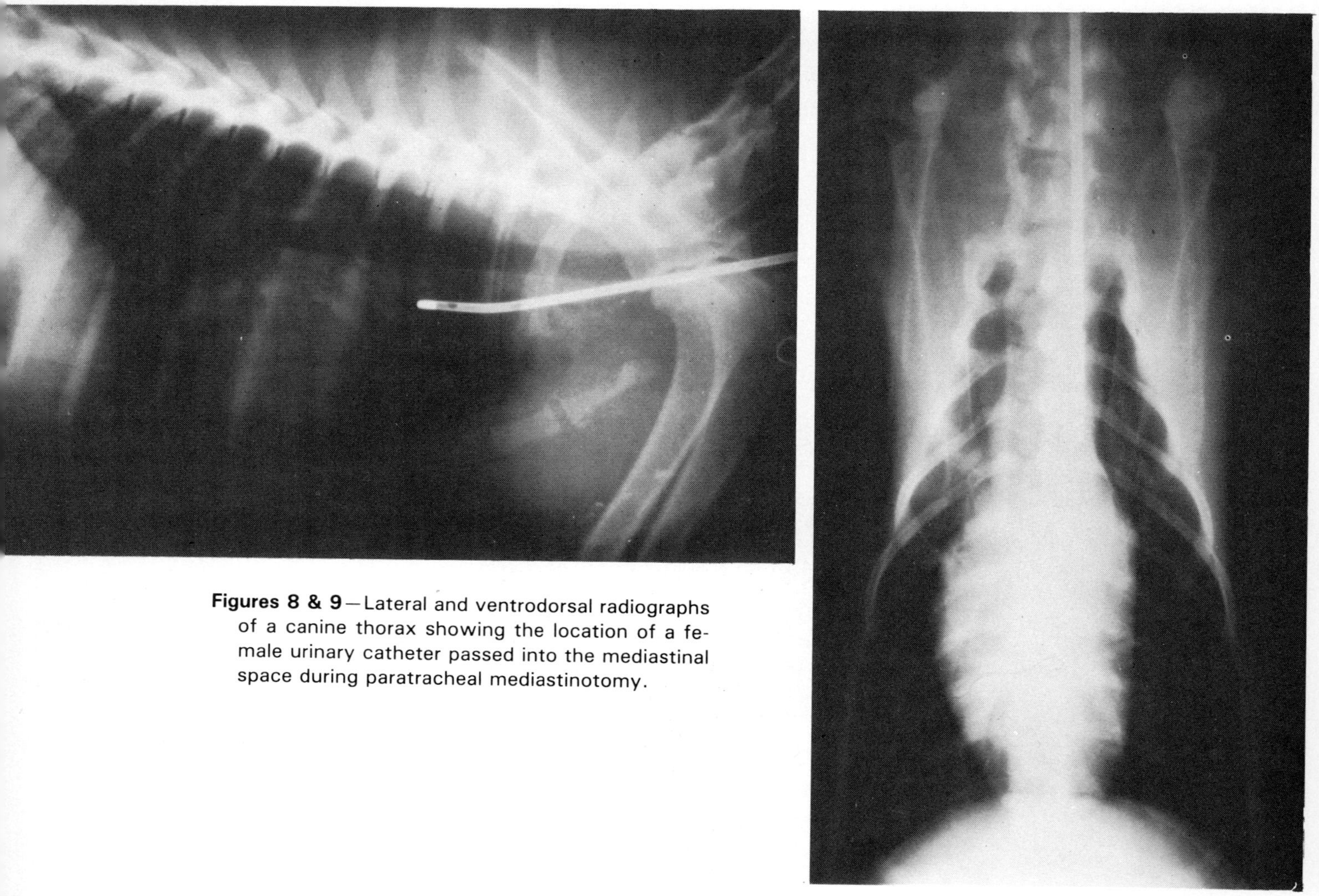

Figures 8 & 9—Lateral and ventrodorsal radiographs of a canine thorax showing the location of a female urinary catheter passed into the mediastinal space during paratracheal mediastinotomy.

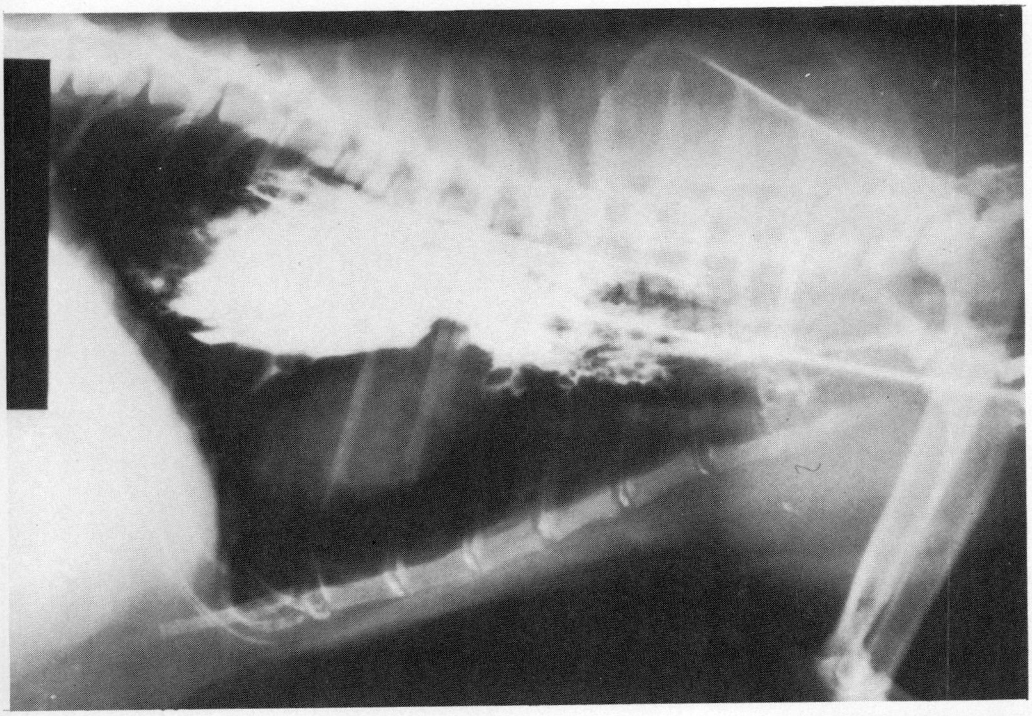

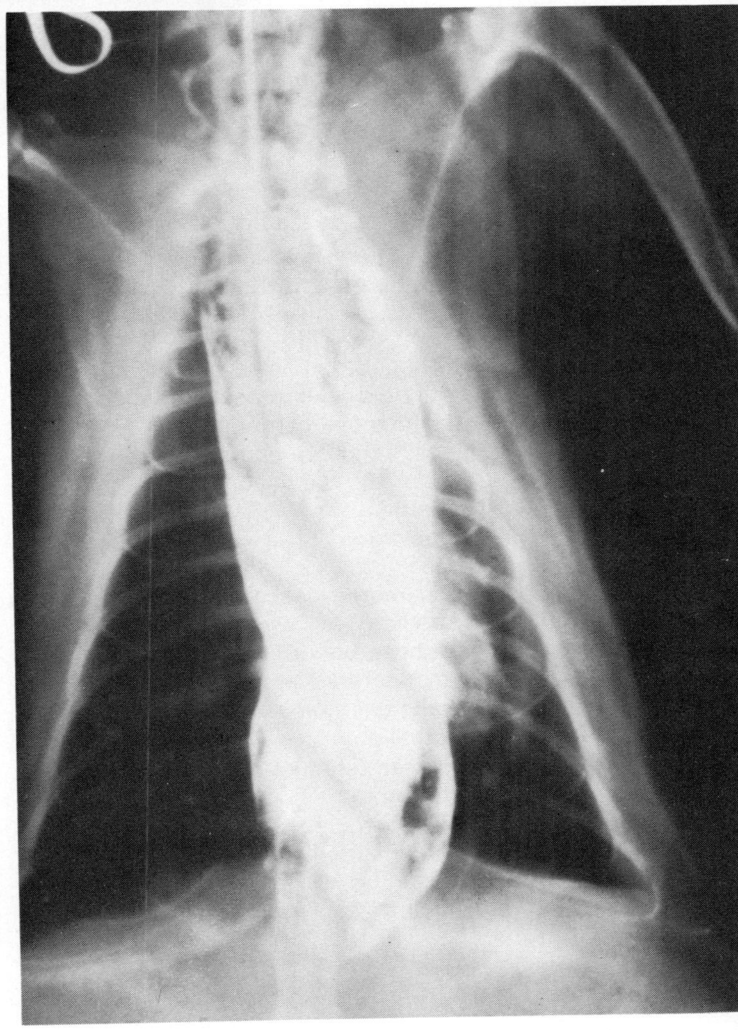

Figures 10 & 11—Lateral and ventrodorsal radiographs of a feline thorax showing the deposition of negative and positive contrast media in the mediastinal space by means of a stainless steel female urinary catheter passed during a paratracheal mediastinotomy. (Note that some of the gas contrast has migrated into the pericardial sac, forming a halo around the heart.)

on the basis of risk or economics. A paratracheal approach to the mediastinal space offers a reasonable way to obtain direct information about the mediastinal space and its contents. The procedure has potential application in diagnosis, in therapy, and in research. When alternatives are considered, the expense and risk are minimal. Performance of paratracheal mediastinotomy is possible in most veterinary hospitals without the need for additional or specialized equipment.

As emphasized by the medical profession, an essential element in the successful use of the procedure is a thorough knowledge of the anatomy and potential complications that exploration of the mediastinum can generate.

REFERENCES

1. Clagett, O.T.: Mediastinoscopy, Good or Evil? *J. Thoracic Cardiovascular Surg. 60*:754; 1970.
2. Foster, E.: Mediastinoscopy: A Review of Anatomical Relationships and Complications. *Ann. Thoracic Surg. 13*:273; 1972.
3. Bhargara, A.K.: Diagnosis of Mediastinal and Heart Base Tumors in Dogs Using Contrast Pleurography. *J. Am. Vet. Radio. Soc. 11*: 56-64; 1970.
4. Dorner, J.L.: Cytologic Examination of Pleural Effusions in the Cat. *Feline Prac. 4*(5):25-31; 1974.

Figures 12 & 13—Lateral and ventrodorsal radiographs of a canine thorax demonstrating mediastinal placement of a fiberoptic scope via paratracheal mediastinotomy. (Note the small biopsy attachment at the tip of the fiberoptic scope on the lateral view.)

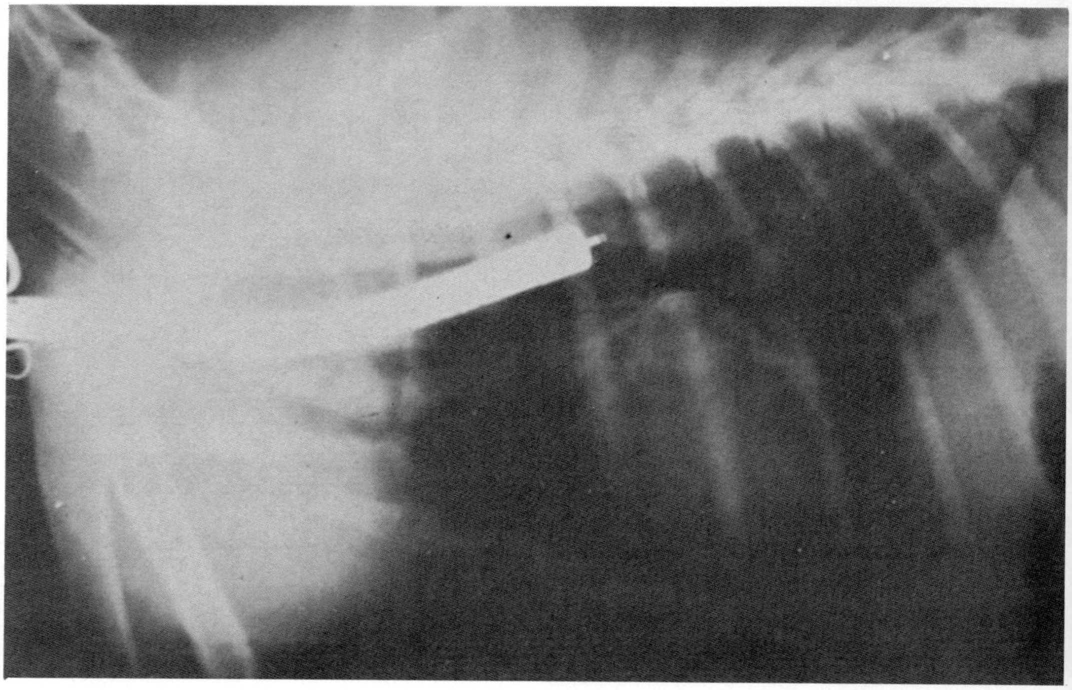

TABLE 1—Diagnosed Lesions in the Mediastinal Space in the Dog and Cat[43]

Neoplastic Lesions

- Undifferentiated adenocarcinoma
- Parathyroid adenoma and carcinoma
- Squamous cell carcinoma
- Thyroid adenoma and carcinoma
- Ovarian adenocarcinoma
- Choristoma
- Myelocytoma
- Mastocytoma
- Fibrosarcoma—secondary to *Spirocera lupi*
- Thymoma
- Heart base tumor
- Chemodectoma
- Hemangiosarcoma
- Mesothelioma
- Undifferentiated sarcoma
- Neurofibroma
- Leiomyosarcoma
- Giant cell anaplastic carcinoma
- Fibroma
- Malignant lymphoma

Non-Neoplastic Lesions

- Teratoma
- Tuberculosis
- Nocardiosis
- Congestion
- Blastomycosis
- Idiopathic granulomas
- Bacterial abscess
- Coccidioidosis
- Bronchogenic cyst
- Granulomatous steatitis
- Lymph node anthracosis
- Reticuloendothelial hyperplasia
- Idiopathic cyst
- Lymphadenitis
- Hemorrhage
- Actinomycosis
- Lymphoid hyperplasia
- Persistent thymus
- Foreign body granuloma
- Congenital anomaly

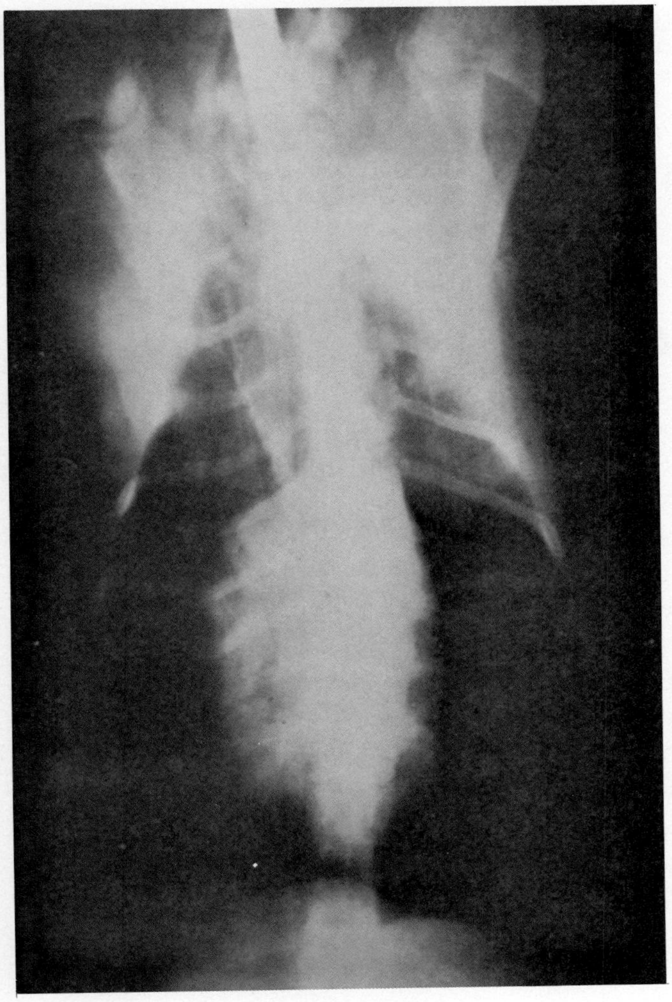

5. Girones, E.M.: Mediastinoscopy for Assessing Mediastinal Spread in Clinical Staging of Carcinoma of the Lung. *Cancer 25*:345; 1970.
6. Jones, B.R.: Pneumomediastinum in Racing Greyhounds. *J. Small An. Prac. 16*:27-32; 1975.
7. Kirschner, P.A.: Mediastinoscopy: Guide to Management of Lung Cancer. *N.Y. State J. Med. 71*:2041; 1971.
8. Nordenstrom, B.: Transthoracic Needle Biopsy. *New Engl. J. Med. 276*:1081; 1967.
9. Robinson, W.C.: Invasive Thymoma in a Dog. A Case Report. *JAAHA 13*:95-97; 1977.
10. Sehic, M.: Pneumomediastinography Technique. *Vet. Archiv. 41* (7-8):163-168; 1971.
11. Schalm, O.W.: Diagnosis of Lymphosarcoma. *Feline Prac. 6*(5): 24-27; 1976.
12. Schalm, O.W.: Pleural Effusions in the Cat. *Feline Prac. 6* (6):41-42; 1976.
13. Tilley, L.P.: Pericardial Mesothelioma with Effusion in the Cat. *JAAHA 11*:60-65; 1975.
14. VonRecum, A.K.: The Mediastinum, and Hemothorax, Pyothorax, and Pneumothorax in the Dog. *JAVMA 171*:531-533; 1977.
15. Rantanen, N.W.: Personal communications. Department of Radiology, Washington State University, Pullman, Wa. 99163; 1979.
16. Deslauriers, J.: Mediastinalpleuroscopy, A New Approach to the Diagnosis of Intrathoracic Diseases. *Ann. Thoracic Surg. 22*(3): 205-209, 1975.
17. Fishman, N.H.: Is Mediastinoscopy Necessary in the Evaluation of Lung Cancer? *Ann. Thoracic Surg. 20*(6):678-686; 1975.
18. Harken, D.E.: A Simple Cervicomediastinal Exploration for Tissue Diagnosis of Intrathoracic Disease. *New Engl. J. Med. 251*:1041; 1954.
19. James, E.C.: Mediastinoscopy and Mediastinal Roentgenology: A Clinical Correlation. *Ann. Thoracic Surg. 18*(5):531-538; 1974.
20. Pearson, F.G.: Mediastinoscopy: A Method of Biopsy in the Superior Mediastinum. *J. Thoracic Cardiovascular Surg. 49*:11; 1965.
21. Sealy, W.: Mediastinoscopy. *Ann. Thoracic Surg. 18*:433; 1974.
22. Stanford, W.: Mediastinoscopy. *Ann. Thoracic Surg. 19*:121; 1975.
23. Widstrom, A.: Palsy of the Recurrent Nerve Following Mediastinoscopy. *Chest 67*(3):365-366; 1975.
24. Trinkle, J.K.: Mediastinoscopy—Experience with 300 Consecutive Cases. *J. Thoracic Cardiovascular Surg. 60*:297; 1970.
25. Fleming, W.H.: Mediastinal Biopsy: Selective or Routine? *Am. Surgeon*, Jan. 1977; pp 74-76.
26. Otto, T.L.: Experience with Mediastinoscopy. *Thorax 27*:463; 1967.
27. Bariety, M.: Twelve Years' Experience with Gas Mediastinography. *Diseases of the Chest 48*:449; 1965.
28. Kreel, L.: Pneumomediastinography by the Transsternal Method. *Clin. Radiol. 15*:219; 1964.
29. Iagergren, H. *et al*: Atrial Triggered Pacemaking Without Thoracotomy: Apparatus and Results in 20 Cases. *Acta. Chir. Scand. 132*:678-695; 1966.
30. Arom, K.V.: Subxiphoid Anterior Mediastinal Exploration. *Ann. Thoracic Surg. 24*(3):289-290; 1977.
31. Carlens, E.: Mediastinoscopy: A Method for Inspection and Tissue Biopsy in the Superior Mediastinum. *Diseases of the Chest 36*:343; 1959.
32. Daniels, A.: A Method of Biopsy Useful in Diagnosing Certain Intrathoracic Diseases of the Chest. *Diseases of the Chest 16*:360; 1949.
33. Stemmer, E.A.: Mediastinoscopy for Undeterminate Pulmonary and Mediastinal Lesions. *J. Thoracic Cardiovascular Surg. 44*:405; 1965.
34. Ward, P.H. *et al*: Mediastinoscopy: A Valuable Diagnostic Procedure for the Evaluation of Lesions of the Mediastinum. *Southern Med. J. 60*:51-56; 1967.
35. Ashbaugh, D.G.: Mediastinoscopy. *Arch. Surg. 100*:568; 1970.
36. Gunstensen, J.: Mediastinoscopy: An Analysis of 320 Consecutive Cases. *Br. J. Surg. 59*:209; 1972.
37. Lallemand, R.C.: Problems in the Management of Mediastinal Tumors. *Post Med. J. 51*:89-96; 1975.
38. Morton, J.R.: Mediastinoscopy Using Local Anesthesia. *Am. J. Surg. 1-2*:696; 1971.
39. Mulder, G.A.: Diagnostic Procedures in Lung Cancer. *Chest 71* (5):629-630; 1977.
40. Paris, F.: Mediastinoscopy in the Surgical Management of Lung Carcinoma. *Thorax 30*:146-151; 1975.
41. Bhargara, A.K.: Radiographic Anatomy of the Pleura. *J. Am. Vet. Radiol. Soc. 10*:61-65; 1970.
42. Bhargara, A.K.: Pleural and Pericardial Fluid Dynamics. *Indian Vet. J. 49*(5):496-499; 1972.
43. Casey, H.W.: Armed Forces Institute of Pathology. Dept. of the Army, Washington, D.C. 20305; Dec. 1979. Personal communication.

Excision of the lung lobe in dogs

Robert L. Leighton, VMD
Clare Gregory, DVM
Department of Surgery
School of Veterinary Medicine
University of California
Davis, California 95616

ALTHOUGH REMOVAL of a lung lobe is well tolerated by dogs, the veterinary literature contains few reports of this surgery. And yet, the almost universal use of gas anesthesia and assisted ventilation, combined with the many well-equipped veterinary hospitals and well-trained veterinarians, leads one to suspect that the procedure is more commonly performed than published.

At the veterinary medical teaching hospital, lung lobectomy has been used to treat lung abscess, tumor, torsion, damage resulting from blunt trauma, lung rupture with pneumothorax, fetal atelectasis, and chronic pneumonia associated with heartworms and cardiac failure. Abscesses of the lung lobe (with and without hypertrophic osteoarthropathy) caused by foxtail awns[1,2] and torsions of the lung lobe[3,4] have been the most common conditions. Diagnosis is achieved primarily by radiography, for which interpretation and techniques have been described.[5] Conditions requiring treatment by lung lobectomy may be acute emergencies, as in cases of severe pneumothorax, or chronic, as in a slowly developing abscess.

Surgical and anesthetic considerations include those done routinely to evaluate the physical state of the animal, severity of the injury, and the degree of respiratory and circulatory compromise. The packed cell volume, plasma protein, and heart are evaluated. If available, blood gas determinations are an aid in determining the need for postoperative oxygen therapy and intensive care. The anesthetist must establish assisted respiration with adequate gas exchange while maintaining or restoring normal blood values and pressures. Fluids and blood are provided via an intravenous catheter. Other monitoring equipment includes an EKG machine, and a device for monitoring indirect blood pressure, a Doppler ultrasound (Parks Electronics Laboratories, Beaverton, Oregon).

Technique for removal of left caudal lung lobe

After the left chest wall is shaved, prepared for aseptic surgery, and draped, the patient is placed in right lateral recumbency. The chest is opened by means of a thoracotomy between the 7th and 8th or 8th and 9th ribs, depending on the shape of the chest and the size of the lung lesion.[6,7] After the wound edges are toweled in, a rib spreader is inserted and expanded widely to expose the left caudal lung lobe (*Figure 1*). The lobe is lifted out and held craniodorsally by an assistant while the surgeon incises the pulmonary ligament (*Figure 2*).

Blunt dissection is used to expose the pulmonary veins, and a doubled silk ligature is tied around them using right-angled hemostatic forceps (*Figure 3*). The vessels are double ligated (*Figure 4*) and sectioned between the ligatures. The lobe is drawn caudoventrally by the assistant, and blunt dissection is used to expose the pulmonary artery. Two doubled ligatures are also drawn around this vessel (*Figure 5*), which is sectioned between the ligatures (*Figure 6*). The exposed bronchus is clamped with small Doyen forceps (cranially) and right-angled forceps (caudally) and sectioned between them (*Figure 7*). (If a tumor or abscess were present, the right-angled forceps would have been applied before manipulation to prevent spread of tumor or abscess material into the bronchus and the rest of the lungs.) Then, the left caudal lobe is removed.

The bronchial stump is oversewn with 3-0 silk in a simple-interrupted or continuous pattern (*Figure 8*). The suture line is tested for leaks by immersing it in saline solution and watching for bubbles when the lungs are inflated. If necessary, additional sutures are added. Fluids, blood clots, and sponges are removed. All ligatures are examined for leakage. The rib spreader and towels are removed, and the thoracotomy is closed. A chest drain is inserted, and as soon as the chest is closed, air is withdrawn. The anesthetist encourages the dog to begin voluntary respiration. The chest drain may be removed 4 to 24 hours after surgery.

Figure 1—The left caudal lung lobe after exposure by means of an intercostal thoracotomy between the 8th and the 9th ribs.

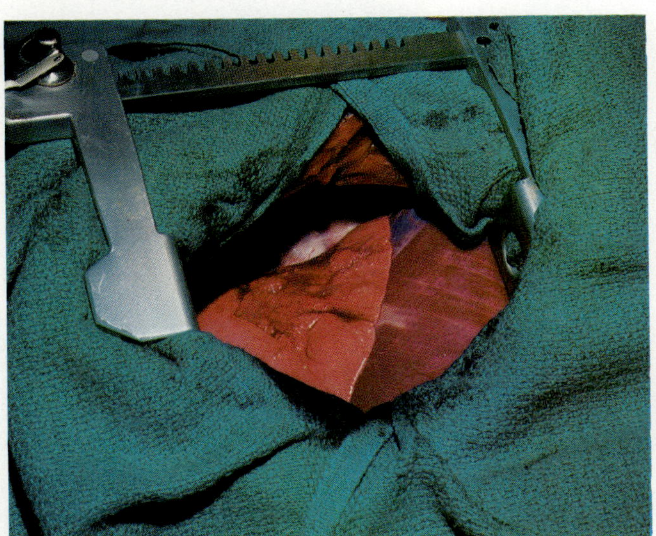

Figure 2—The left caudal lung lobe is retracted craniodorsally to expose the thin, membranous, pulmonary ligament.

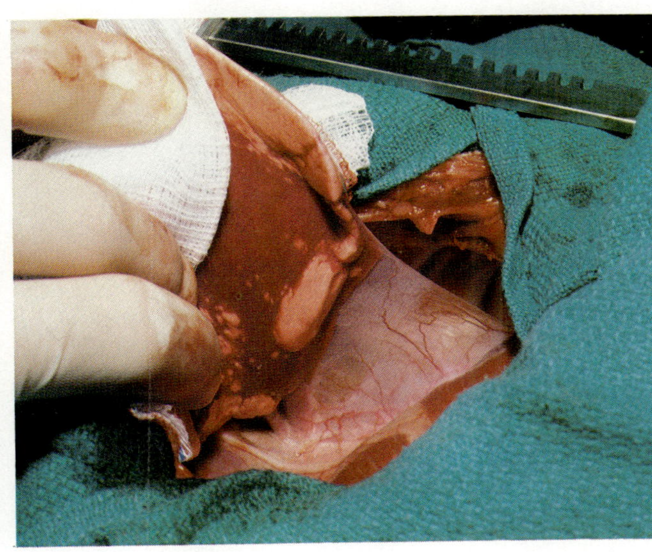

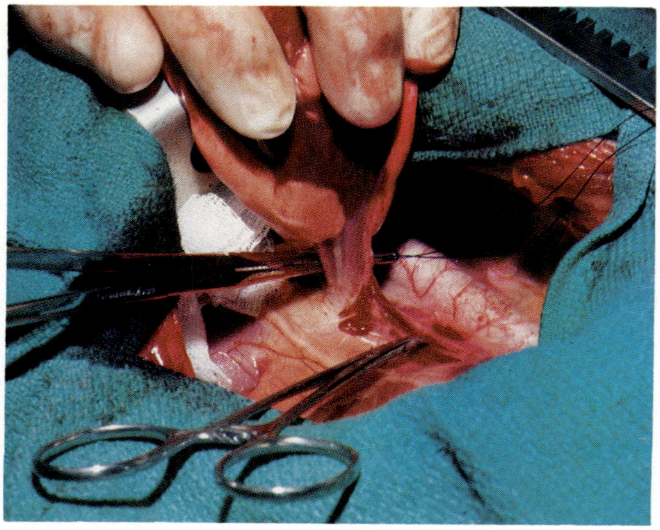

Figure 3—A right-angled hemostat is used to pass a doubled ligature around the pulmonary venous vessels.

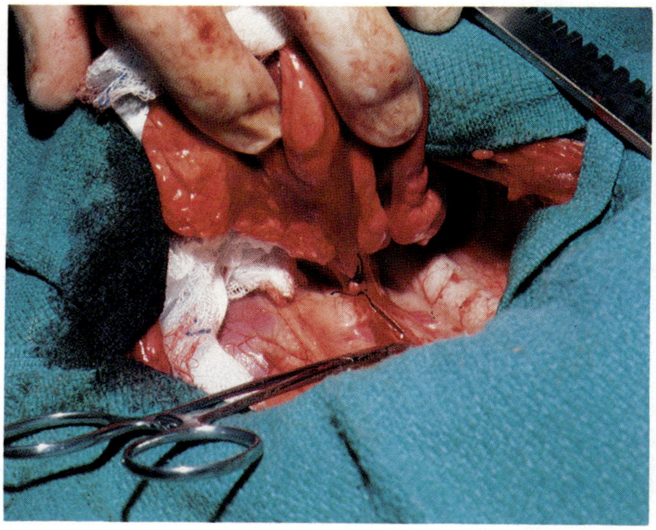

Figure 4—The pulmonary veins have been double ligated with 2-0 silk before transection between the ligatures.

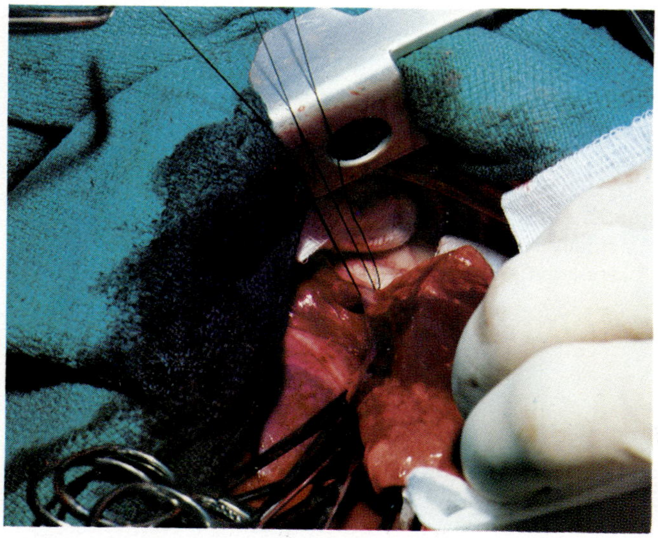

Figure 5—The left caudal lung lobe is held caudoventrally to expose the pulmonary artery, and a doubled ligature of 2-0 silk is drawn under it using a right-angled hemostat.

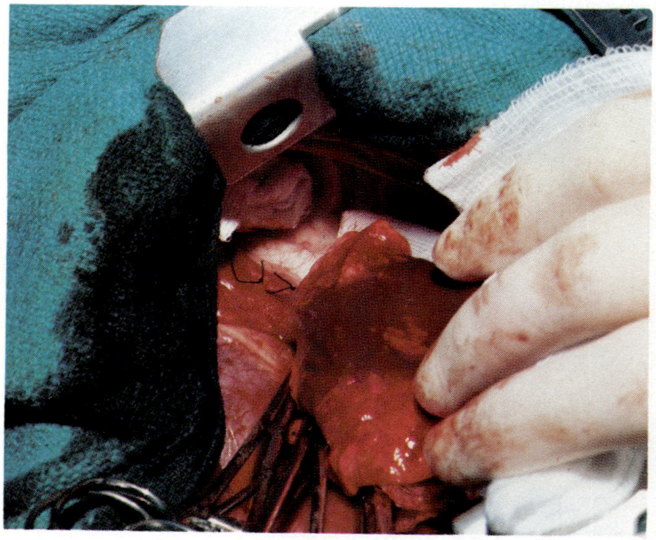

Figure 6—The pulmonary artery is sectioned between the ligatures, and the bronchus is exposed.

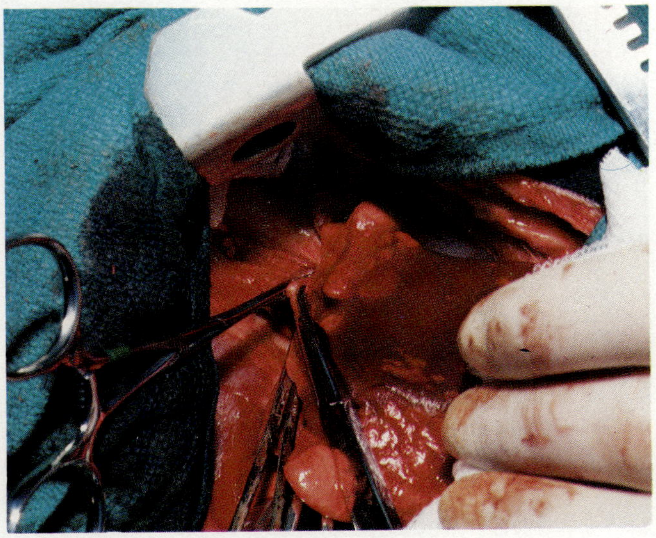

Figure 7—The exposed bronchus before sectioning between the small Doyen clamp (cranially) and the right-angled forceps (caudally), permitting removal of the left caudal lung lobe.

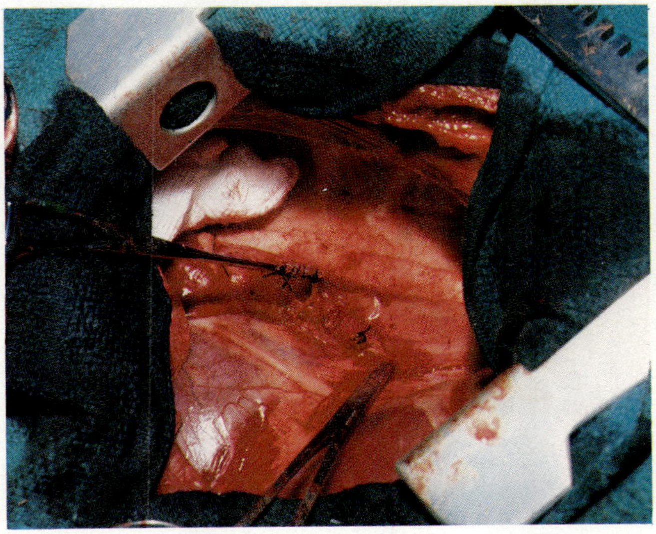

Figure 8—The exposed bronchial stump is oversewn with 3-0 silk suture.

Comments

Dogs usually recover from the surgery quickly and adapt readily to the loss of a lung lobe. The cranial lobes and their subdivisions are removed in a similar manner, except for an alteration in the site for thoracotomy.[8] Large intrathoracic masses are best removed via a sternotomy incision. The procedure described here is also used for removal of the right lung lobe.

REFERENCES

1. Leighton, R.L.; Olson, S.: Hypertrophic Osteoarthropathy in a Dog with a Pulmonary Abscess. *JAVMA 150*:1516-1520; 1967.
2. Brodey, R.S.: Hypertrophic Osteoarthropathy in the Dog. A Clinicopathologic Survey of 60 Cases. *JAVMA 159*(10):1242-1256; 1977.
3. Lord, P.F. *et al*: Lung Lobe Torsion in the Dog. *JAAHA* 9(5):473-482; 1975.
4. Alexander, J.W. *et al*: Torsion of the Diaphragmatic Lobe of the Lung Following Surgical Correction of a Patent Ductus Arteriosus in a Dog. *VM/SAC 69*(5):595-597; 1974.
5. Suter, P.F.; Gomez, J.A.: *Diseases of the Thorax—Radiographic Diagnosis*. Venture Press, Davis, Calif., 1981.
6. Lipowitz, A.J.; Schenk, M.D.: Surgical Approaches to the Abdominal and Thoracic Viscera of the Dog and Cat. *Vet. Clin. N. Am.* 9 (2):185-194; 1979.
7. Hoffer, R.E.: Thoracic Exposures and Closure. In *Atlas of Small Animal Surgery*, 2nd ed. C.M. Mosby, St. Louis, Mo., 1977; pp 11-24.
8. Arnoczky, S.P.; O'Neil, J.A.: Lung Lobectomy. *Vet. Clin. N. Am.* 9(2):219-227; 1979.

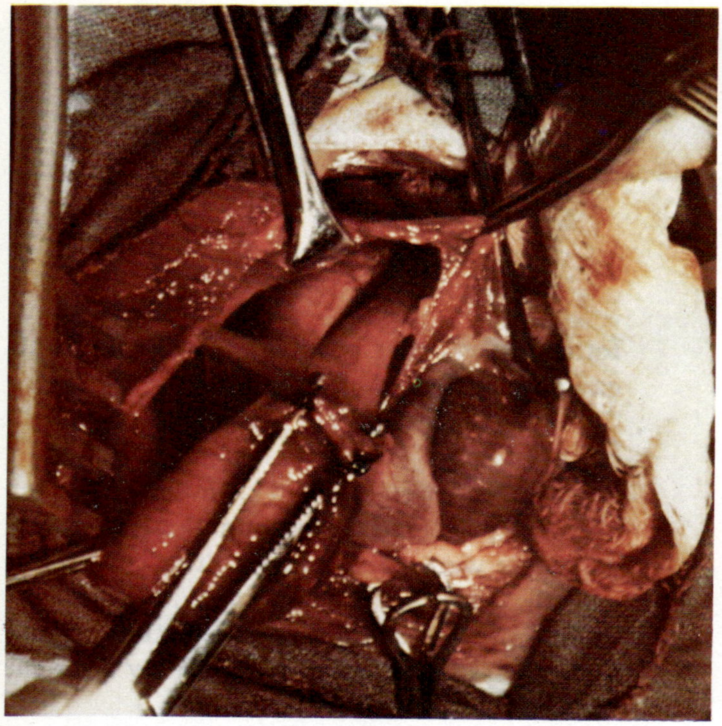

Figure 7—The ligamentum arteriosum has been elevated with a hemostat and ligated.

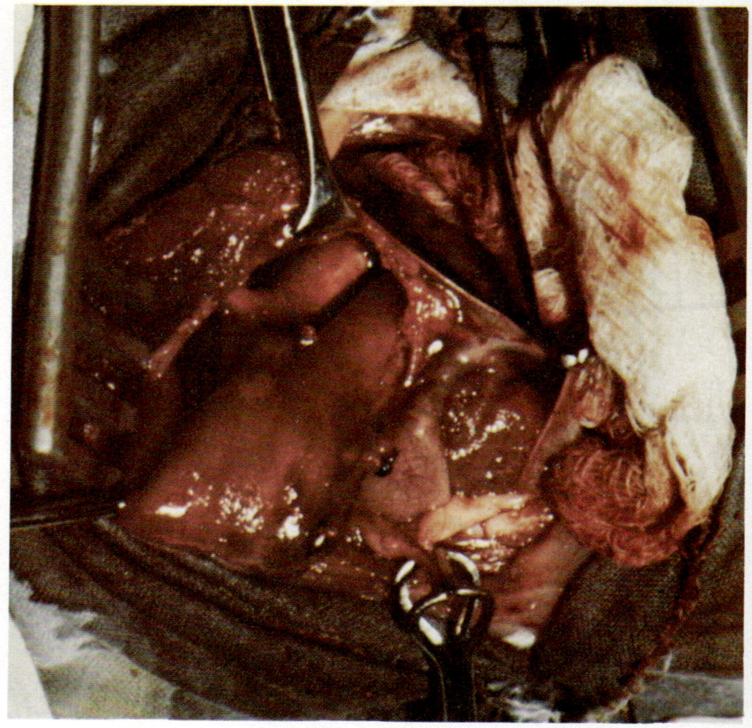

Figure 8—The esophagus has been freed from the vascular ring by transection of the ligamentum arteriosum.

On the second postoperative day, a bland liquid diet was started. By the fifth day, the cat was eating canned cat food with water added. Regurgitation has not recurred.

A postoperative radiograph showed continued, but less extensive, distension of the esophagus. Ovariohysterectomy was recommended to prevent possible genetic transmission of an undesirable trait.

REFERENCES

1. Ettinger, S.J.; Suter, P.F.: Diseases of the Great Vessels. In *Textbook of Veterinary Internal Medicine*, vol. 2 (S.J. Ettinger, ed.). W.B. Saunders Co., Philadelphia, Pa., 1975.
2. Liu, S.K.: Pathology of Feline Heart Disease. In *Current Veterinary Therapy V* (R.W. Kirk, ed.). W.B. Saunders Co., Philadelphia, Pa., 1974.
3. Jessop, L.: Persistent Right Aortic Arch in the Cat Causing Esophageal Stenosis. *Vet. Rec.* 72:3; 1960.
4. Core, S.H.; Dominy, W.R.: Surgical Correction of a Persistent Right Aortic Arch in a Cat. *VM/SAC 74*:822; 1979.
5. Guffy, M.M.: Esophageal Disorders. In *Textbook of Veterinary Internal Medicine*, vol. 2 (S.J. Ettinger, ed.). W.B. Saunders Co., Philadelphia, Pa., 1975.

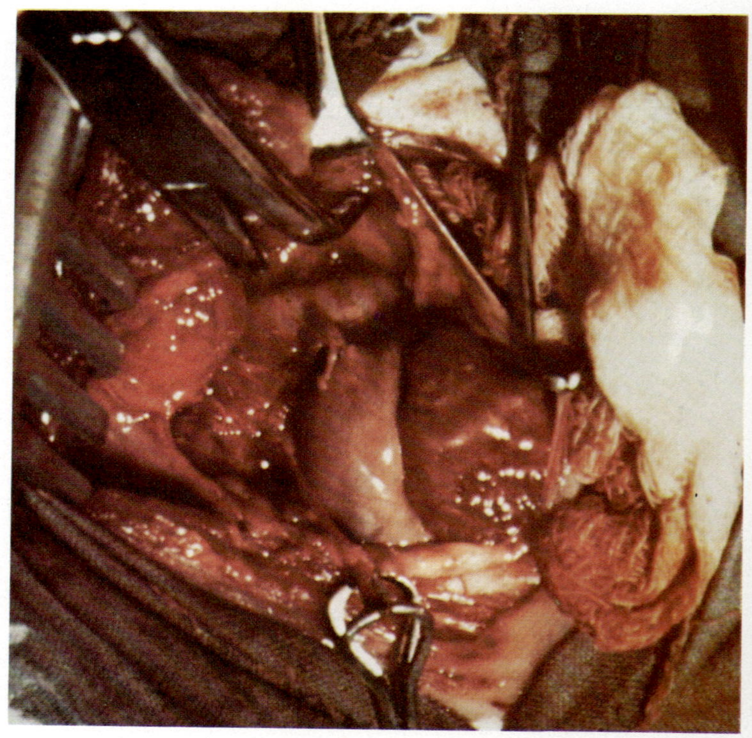

Figure 9—The esophagus is reflected dorsally to reveal the trachea, which is also contained in the ring.

Esophagomyotomy for treatment of canine megaesophagus

Robert L. Leighton, VMD
Department of Surgery, School of Veterinary Medicine
University of California, Davis, California 95616

Both congenital and acquired forms of megaesophagus are recognized in dogs. Puppies with the congenital form regurgitate solid food soon after weaning. The acquired form appears in mature animals—often after a period of stress.

Affected animals usually are presented because of vomiting. The vomitus appears never to have reached the stomach; it does not have a typical sour odor and contains a considerable amount of foamy saliva. Because an inadequate amount of food enters the digestive tract, an affected dog soon loses weight and condition.

Radiographs of the esophagus aid in diagnosis and can be used to rule out a persistent right aortic arch or other constricting anomalies at the base of the heart. The entire esophagus may be affected or, more commonly, only the portion caudal to the heart. The affected part is flaccidly dilated and does not constrict sequentially or transmit stimuli. Swallowed food accumulates in the dilated portion of the esophagus until it is filled. The food then is regurgitated. There is no stimulus to cause opening of the normally constricted musculature at the cardia.

The cause of megaesophagus is unknown. It is notable that injury to the nucleus ambiguus results in a similar lesion in the esophagus. The congenital form seems to have some hereditary or familial basis. It is seen more commonly in certain breeds and bloodlines and, occasionally, in littermates.

Medical treatment involves altering the diet and feeding the dog in an upright position so that gravity will aid in moving food into the stomach. Sometimes, a dry food is more effective than a moist one. Patients with the acquired form are seldom amenable to such management. However, in congenital cases, considerable improvement has been reported after several months of medical treatment. Although bougienage is used in human patients with achalasia, it is of little value for treating canine patients with megaesophagus because the

Figure 1—The esophageal hiatus is exposed via a left intercostal thoracotomy between the eighth and ninth ribs. The left caudal lung lobe has been packed off cranially.

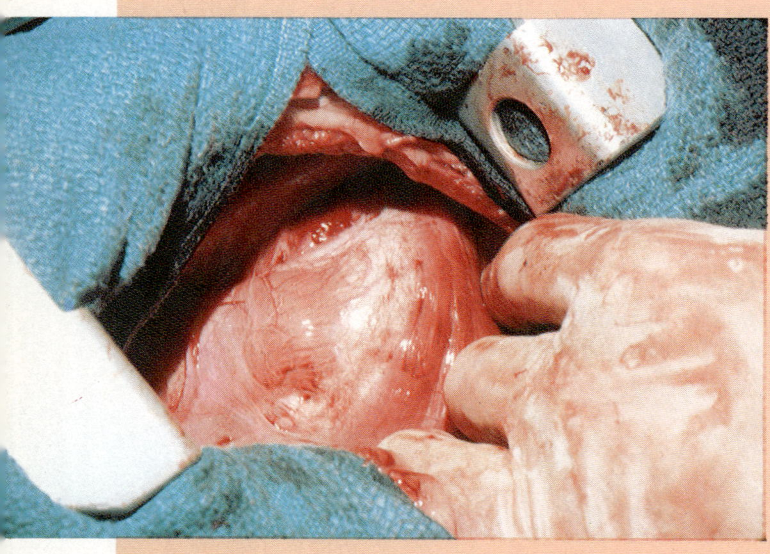

Figure 2—A piece of umbilical tape is used to retract the esophagus, which has been freed from surrounding tissues. The dorsal and ventral vagal branches are undisturbed.

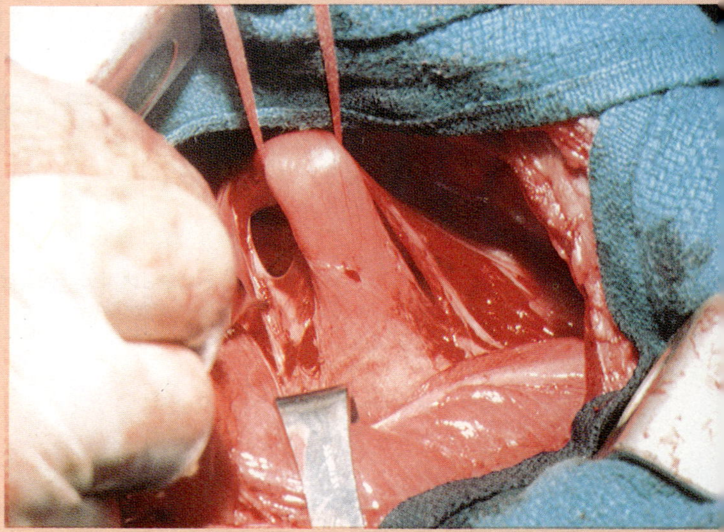

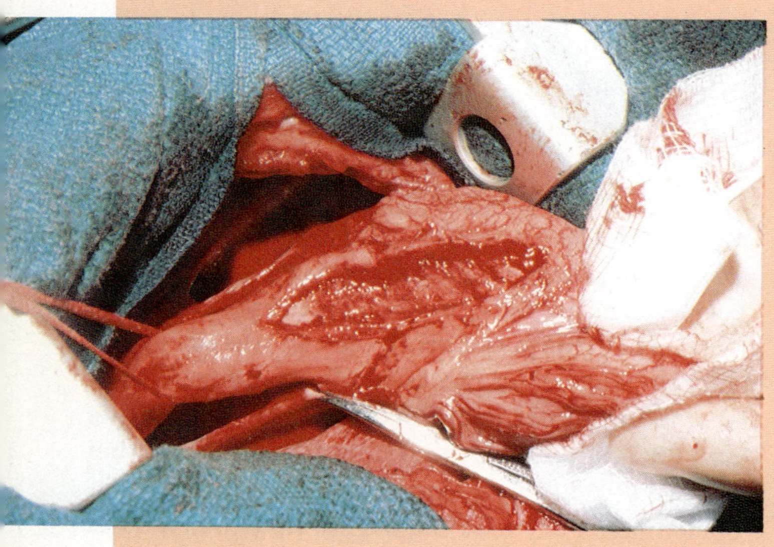

Figure 5—A longitudinal incision is made through the muscularis of the stomach and esophagus.

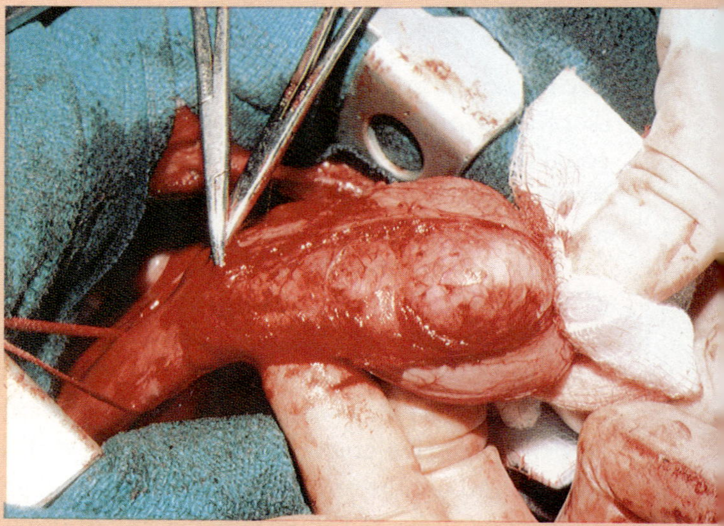

Figure 6—Continued dissection has severed the muscle fibers, allowing the mucosa of the esophagus and stomach to bulge.

Figure 3—The cardia of the stomach is prolapsed through a left-side hiatal incision.

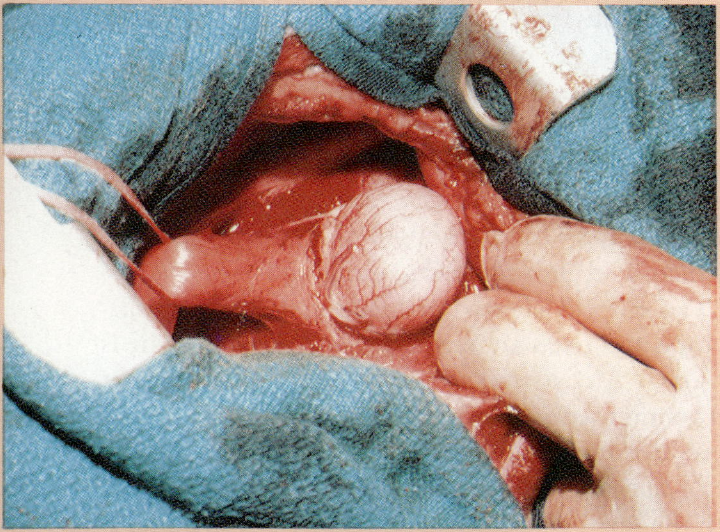

Figure 4—An assistant holds the stomach and esophagus in position.

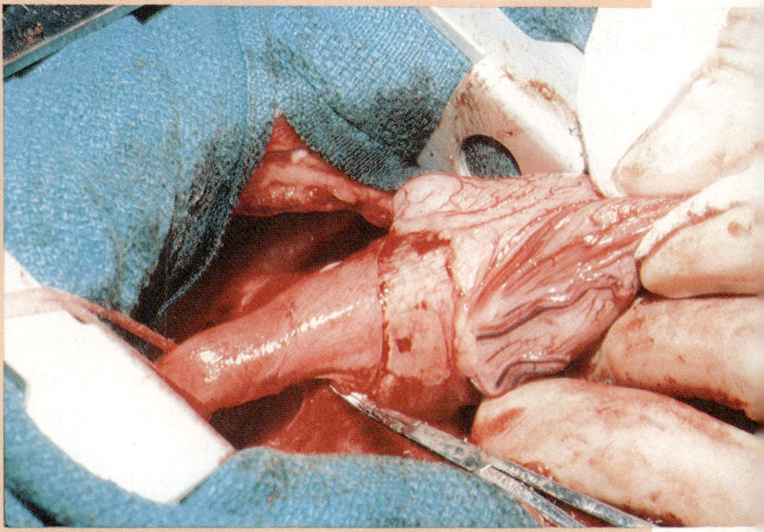

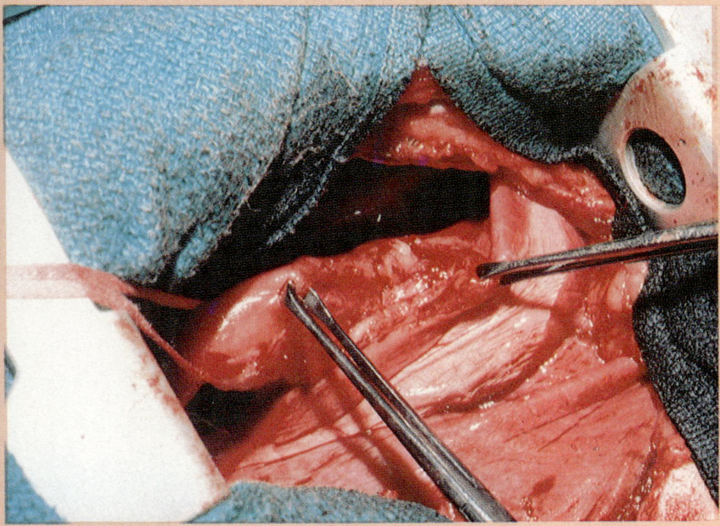

Figure 7—The most cranial portion of the incision in the muscularis of the esophagus will be sutured to the center of the hiatal incision in the diaphragm.

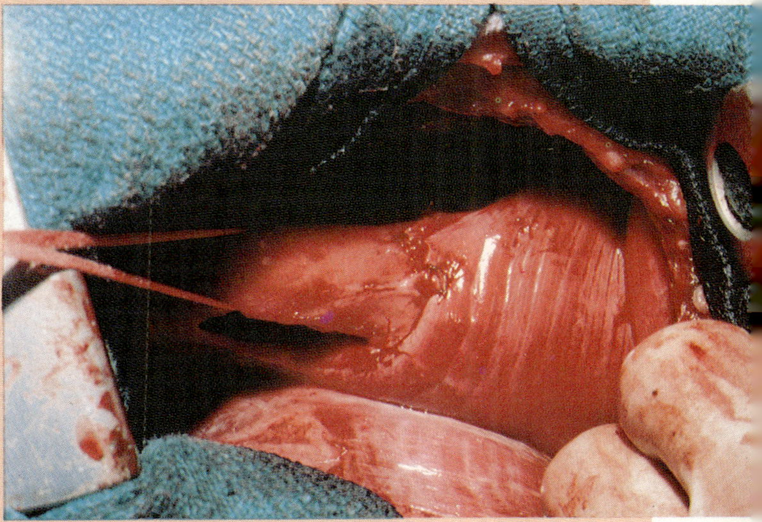

Figure 8—Closure of the hiatal incision is achieved by suturing it to the muscularis of the esophageal incision with 2-0 chromic catgut.

conditions are dissimilar. Inhalation of ingesta frequently results in pneumonia.

Esophagomyotomy is done to release the constricted musculature at the cardia, thus facilitating passage of food from the dilated esophagus into the stomach—especially when the dog is fed in an upright position.[1] The surgery is more often successful in acquired cases than in congenital cases. Some veterinarians think esophagomyotomy is of no value. Certainly, in cases where the entire esophagus is congenitally affected, results will be disappointing.

Surgical technique

After the esophagus is emptied, the dog is placed in right lateral recumbency. The left chest wall is shaved, prepared for aseptic surgery, and draped between the eighth and ninth ribs.

The edges of the incision are toweled-in and a rib speculum inserted. The left caudal lobe of the lung is packed off cranially, and the esophageal hiatus is exposed (*Figure 1*). After the esophagus is isolated from its mediastinal tissues, a piece of umbilical tape is drawn around it to aid in retraction. Injury to the dorsal and ventral vagal trunks is avoided (*Figure 2*). Using a scalpel, the surgeon makes a small incision at the esophageal hiatus. This is then enlarged with scissors. The cardia of the stomach is exposed (*Figure 3*). Next, more of the stomach is withdrawn and held by an assistant (*Figure 4*). A longitudinal incision, the same length as the incision in the esophageal hiatus, is made through the muscularis of the stomach and esophagus (*Figure 5*). Continued delicate dissection is done to sever all the muscle fibers and allow the mucosa to bulge out from the stomach. Numerous blood vessels will require ligation or cauterization. The esophageal mucosa is much thinner than the gastric mucosa (*Figure 6*). Inadvertent punctures may be closed with 4-0 silk suture.

The incision in the esophageal hiatus is closed by suturing the esophageal muscularis to it, beginning with a suture placed from the most cranial aspect of the incision in the esophageal muscularis to the center of the hiatal incision (*Figure 7*). The remaining portion of the hiatal incision is closed using 2-0 chromic catgut (*Figure 8*). The technique is advantageous because it securely closes the hiatal incision while relocating the exposed mucosal area abdominally. This is thought to reduce reflux of stomach acid into the distal esophagus.

The chest is cleared of blood clots, the umbilical tape and pack are removed, and the lung lobe is replaced. Any atelectasis is corrected by inflation and gentle massage with a moistened, gloved finger. Chest closure is done routinely. Food is withheld for 24 hours and then is allowed in small amounts with the dog in an upright position. This regimen is continued for several weeks or longer.

REFERENCE

1. Guffy, M.M.: Esophageal Disorders. In *Textbook of Veterinary Internal Medicine.* (S.J. Ettinger, Ed.) W.B. Saunders, Philadelphia, Pa., 1975; p 1101.

Small Animal Surgery

ABDOMEN

Peritoneopericardial hernia in a dog

Robert L. Leighton, DVM
Department of Surgery
School of Veterinary Medicine
University of California
Davis, California 95616

The clinical diagnosis and successful surgical correction of a congenital peritoneopericardial hernia in a 1-year-old male Great Dane are described. The surgical approach was via an abdominal midline celiotomy.

THE FIRST clinical diagnosis of peritoneopericardial diaphragmatic hernia in dogs was made in 1951.[1] Although the condition is considered rare,[2-7] the literature before 1951 and more recently contains a number of reports of peritoneopericardial hernia as a postmortem finding.[1,4-6,8] The condition is often an incidental finding[8] because overt signs are usually few except when a liver lobe is affected[2] or acute gastric dilatation supervenes.[9]

The hernia has been repaired by means of an abdominal midline celiotomy, thoracotomy, or a ventral transverse thoracotomy.[2-4,7,8,10,11] In some instances difficulty in repositioning some of the herniated viscera was encountered because of strong adhesions.[1,10]

Peritoneopericardial hernia is presumed to be congenital because of its occurrence in littermates,[12] the absence of any history of trauma, and the smooth confluence of pericardium with peritoneum. The mechanism by which the diaphragm develops and the interruption of that development that causes the hernia have been well described.[1]

Figure 1—Entry into the abdomen was by a midline celiotomy.

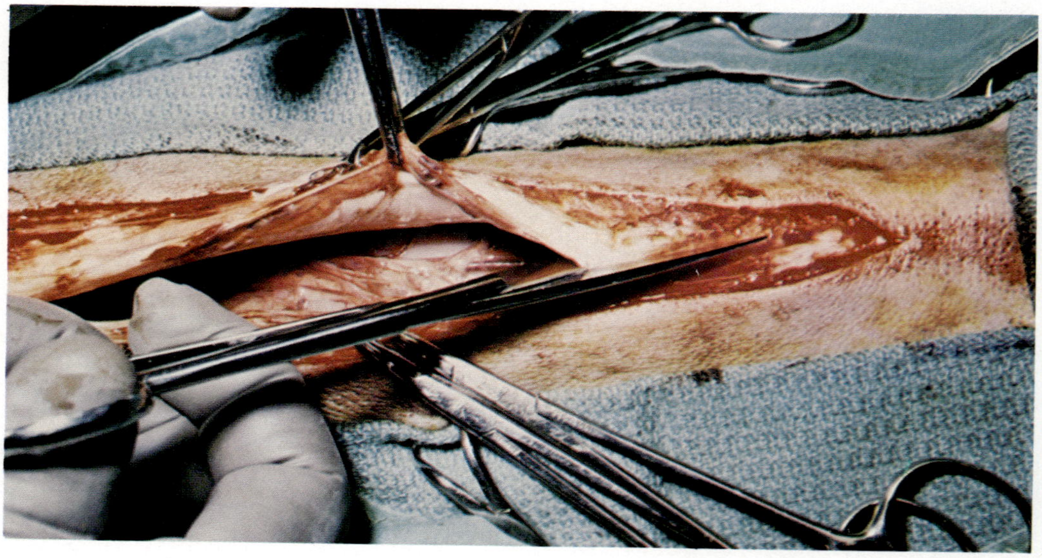

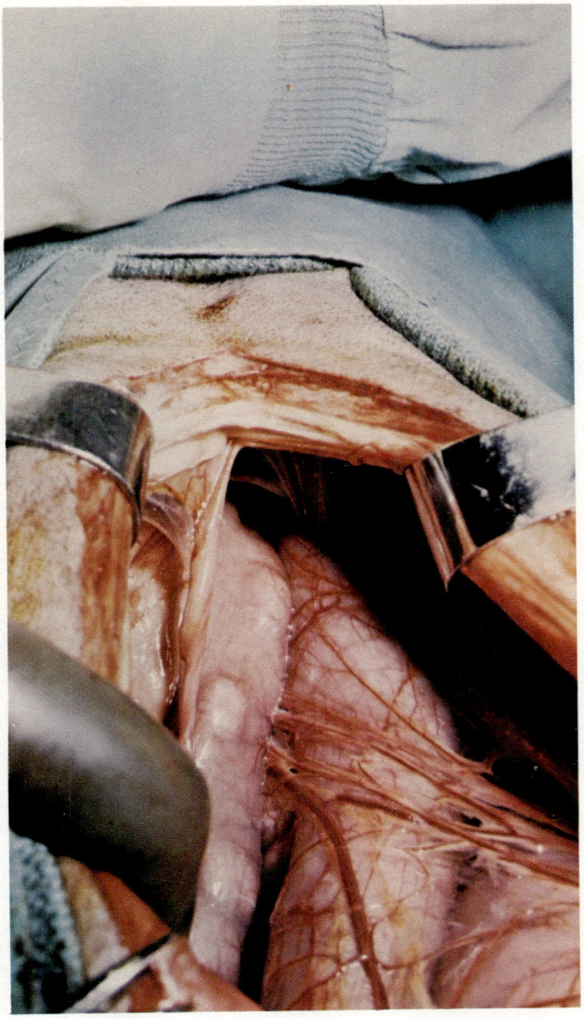

Figure 2
The hernia contained small intestines and about one-half of the liver.

Case Report

On October 20, 1973, a 1-year-old male brindle Great Dane was presented at the Veterinary Medical Teaching Hospital for repair of a diaphragmatic hernia. The referring veterinarian had diagnosed peritoneopericardial hernia when he saw on a radiograph, coils of small intestine surrounding the heart.

During the previous June, the dog had experienced partial intestinal obstruction after eating bones. Since that time the dog had not been well. No definite clinical signs were observed other than failure of the animal to thrive despite excellent food and care.

The vague signs and diagnosis incidental to a radiographic examination are typical of this condition. The heart wounds were muffled. No respiratory difficulty was observed. Some tapeworm segments were seen in the feces (Dipylidium). Results of all other laboratory tests were within normal limits. No electrocardiographic studies were done.

Surgical Procedure

The dog, which weighed 90 lb (40.9 kg), was premedicated with 90 mg meperidine hydrochloride (Demerol® —Winthrop), Methohexital sodium (Brevital® Sodium—Eli Lilly) was given through an intravenous catheter in the right cephalic vein. An endotracheal tube was inserted for induction of anesthesia, and methoxyflurane (Metofane—Pitman-Moore) was used to maintain anesthesia.

The ventral caudal chest and the abdominal area were shaved and prepared for aseptic surgery. The dog was placed in dorsal recumbency.

A ventral midline incision was made through the skin and subcutaneous tissues from the xiphoid to 6 cm caudal to the umbilicus. The abdomen was entered by incising the linea alba (*Figure 1*).

A midline gap in the diaphragm was found, through which most of the small intestines and about half of the liver protruded into the thorax (*Figure 2*). The small intestines were easily withdrawn (*Figure 3*) and replaced in the abdominal cavity. The portion of the liver in the thorax was returned to the abdominal cavity with moderate difficulty. It appeared somewhat shrunken and darker brown than the rest of the

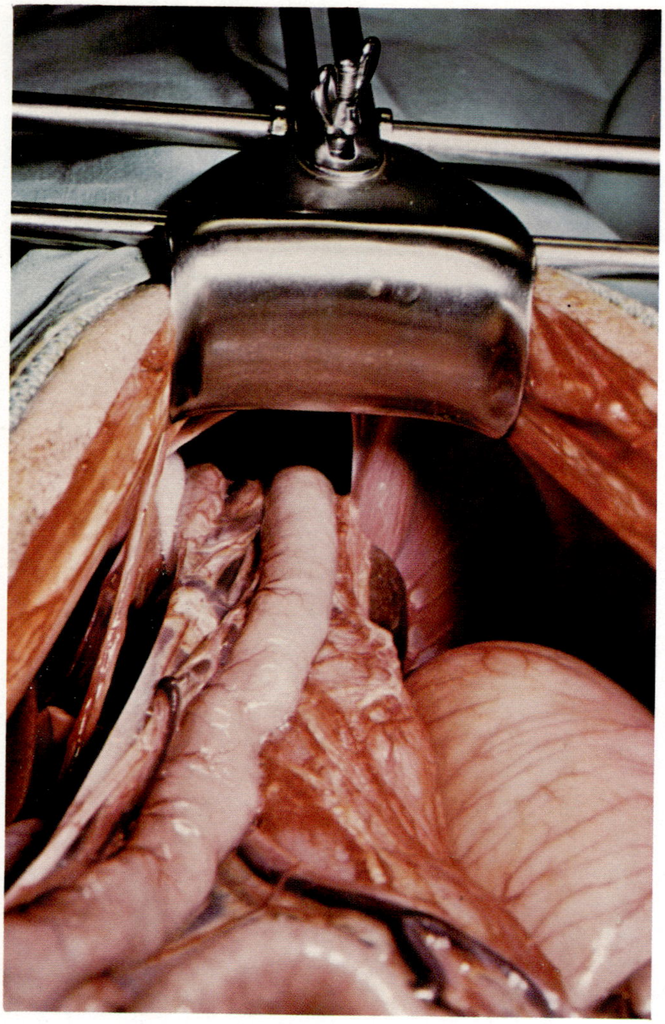

Figure 3
The herniated small intestines were easily removed from the thoracic cavity.

Figure 4
One omental adhesion was ligated and cut free. Note the appearance of the surface of the portion of the liver that had been herniated.

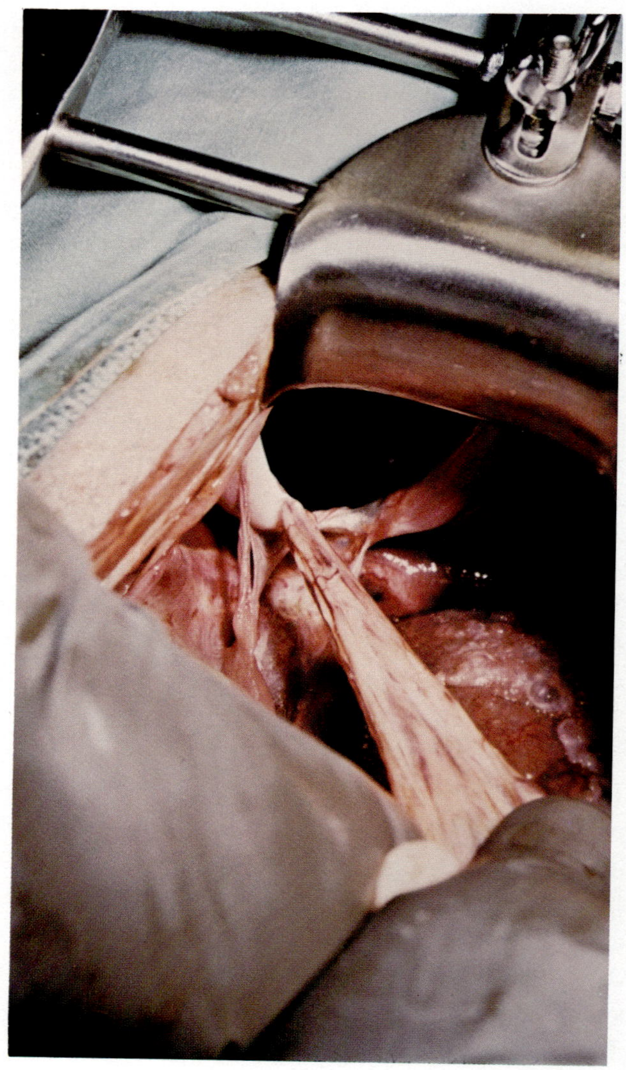

liver, and small bubbles covered its surface. One omental adhesion was ligated and cut (*Figure 4*).

The lining of the pericardial sac was smoothly contiguous with the peritoneum. Although respiration was assisted after the abdomen was entered, true pneumothorax did not develop and the lungs could not be seen. Air entering through the hernia filled only the enlarged pericardial space.

The hernia was closed with simple interrupted sutures of 0 chromic catgut (*Figure 5*). Just before the last stitch next to the xiphoid was tightened, the lungs were expanded to capacity. This compressed the enlarged pericardial space, evacuating the air it contained. This procedure obviated the need for a chest drain (*Figure 6*).

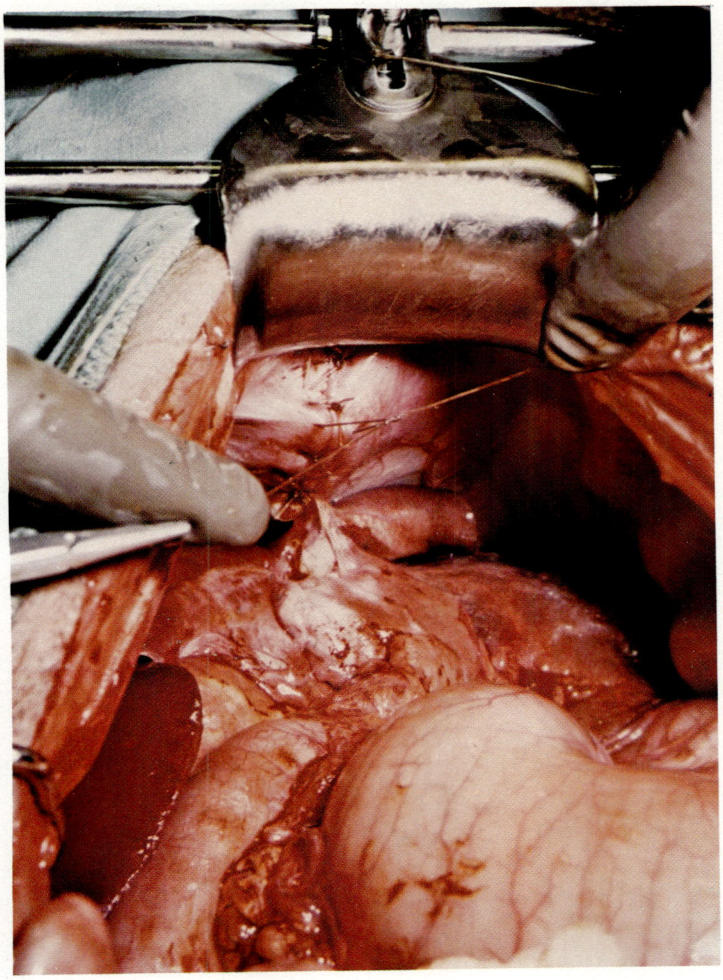

Figure 5
The hernia was closed with simple interrupted sutures of 2-0 chromic catgut.

The abdomen was closed with simple interrupted sutures of 2-0 chromic catgut placed through the abdominal fascia and peritoneum. The subcutaneous tissue was closed with the same material. To reduce potential dead space, the subcutaneous sutures included a bite into the abdominal fascia. The skin was closed with simple interrupted sutures of 30 Vetafil® (S. Jackson).

Recovery was rapid and uncomplicated except for diarrhea on one postoperative day. The dog was hospitalized 10 days.

Discussion

Peritoneopericardial hernias also occur in species other than dogs.[8,13] In our clinic the condition is much more common in cats than in dogs.

Affected animals rarely show severe signs of disease. Postmortem reports and diagnostic findings are often incidental. Auscultation discloses borborygmi and diminished heart sounds. Although diagnosis is enhanced by contrast radiographs showing the intestinal loops in the pericardial area, such radiographs are not essential (*Figure 7*).

Surgical approaches used are intercostal, ventral transverse thoracotomy, and midline abdominal. Our surgical approach to diaphragmatic hernias has been the midline with the option of

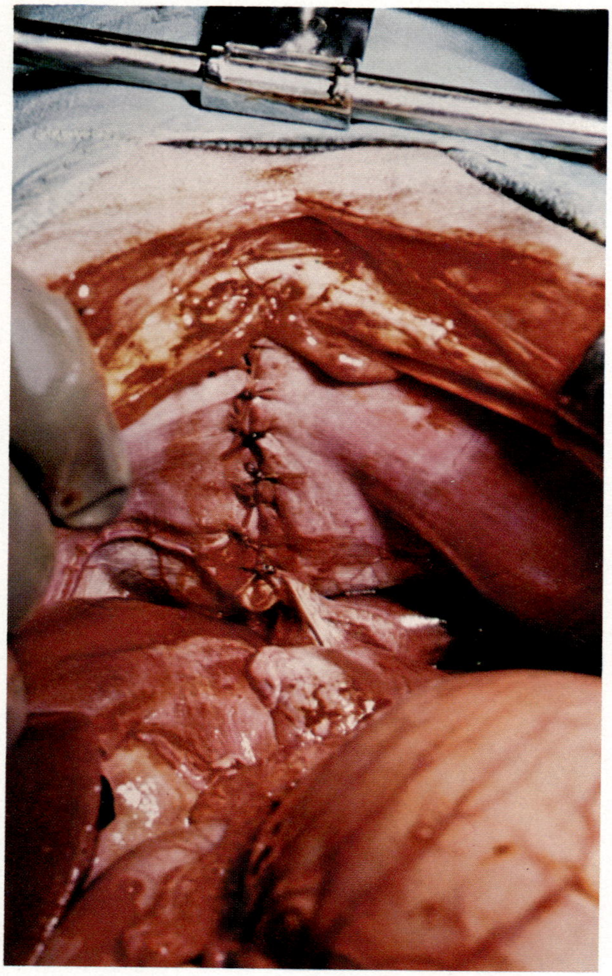

Figure 6

The final closing suture was placed with the lungs expanded. This emptied the pericardial space of air.

Figure 7

Radiograph of a case of peritoneopericardial hernia. The stomach and the small intestine are outlined by radiopaque medium in the pericardial sac.

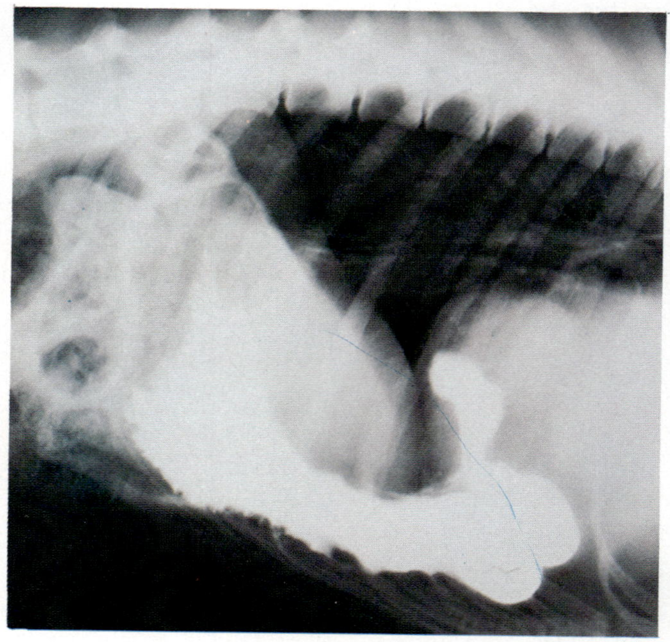

partial sternotomy if required. If the hole in the diaphragm is of long standing and is constricting the viscera, it can be enlarged to ease repositioning of the viscera. The enlarged hole is easily repaired.

When the dog in this case was returned for a checkup more than three and one-half years after surgery, it was in excellent health.

Surgical repair of peritoneopericardial hernia should entail no greater difficulties than repair of traumatically-induced hernia.

REFERENCES

1. Pommer, A.: Hernia Diaphragmatica Pericardialis Bei Hunden. *Wein. tierarztl. Monatssch.* *38*(8):497-507; 1951.
2. Amman, K.: Angeborener Zwerchfell Herzbeutlbroch Beim Hund. *Kleintier-Praxis.* *5*:121-123; July 1968.
3. Bolton, G.R. *et al:* Congenital Peritoneopericardial Diaphragmatic Hernia in a Dog. *JAVMA* = = (5):723-730;1969.
4. Detweiler, D.K. *et al:* Diagnosis and Surigcal Correction of Peritoneopericardial Diaphragmatic Hernia in a Dog. *JAVMA* *137*(3):177-182; 1960.
5. Finn, J.P.; Martin, C.C.: Diaphragmatic Pericardial Hernia. *J. Small Anim. Pract.* *10*:259-300; 1969.
6. Rajan, A. *et al:* Congenital Diaphragmatic Hernia in a Dog. *Kerala J. Vet. Sci.* *5*(1):78-81; 1975.
7. Reed, J.H.; Pennock, P.W.: Concurrent Ventral and Pericardial Diaphragmatic Hernias in two dogs. *MVP 52*(2):47-49; Feb. 1971.
8. Baker, G.J.; Williams, C.S.F.: Diaphragmatic Pericardial Hernia in the Dog. *Vet Record 78*(17):578-583; 1966.
9. Verine, H.; Perot, F.: Hernie Diaphragmatique Congenitale Chez un Chien. *Bull. Soc. Sci. Vet. et Med. Comparee, Lyon* *73*:143-147; 1971.
10. Bjorck, G.R.; Tigetschiold, A.: Peritoneo-pericardial Diaphragmatic Hernia in a Dog. *J. Small Anim. Pract.* *11*:585-590; 1970.
11. Butler, H.C.: Repair of Congenital Diaphragmatic Hernia. *JAV-MA 36*(11):559-560; 1960.
12. Feldman, D.B. *et al:* Congenital Diaphragmatic Hernia in Neonatal Dogs. *JAVMA 153*(7):942-944; 1968.
13. Wilson, G.P. III *et al:* A Review of 116 Diaphragmatic Hernias in Dogs and Cats. *JAVMA 159*(9):1142-1145; 1971.

PARTIAL COLECTOMY

in the treatment of recurrent obstipation/megacolon in the cat

Stanley Fellenbaum, DVM
North Haven Animal Hospital
386 Washington Avenue
North Haven, Connecticut 06473

Two cases of recurrent obstipation in the cat were treated by partial colectomy. The resected segment of the colon extended from the ileum, proximal to the ileocecocolic junction, to the descending colon, cranial to the pelvic brim. A second partial colectomy was performed on one cat because of a recurrence of severe obstipation one year after the initial surgery. Both cats have apparently normal bowel function, six months after surgery in one case and one year after surgery in the other.

RECURRENT OBSTIPATION with extreme dilatation of the colon and stretching of the tube by fecal concretions occurs occasionally in the cat. A summary of the etiology and related terminology has been published.[1]

In the cat, the concretions may or may not have a matrix of grass or hair, or both; but often such a matrix is involved. When filled with concretions, the colon can be readily palpated and might seem to fill most of the abdomen. Digital palpation via the anus may indicate the rectum[2] is empty. However, the rectum sometimes contains small amounts of liquid feces that have passed through the colon, past the concretions. The rectum can be empty except for a concretion at its most caudal aspect. When this is the case, mobility of the concretion is blocked caudally by the anal sphincter and is limited anteriorly by the posterior end of the pelvic canal.

Case Histories

Two case histories are reported in this paper. In both cases the cat had recurrent, life-threatening obstipation which was not responsive to conservative treatment or prophylaxis.

Case No. 1

Because of obstipation, a 3-year-old ovariohysterectomized Siamese cat was presented three times in eight months. On each of these occasions treatment at the hospital consisted of intravenous fluids with steroids, vitamin B_{12}, B complex, and antibiotics. Under anesthesia induced with nitrous oxide and halothane, high enemas of soapy water were given and the obstipations

Figure 1
Radiograph taken immediately following the first partial colectomy (*Case 1*).

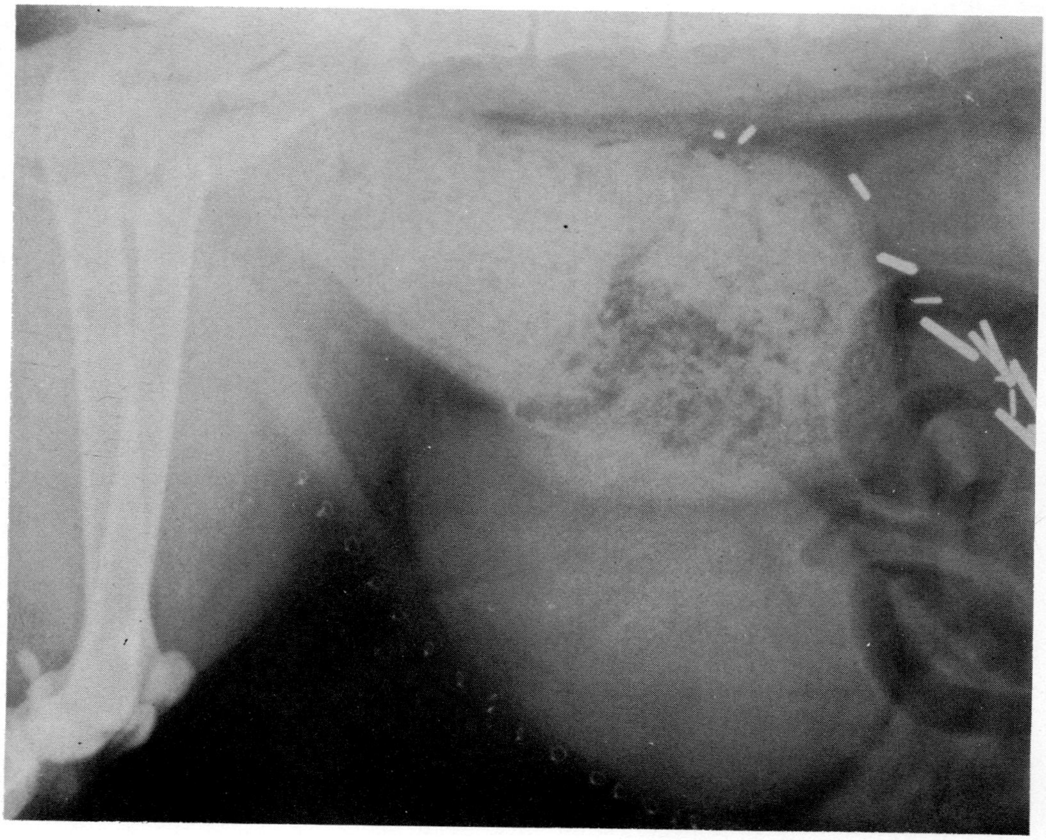

Figure 2
Radiograph taken four days after the second colectomy (*Case 1*) performed one year after the first. Barium was administered by mouth and the radiograph was taken 12 hours later.

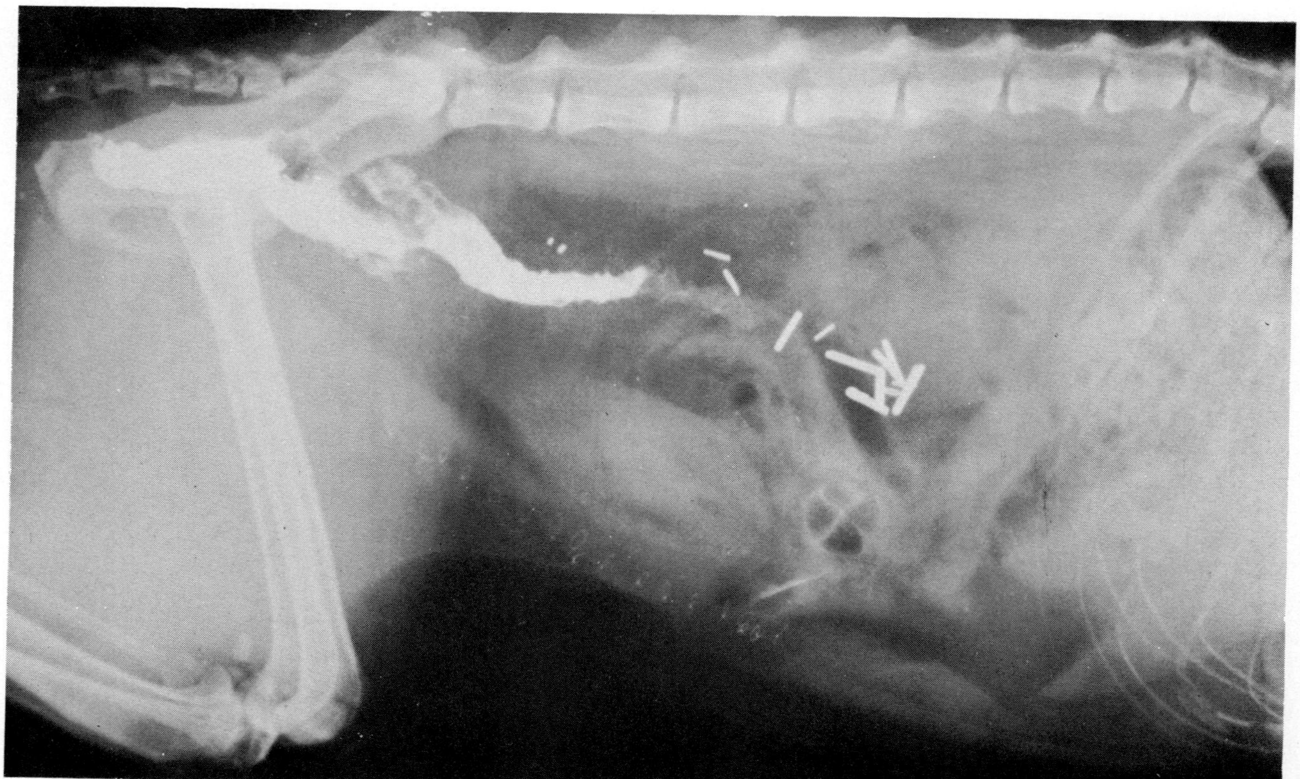

were relieved by mechanically breaking up the concretions by manipulation of the abdomen and the use of a rectal irrigator.

Home care after treatment at the hospital consisted of the following:

1. A petrolatum-based, vitamin-supplemented laxative (Laxatone® —Evsco) given twice daily.
2. 1 ml of an extract of senna fruit (Senokot® —Purdue Frederick, or Casafru® Fluid—Lakeside) given twice daily to soften the feces and stimulate the colon.

Partial colectomy (described later in this report) was performed in a few days after the third episode of obstipation (*Figure 1*). During the three months immediately preceding surgery, the cat's weight had dropped from 13 lb 11 oz (6.2 kg) to 11 lb 7 oz (5.2 kg).

Eight months postoperatively, the cat was again presented because of constipation. A hard stool, palpable in the remaining rectum, was expelled after administration of a routine enema.

One year postoperatively, the obstipation recurred. A radiograph was taken, and while the animal was anesthetized an enema was given and an additional segment of the rectum was resected. Four days later, a barium suspension was administered by mouth. A radiograph taken 12 hours after administration of the barium showed no retention of feces (*Figure 2*).

When reexamined one and one-half months after the second colectomy, the cat was having daily bowel movements, the stools occasionally being soft. A radiograph was taken five hours after oral administration of a barium solution (*Figure 3*).

This cat continues to have normal daily bowel movements approximately six months after surgery. Stools are occasionally soft.

Case No. 2

An aged, castrated, domestic short-hair red tabby was first presented because of obstipation in 1972. When seen again the next year the cat was showing

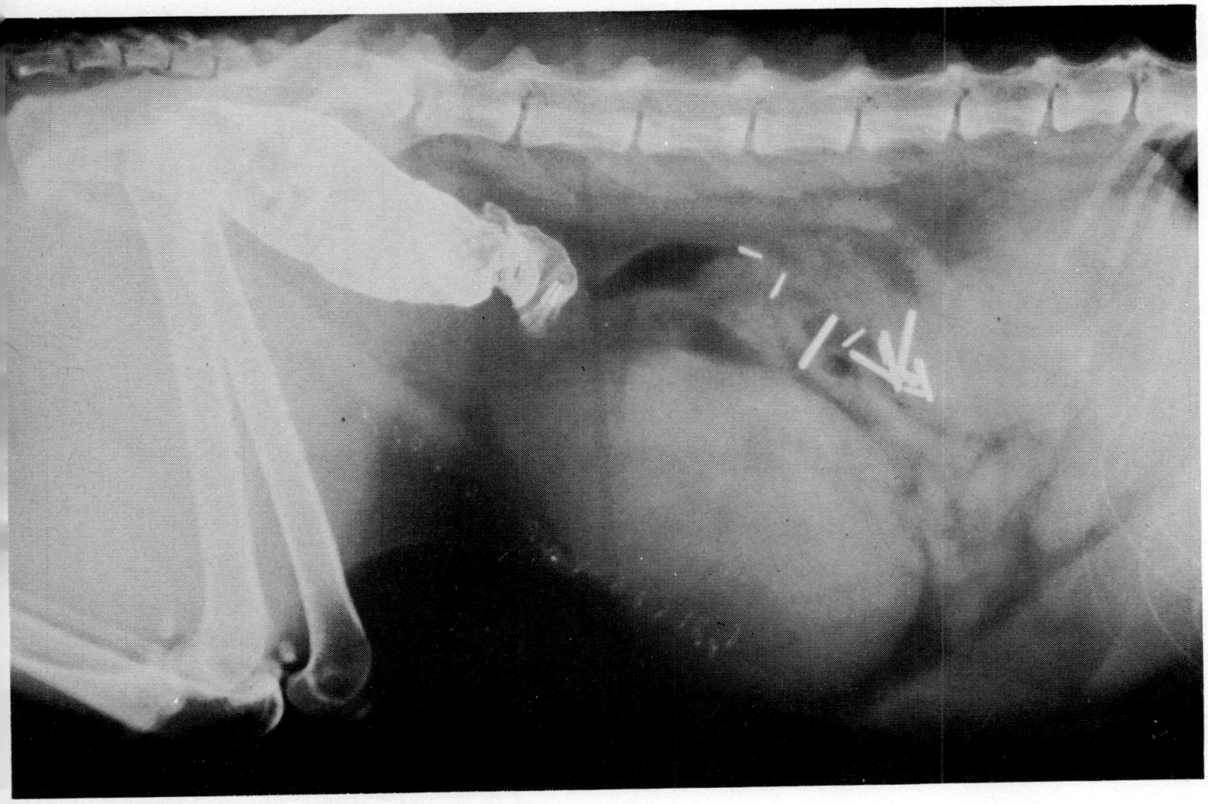

Figure 3
Radiograph taken one and one-half months after the second colectomy (*Case 1*) and five hours after oral administration of barium.

signs of cardiovascular disease, a bruit being noted over the left atrioventricular valve. Obstipation recurred twice during 1975.

In April and May of 1977 the cat was again presented because of obstipation. Treatment was essentially the same as that given in Case No. 1. Between April 4 and May 11, even though treatment with the petrolatum-based laxative and fruit extract syrup was being given, the cat had few bowel movements and feces were scanty. When the cat was presented with obstipation on May 11, it was depressed, anorexic, and dehydrated; its weight had fallen from 11 lb 14 oz (5.3 kg) to 9 lb 14.5 oz (4.4 kg). Partial colectomy was performed a few days later (*Figure 4*).

Colon function in this cat is apparently normal one year after surgery.

Surgical Procedure

The procedure for colectomy was the same in both cats. Before surgery, packed cell volume, blood urea nitrogen, and plasma protein concentration were determined and urinalysis was performed.

An indwelling jugular catheter was inserted and the patient was anesthetized with an appropriate combination of a short-acting barbiturate, nitrous oxide, and halothane. A venoclysis solution was administered during surgery.

A posterior midline abdominal incision was made. While the jejunal vessels and colic vessel were carefully preserved, the ileum was mobilized by applying hemostatic clips (Versa-Clips™—Pitman-Moore) to the terminal ileocecal vessel and severing, up to the last jejunal vessel, the mesenteric attachment to the terminal ileocecal vessel.

A straight Fergusson angiotribe was applied across the ileum, just proximal to the cecum, and the ileum

Figure 4—Radiograph taken four months postoperatively (*Case 2*). Barium, given by mouth 15 hours previously, delineates the terminal ileum, terminal colon, and rectum.

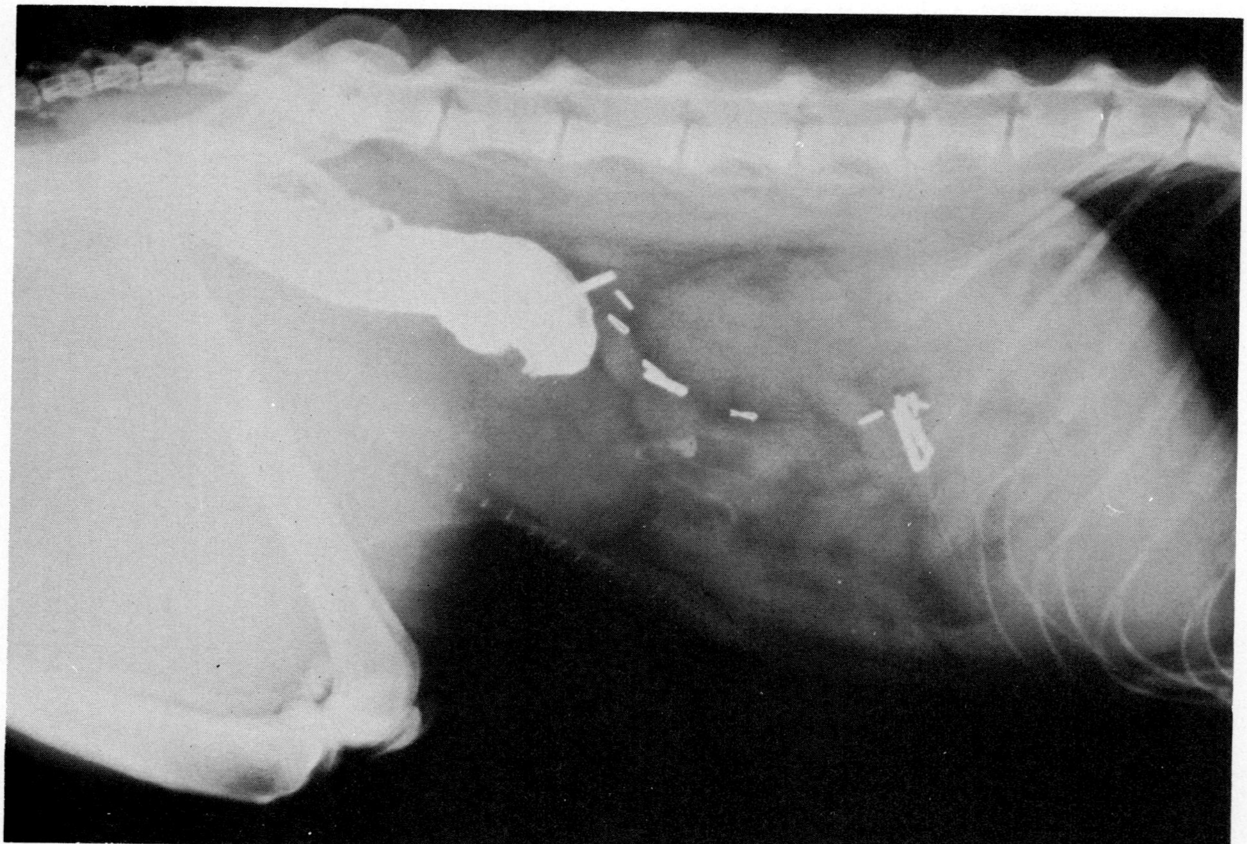

was severed by cutting with a scalpel along the proximal surface of the clamp. The severed artery in the mesenteric attachment was ligated and the end of the ileum was inverted. Then, the distal end of the intact proximal ileum was closed with interrupted sutures.

Any fecal matter remaining in the colon was manipulated into the segment between the ileocecal valve and the descending colon. The lymph nodes and the anastomosing vasculature of the colon were preserved in the mesocolon. Terminal vessels in the colon were ligated with Versa-Clips, and the mesocolon was severed distal to the clips. With enough of the descending colon preserved for anastomosis, the colon was cross-clamped with a straight Fergusson angiotribe. To complete the resection, the rectum was resected with a sharp scalpel along the distal edge of the angiotribe.

The remaining distal colon was cleaned by flushing with a warm isotonic saline solution, and the open proximal end was closed with interrupted through-and-through sutures of 4-0 silk placed through all layers. Excess mucosa was removed where necessary.

While proximal and ventral traction was applied to the remaining descending colon, the distal ileum and remaining colon were joined by means of a two-layered side-to-side anastomosis. Protruding rectal mucosa was resected.

Postoperative Complications

The cat in Case No. 1 became hypothermic and was in a shock-like state for several hours after surgery. In the second case an apparent bacteremia developed one week postoperatively. Both of these complications responded to appropriate therapy.

Discussion

Both cats drank more water after surgery and both urinated more frequently. In Case No. 2 the BUN was 30 mg/100 ml before surgery, and the urine specific gravity was 1.045. This animal's diet had consisted of meat and fish, and the elevated BUN was considered a reflection of the diet, and thus normal. Increased intake of water by these cats is consistent with one of the objectives of the surgery: to prevent feces from dehydrating the colon. "Its (large intestine) most important function is the dehydration of its fecal contents."[3]

No apparent sequelae have developed in these cats, although the closure of the intact sphincter may prevent the regurgitation of cecal and colonic material into the terminal ileum.[4] During the second resection in the first cat, the surgically produced ileocolic junction could be seen and palpated. It very much resembled a functional ileocecocolic valve.

Few attempts at surgical treatment of obstipation/megacolon in the cat have been documented. Personal experience with removal of a longitudinal segment of the colon has not been satisfactory. The experience of other surgeons has been similar, in that the beneficial results of the surgery seem to be only temporary.[5,6] Success has been reported in one case in which 70% of the colon, including the transverse and descending colon, was removed and an end-to-end anastomosis was performed.[7] That patient was reported to be well nine years after surgery, and the procedure is being successfully used by other practitioners.[8]

Conclusion

The two cases of recurrent obstipation/megacolon in cats reported in this paper were of life-threatening proportion and did not respond to conservative therapy. Both cats were salvaged by partial colectomy and anastomosis of the ileum to the descending colon. Although further experience with the procedure may necessitate alteration of some details, the described procedure appears to restore normal colonic function in cases of recurring obstipation in the cat. The procedure is also indicated in cases of colonic neoplasms and non-salvageable injuries of the colon.

REFERENCES

1. Lorenz, M.D.: Disorders of the Large Bowel; in *Textbook of Veterinary Internal Medicine*, Vol. 2 (S.J. Ettinger, ed.). W.B. Saunders Co., Philadelphia, Pa., 1975; p 1193.
2. Use of the word *rectum* is after Sisson and Grossman, *Anatomy of the Domestic Animals*, 3rd ed., revised. W.B. Saunders Co., Philadelphia, Pa. This usage selects the plane of the pelvic inlet as the division between the colon and rectum. "The rectum is the terminal part of the bowel; it extends from the pelvic inlet to the anus."
   The same usage is maintained in *Anatomy of the Dog*, Miller, M.E. *et al.* W.B. Saunders Co., Philadelphia, Pa., 1965.
3. Miller, M.E. *et al*: *Anatomy of the Dog*. W.B. Saunders Co., Philadelphia, Pa., 1965.
4. Hill, K.J.: Gastrointestinal Motility; in *Dukes' Physiology of Domestic Animals*, 8th ed. (M.J. Swenson, ed.). Comstock Pub. Assoc., Ithaca, N.Y., 1970; p 363.
5. Dann, R.J., DVM, Ridgefield, Conn. Personal communication.
6. Dietzman, V.: Congenital Megacolon. *M. h Vet. Med.* *23*(9):349-352; 1968.
7. Yoder, J.T. *et al*: Partial Colectomy for Correction of Megacolon in a Cat. *VM/SAC 63*:1049-1052; November, 1968.
8. Yoder, J.T., DVM, Des Moines, Iowa. Personal communication.

Traumatic subcapsular splenic cystic hematoma in the dog / a case study

Samuel Pollock, DVM
South Orange Animal Hospital
66 Valley Street
South Orange, New Jersey 07079

Victor T. Rendano, VMD
New York State College of Veterinary Medicine
Cornell University
Ithaca, New York 14853

Bernard M. Wagner, MD
Overlook Hospital
Columbia University
Summit, New Jersey 07901

Joseph M. Fell, DVM
Animal and Bird Hospital
467 South Street
Morristown, New Jersey 07960

Figure 1A — Lateral radiograph of the abdomen. A homogenous, soft-tissue mass with definable borders is located in the middle of the abdomen. The intestines are displaced by the mass.

Figure 1B (*right*) — Ventrodorsal view of the chest and abdomen.

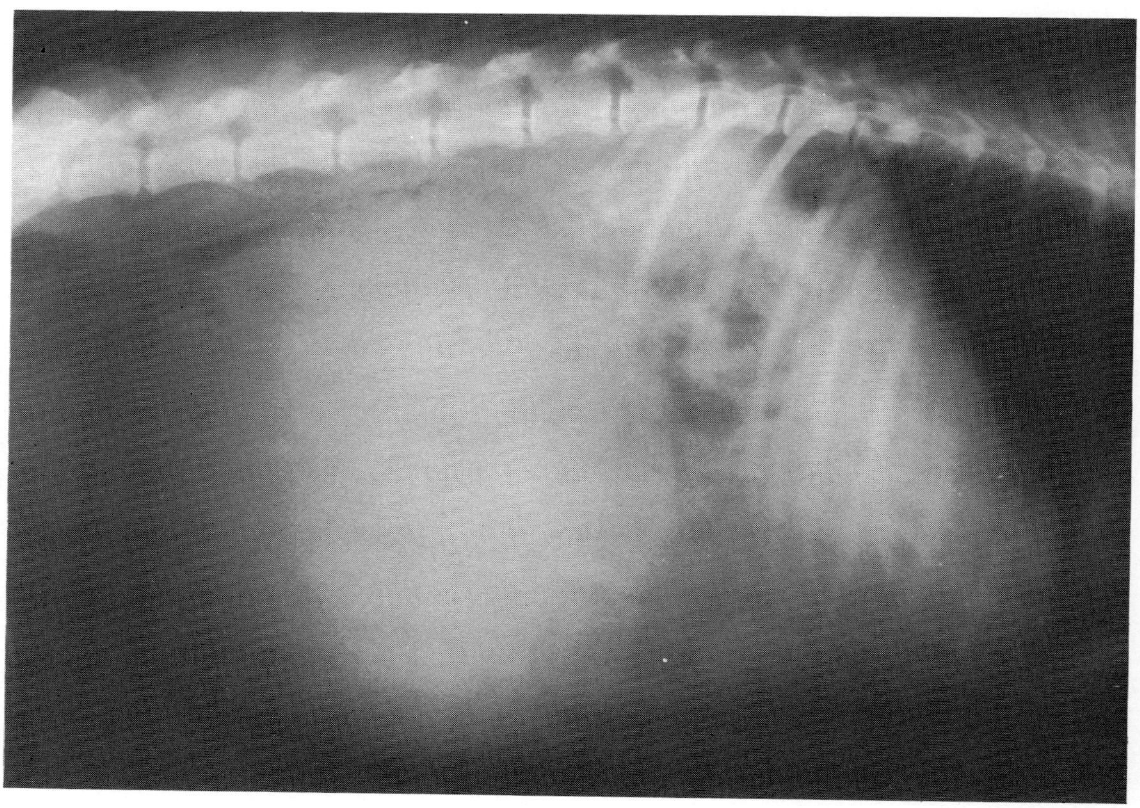

RUPTURE OF THE SPLEEN in the dog is common after automobile injuries or sudden blows over the left side of the abdomen. Evidence of an old injury to the spleen is commonly seen after laparotomy or during necropsy. Occasionally, the spleen is found in two or three fragments. In some instances, autotransplantation of splenic tissue to adjacent peritoneal surfaces occurs, resulting in the formation of small red nodules. This condition is known as *splenosis.* These observations indicate that animals can survive severe splenic trauma without surgical intervention.

Delayed rupture of the spleen in the dog is considered rare. However, in man one of every six cases of splenic rupture occurs one to 30 or more days after the initial trauma. Subcapsular hemorrhage results in progressive formation of hematoma and subsequent stretching and rupture of the capsule.[1]

The following report describes a case of delayed splenic subcapsular hematoma in a dog.

Case Report

A 13-year-old ovariohysterectomized Golden Retriever was presented because of anorexia, apathy, loss of weight, and abdominal distention. The owner first noticed these signs several weeks before the dog was examined, but attributed them to the animal's advanced age and lack of children and other dogs for play.

Upon palpation, a firm mass was found that seemed

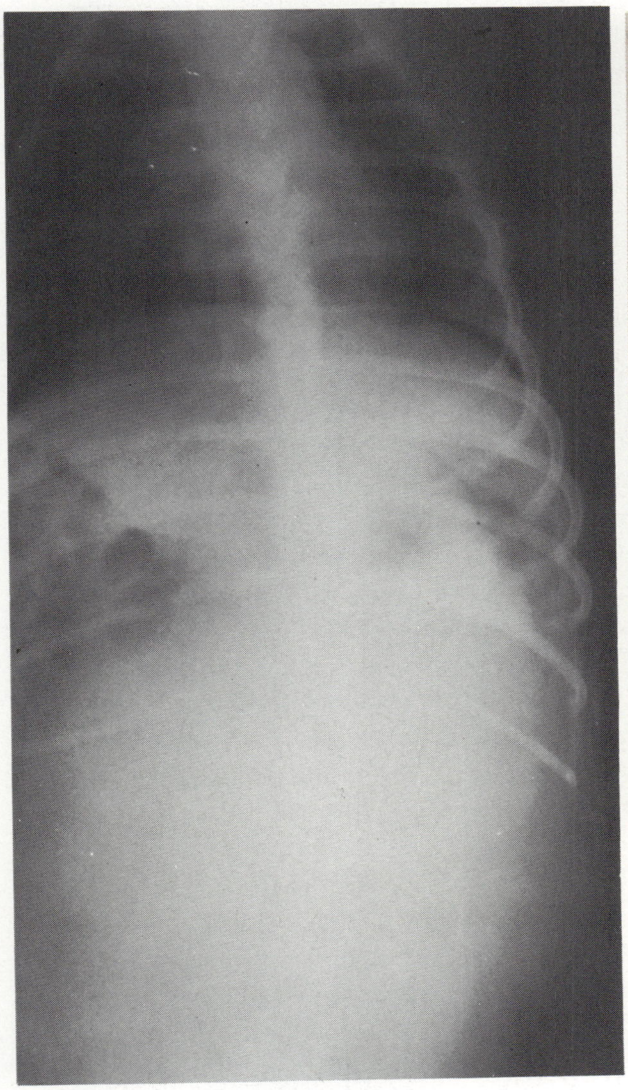

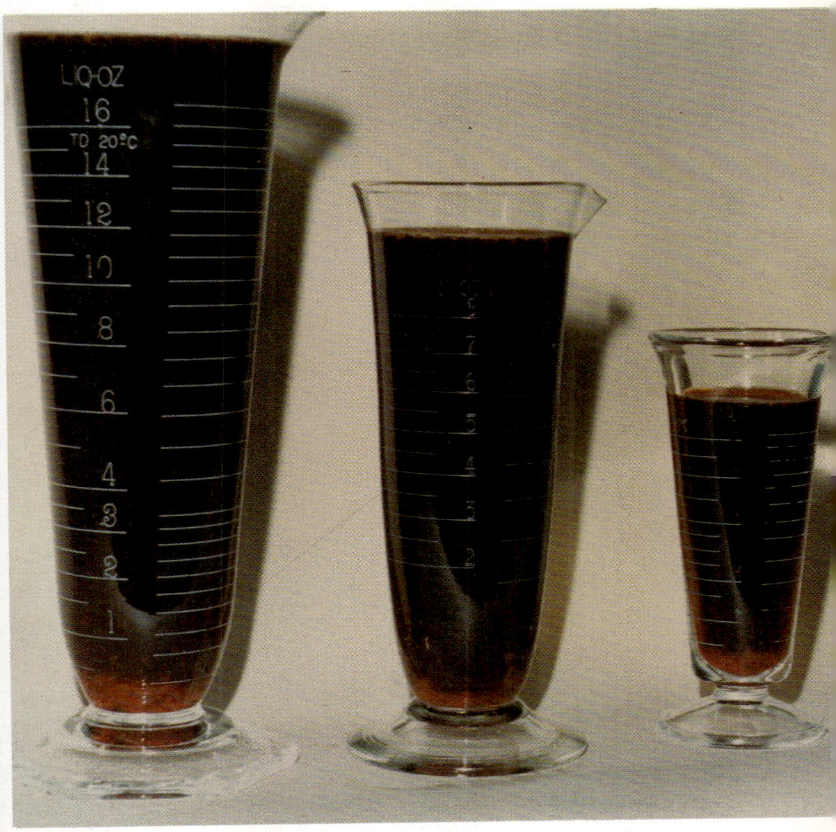

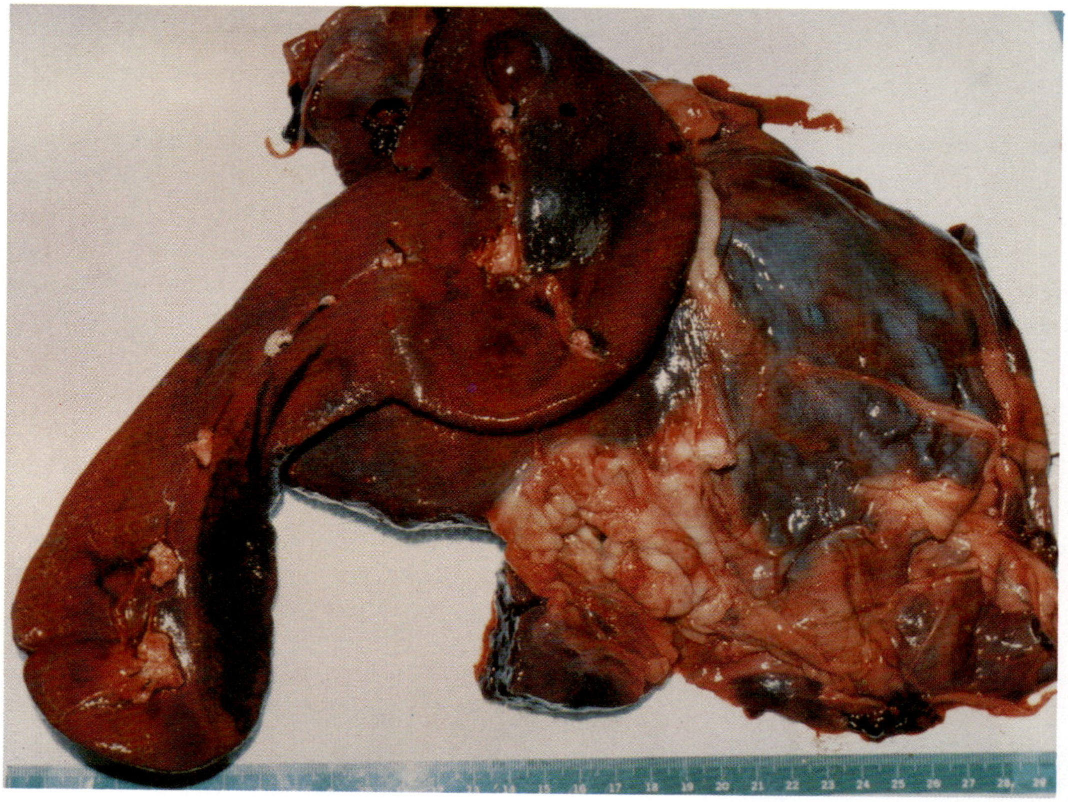

Figure 3
Visceral surface of the spleen with the cystic mass enveloped by omentum.

Figure 4
(*far right*)
Spleen and cyst after aspiration of fluid.

to occupy the entire abdomen. Radiographs showed a homogenous soft-tissue density with definable borders in the mid-portion of the abdomen. The intestines were displaced by the mass (*Figures 1A & B*).

Permission was obtained to perform an exploratory laparotomy.

Surgical Procedure

Morphine and atropine were given before anesthesia was induced with Surital® (Parke-Davis). Anesthesia was maintained with Metofane™ (Pitman-Moore) via tracheal intubation. During surgery 500 cc lactated Ringer's solution was administered intravenously.

A mid-ventral incision was made from the xiphoid to the pubis. A large mass encased in omentum could be seen filling the entire abdomen. When the mass was palpated it appeared to have a cystic structure which, on needle aspiration, was found to be serosanguineous fluid.

The nozzle of a suction apparatus was inserted into the mass through a stab wound, and a liter of fluid was aspirated (*Figure 2*). The growth was rotated and a portion of the mass was identified as the spleen (*Figure 3*). When removed, the spleen with attached cystic structures weighed 5 lb (*Figure 4*).

The abdomen was closed in layers. The peritoneum was closed with No. 3 Dexon® (American Cyanamid) sutures, the muscle and fascia with interrupted No. 3 siliconized silk, the subcutaneous tissue with No. 3 Dexon, and the skin with interrupted No. 4 nylon using a suturator.

Postoperative radiographs were taken of the mass and the patient (*Figures 5 & 6*).

When informed of the findings, the client recalled that three years earlier, while she had been out of town, her dog was hit by a car. The dog was hospitalized over a weekend and released without radiographs or diag-

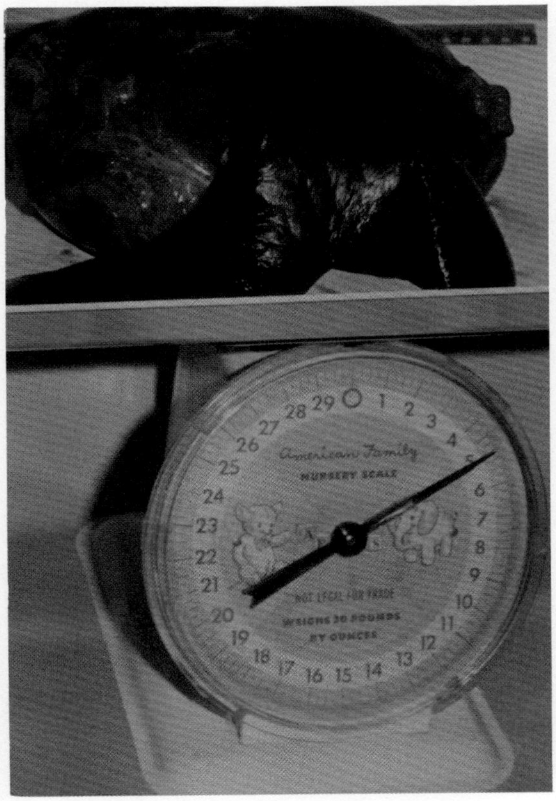

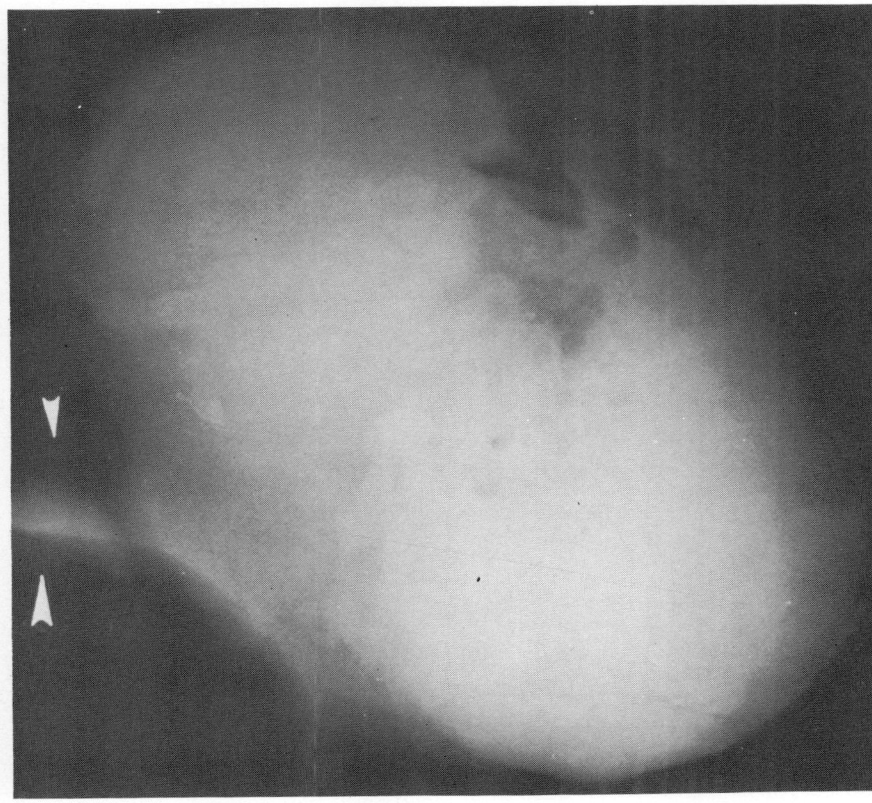

Figure 5
Radiograph of the mass after surgical removal and aspiration of fluid. Note the lobed nature of the mass and the uninvolved portion of the spleen (*arrows*).

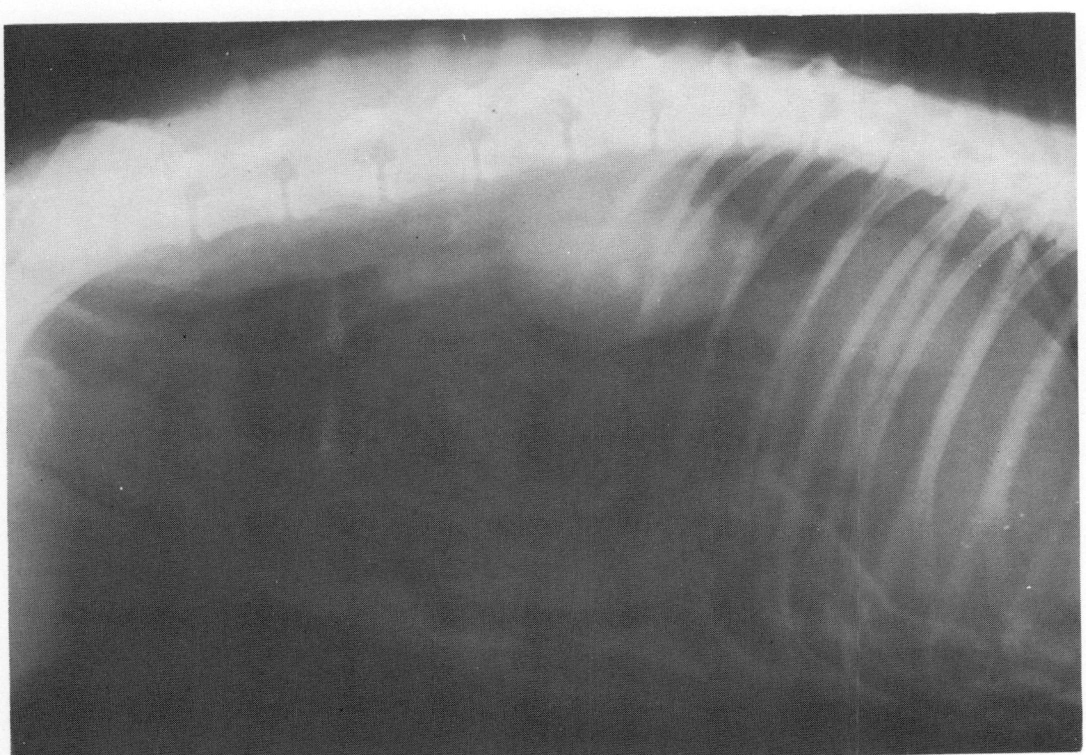

Figure 6
Postoperative lateral radiograph of the abdomen. The intestines have returned to their usual anatomic location. Free gas is present, improving visualization of some of the organs.

nostic laboratory tests. From that time the patient's general condition seemed to deteriorate gradually.

The patient's apathy and anorexia may have been related to pressure exerted on other abdominal organs by the cystic splenic mass. These signs were no longer present when the animal was evaluated three months postoperatively.

Upon pathological examination of the splenic mass, subcapsular hematomas due to trauma were found.

When the spleen was examined microscopically, normal splenic tissue could not be identified. There was extensive formation of blood clots associated with cystic, mucoid degeneration. A thin fibrous capsule surrounded the tissue. Strands of fibro-fatty connective tissue suggestive of omental adhesions were attached to the capsule at focal points.

Discussion

The pathogenesis of the lesion was probably the result of trauma to the spleen, with acute and chronic hemorrhage into the parenchyma and capsule. With progressive bleeding the spleen is expanded and the parenchyma compressed. Compression results in pressure atrophy of the splenic cellular elements. Continual formation of clotted blood at different intervals results in blood clots, cysts, and mucoid, gelatinous amorphous masses.

As blood clots and fibrin contracts, blood loses its water component. However, as the osmotic gradient with the surrounding tissue changes, fluid is introduced and a cystic mass develops. The process is best known in the brain, where an intracerebral hemorrhage evolves into a cystic encephalomalacia. Due to chronic bleeding, the spleen in this case was converted into a huge sac containing blood and blood degradation products (*Figure 7*).

In man, the spleen may rupture spontaneously in the course of splenomegaly due to disease or secondary to trauma. Traumatic rupture is due to nonpenetrating injuries to the abdomen or the lower left side of the thoracic cage. The rupture may be immediate or delayed.

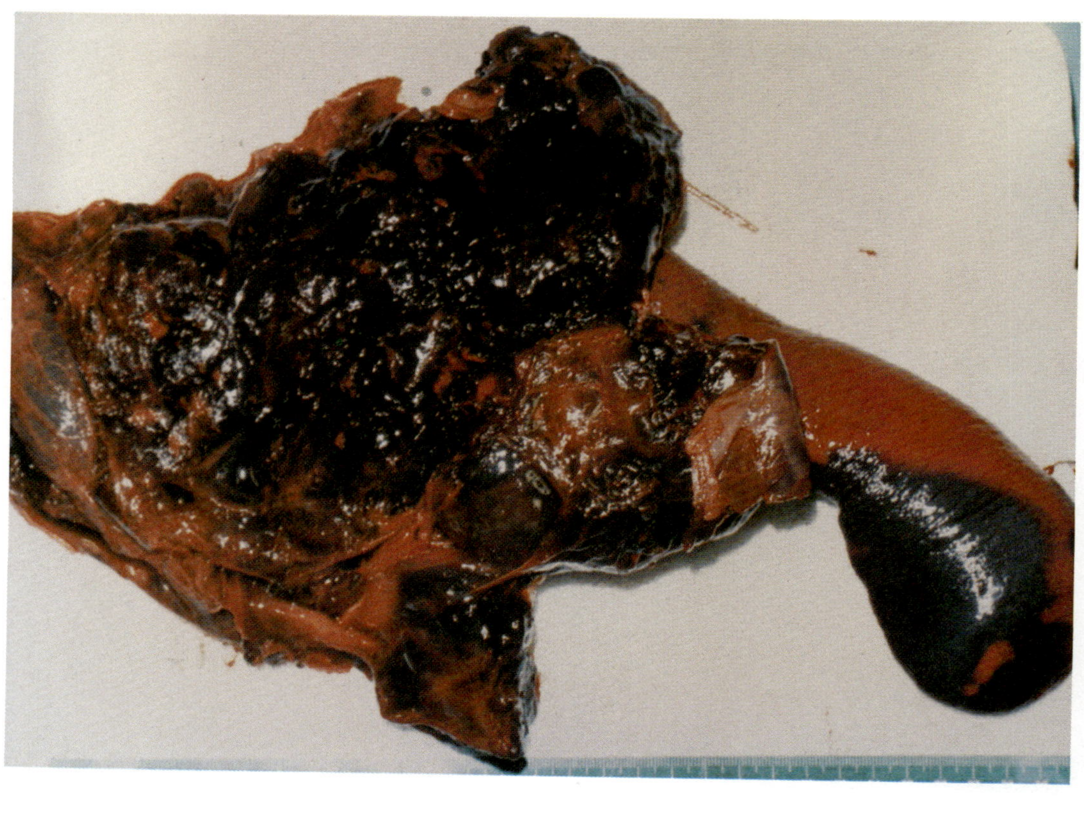

Figure 7
A section of the cystic mass with clots and blood degeneration.

Spontaneous rupture occurs as a complication of acute febrile diseases associated with splenomegaly. Malaria and infectious mononucleosis in man are the most common causes. Signs of peritoneal irritation accompanied by shock and evidence of concealed hemorrhage in the course of an acute illness are indicative of this complication and warrant prompt exploration.

Traumatic rupture is accompanied by prompt evidence of peritoneal irritation and blood loss. In the hours immediately after injury, the signs may consist of only pain in the left upper quadrant or left shoulder, or an inability to stand straight.

Tell-tale contusions or abrasions on the left side of the trunk may help the practitioner locate the site of injury. As loss of blood continues, abdominal rigidity and tenderness become increasingly diffuse. Signs of hemorrhage occur, with elevated pulse, lowered blood pressure, decreasing hemoglobin and red cell count, and leukocytosis. Diagnosis may be corroborated by aspiration of blood from the peritoneal cavity, although a negative aspiration does not exclude the diagnosis. Prompt replacement of blood should always be performed, followed by splenectomy. During surgery, adjacent viscera should be inspected for signs of injury.

Delayed rupture is caused by the sudden collapse of a contained subcapsular rupture. The patient may appear to be uninjured for 48 hours or longer after trauma. Signs of delayed rupture are sudden onset of pain, peritoneal irritation, and shock.

In man, diagnosis can be made via radiographs that show loss or enlargement of splenic outline and indentation or displacement of gastric outline with downward displacement of the splenic flexure of the colon. Also present may be elevation and fixation of the left hemidiaphragm, fracture of the lower ribs, downward displacement of the left kidney, loss of outline of the left kidney and psoas muscle, and widening of the left paravertebral shadow.

If a ruptured spleen is either suspected or confirmed, splenectomy should be performed before intraperitoneal rupture and shock occur.[2]

REFERENCES

1. Brody, R.S.: *Canine Surgery* (Archibald, J., ed). American Veterinary Publications, 2nd ed., 1974; pp 816-818.
2. Blaustein, Ancel, M.D.: *The Spleen*. The Blakiston Division—McGraw Hill Book Co., 1963: pp 208-209.

removal of a THECOMA IN A POODLE

Roy T. Faulkner, BS, DVM, Clinical Investigation Service
Dwight David Eisenhower Army Medical Center, Fort Gordon, Georgia 30905

Ovarian tumors in dogs are common.[1] In the bitch, the two types of germ-cell tumors most frequently seen are the dysgerminoma and the teratoma.[1] The granulosa cell tumor is the most commonly reported sex cord-stromal neoplasm.[1] Granulosa cell tumors, dysgerminomas, and teratomas have been reported in the recent literature.[2-4] However, there appears to be lack of reports describing ovarian thecomas.

Case Report

A 10-year-old female toy Poodle was presented because of depression and vomiting. The owner said that the dog had a cesarean section four years earlier and that no estrus had been observed within the past 18 months.

The dog was in good condition and was normally hydrated. Pulse, temperature, and respiration were normal. Upon abdominal palpation, a large, firm, round, mobile mass was found within the left abdominal cavity. A blood sample was drawn for a complete blood count (CBC) and blood chemistry analyses (SMA-6 and SMA-12). Radiographs of the abdomen were taken.

The blood evaluations showed moderate leukocytosis (23,900 WBC), with absolute neutrophilia (90%), relative lymphopenia (6%), and absolute eosinopenia (0%). The SMA-6 and SMA-12 profiles were within normal limits except for a slight elevation in serum lactic dehydrogenase (230 mU/ml).

A mass approximately 8 cm × 10 cm, caudal to the left kidney within the left abdominal cavity, was seen in the abdominal radiographs (*Figure 1*). The mass displaced the descending colon to the right. A tentative diagnosis of ovarian neoplasm was made and the dog was scheduled for an exploratory laparotomy.

Surgical Procedure

General anesthesia was induced with 2.5% sodium pentothal, given intravenously, and maintained with a mixture of nitrous oxide, halothane, and oxygen. Premedication consisted of atropine sulfate at a dosage of 0.02 mg/lb. Lactated Ringer's solution at 10 ml/lb was given throughout the procedure. The patient was placed on a warm-water, circulating heating pad and the electrocardiogram was continuously monitored on an oscilloscope-type cardiac monitor (American Optical).

The exploratory celiotomy was performed through a ventral midline incision. A Balfour abdominal retractor padded with moist gauze sponges was positioned within the abdomen. The mass was exposed and identified as a left ovarian tumor. It was freely mobile except for a few omental adhesions on its cranial aspect. These adhesions were isolated, ligated between ties of 3-0 silk, and divided until the neoplastic ovary was completely freed. A routine ovariohysterectomy was performed. The abdomen was examined and no signs of metastasis were seen. The abdomen was washed several times with warm, sterile, physiologic saline solution and closed in a routine manner.

The patient was discharged the next day. Ten days later, when the sutures were removed, the dog was doing well. It has had no further problems during the past nine months.

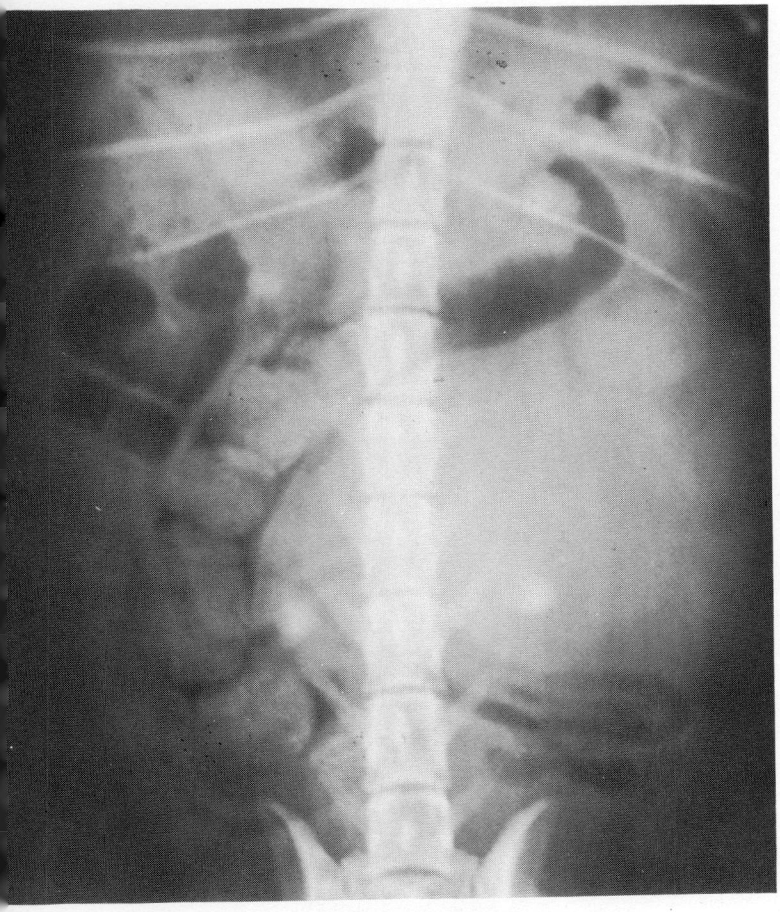

Figure 1—Abdominal radiograph. The ovarian neoplasm and displacement of the descending colon are seen.

Pathology

The excised ovarian neoplasm, 8 cm × 10 cm, was firm and light gray. Its center contained a colorless fluid. Histologically, the tumor was diagnosed as a malignant ovarian stromal neoplasm consistent with thecoma.

Discussion

Most ovarian tumors can be classified into three groups: epithelial, germ cell, and sex cord-stromal.[1] Granulosa cell tumors, thecomas, and luteomas are considered sex cord-stromal tumors. Granulosa cell tumors are of sex cord origin, whereas thecomas are considered to originate in ovarian stromal cells.[1] Luteomas may develop from either one of these types of tumors.[1]

The client in this case reported that the dog had not shown signs of estrus for 18 months. Many sex cord-stromal tumors have the ability to produce estrogen or progesterone, or both.[1] Estrogen, testosterone, and progesterone were reportedly found in the tumor fluid of three mares with granulosa cell tumors.[5]

Thecomas are generally considered benign and they grow by expansion, without metastasis.[1] In this case the neoplasm was histologically regarded a malignant thecoma of stromal origin. At surgery, no areas of metastasis were seen. No signs of metastasis or other problems have been noted nine months after surgery.

ACKNOWLEDGMENT

The author expresses appreciation to Dr. Lloyd Rothouse, Dwight David Eisenhower Army Medical Center, Fort Gordon, Georgia, and to Dr. Michael Elwell, United States Army Research Institute of Infectious Diseases, Fort Detrick, Maryland, for their histologic examination.

REFERENCES

1. Nielsen, S.W. *et al:* XV. Tumours of the Ovary. *Bull. World Health Organ. 53:*203; 1976.
2. Allen, H.L.; Franklin, G.A.: Malignant Granulosa Cell Tumor in a Bitch. *JAVMA 166:*447; 1975.
3. Buergelt, Claus-D: Dysgerminoma in Two Dogs. *JAVMA 153:*553; 1968.
4. Crane, S.W. *et al:* Malignant Ovarian Teratoma in a Bitch. *JAVMA 167:*72 1975.
5. Stickle, R.L. *et al:* Equine Granulosa Cell Tumors. *JAVMA 167:*148; 1975

Surgical Removal of a BB Shot from the Abdominal Aorta of a Cat

Charles R. Horton, DVM
Bill J. Renfroe, DVM
North Parkway Animal Hospital
931 Cook Avenue N.W.
Huntsville, Alabama 35801

A 3-YEAR-OLD domestic short-hair cat was presented because of bilateral posterior paresis. The owner suspected the cat had been hit by a car since it was found lying in the street. The injury had occurred approximately 12 hours before the cat was presented.

Examination

The only external injury was a small puncture wound in the right thorax. The respiratory and heart rates were rapid. The cat was in considerable pain and resisted palpation of the rear legs and abdomen. Both rear legs were ischemic (*Figure 1*), and no femoral pulse could be palpated. Only a slight toe pinch reflex could be elicited. Firm, edematous masses could be palpated in the popliteal areas of both legs.

Figure 1
Comparison between ischemic rear foot pads and well-perfused front foot pads.

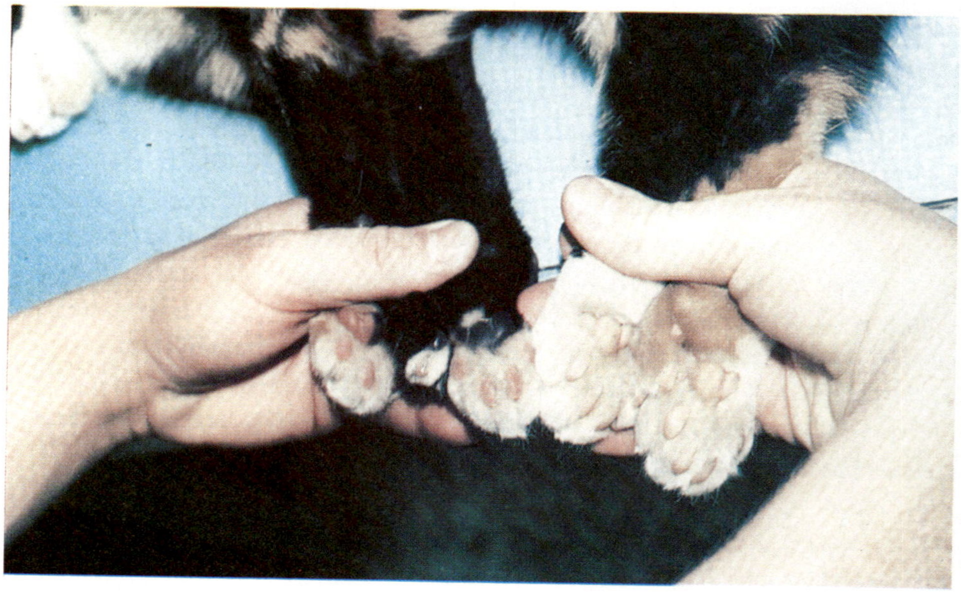

An intravenous injection of 10 mg ketamine hydrochloride (Ketaset®—Bristol) was administered and radiographs were taken. A metallic density in the area of the abdominal aorta was seen in the lateral and ventrodorsal views of the abdomen (*Figures 2 & 3*). All evidence suggested that the metallic object was impairing aortic circulation to the caudal extremities. The owners agreed to our request to perform exploratory surgery.

Surgical Procedure

The animal was intubated and anesthesia was maintained with methoxyflurane (Metofane®—Pitman-Moore). A laparotomy was performed through a ventral midline incision. The aorta was exposed by packing the abdominal viscera anteriorly and laterally with gauze sponges soaked in saline solution. The metallic object could be easily palpated within the aorta, just anterior to the orgin of the caudal mesenteric artery.

The aorta was encircled with umbilical tape proximal to the obstruction. An assistant placed forceps over the umbilical tape and applied pressure sufficient to impede the blood flow through the aorta. This allowed an arteriotomy to be performed. A BB shot was removed from the aorta.

The aorta was sutured with three simple interrupted sutures of 4-0 silk. An absorbable gelatin sponge (Gelfoam®—Upjohn) was applied to the incision to induce clotting. After hemostasis was achieved, the abdomen was closed with 2-0 chromic gut and the skin was sutured with Vetafil® (S. Jackson).

The cat was given dexamethasone (Azium®—Schering) and a penicillin-streptomycin combination (Distrycillin®—Squibb) and placed in an infant warmer. After a prolonged recovery period of 10 hours, the cat began to respond. It was eating by the second day after surgery. Swelling in the popliteal area persisted for more than a week, but gradual restoration of function accompanied the reduction in swelling.

Two weeks postsurgically the cat was ambulatory but could not fully extend the hock joint. Nine weeks postsurgically the legs were clinically normal, although the distal third of the tail had no voluntary movement and was insensitive to stimulus. Five months postsurgically the cat was asymptomatic.

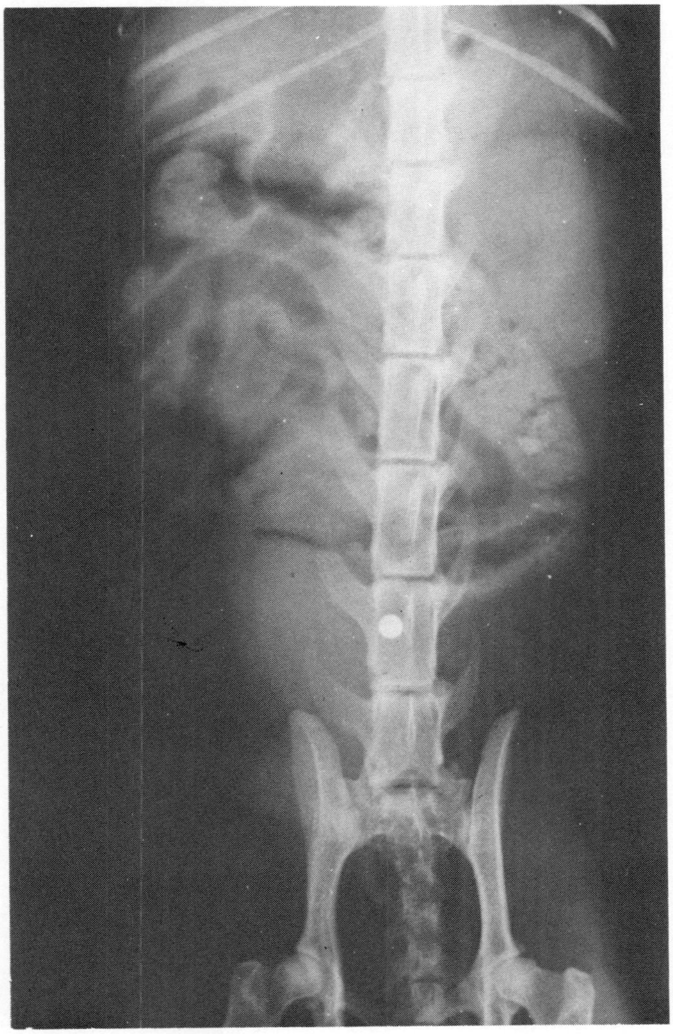

Discussion

Since the wound in the right thorax was the only lesion found, the BB must have entered the cat's body at that point (*Figure 4*). The course of the BB after it entered is a matter of speculation. Since it had lodged in the abdominal aorta, the pellet must have entered the left atrium, the left ventricle, or the thoracic aorta itself. In all probability it entered through the apex of the thick-walled ventricle. Entry by any other route would probably have caused fatal hemorrhage.

ACKNOWLEDGMENT

Gratitude is expressed to Dr. James Milton and other members of the staff at Auburn University for their advice in the preparation of this article.

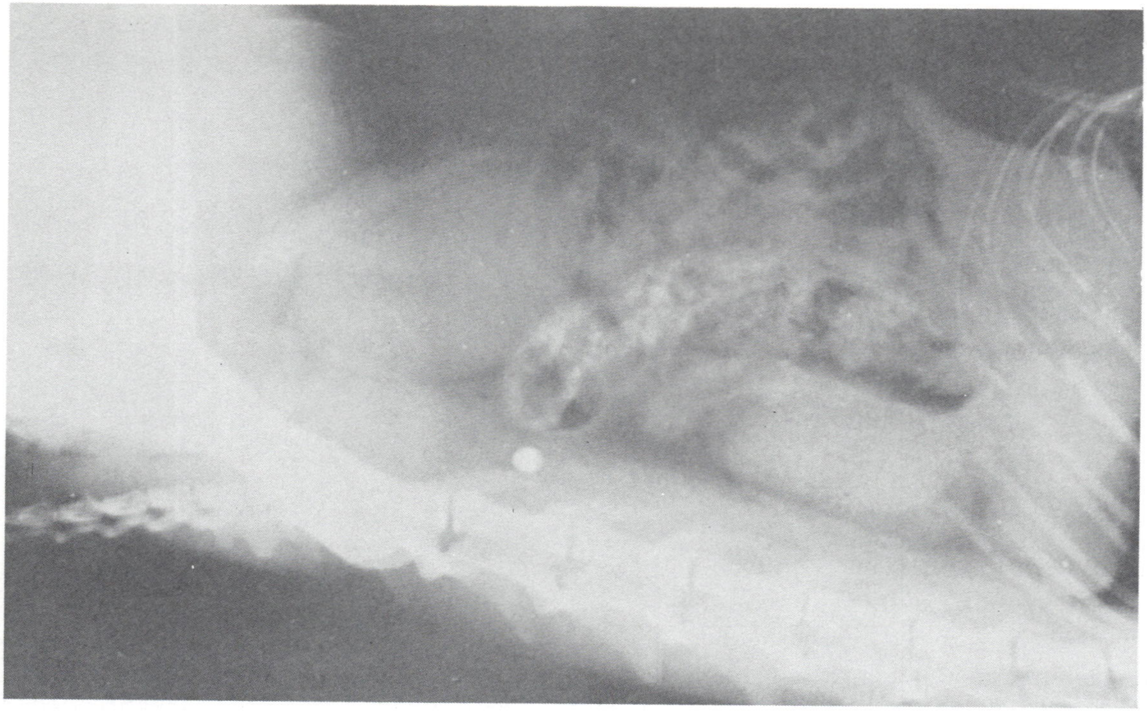

Figures 2 & 3—Lateral and ventrodorsal views of the abdomen showing the location of the BB shot in the aorta.

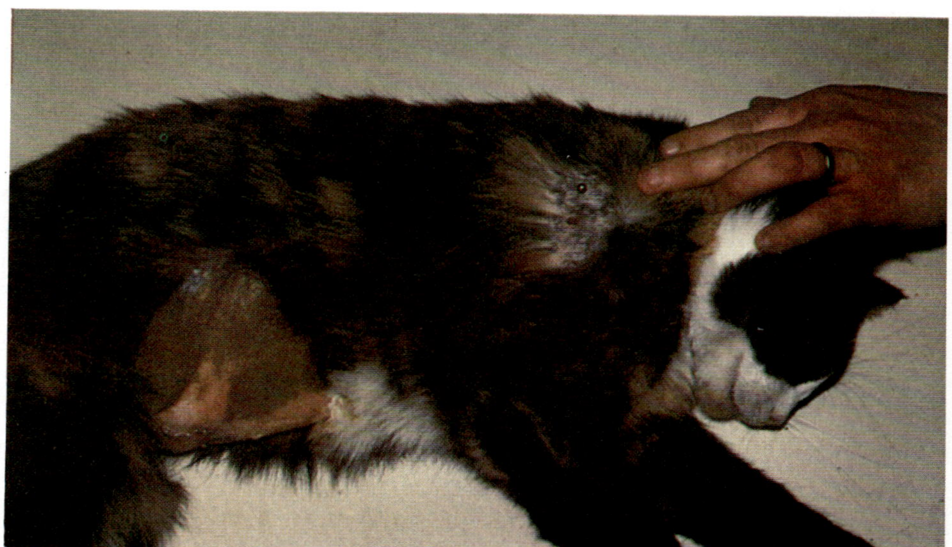

Figure 4
Postsurgical view showing the BB shot after its removal from the aorta, and the entry wound on the right thorax.

The sutureless nephrotomy closure

A photographic essay

G. Robert Weedon
Junior Veterinary Student
Stephen Birchard, DVM
Resident, Small Animal Surgery
School of Veterinary Medicine
Purdue University
West Lafayette, Indiana 47907

PROCEDURES FOR NEPHROTOMY are well documented in veterinary literature, as are various suture techniques for closing the nephrotomy incision.[1,2] In this paper we describe and illustrate sutureless closure, an alternative method. The sutureless closure has been described in human as well as veterinary literature,[3,4] but has not as yet gained wide acceptance. The conclusion from one study was that sutureless closure is the preferred technique.[4]

Figure 1
The kidney is exposed and isolated from the abdominal cavity, and the vessels are separated from the ureter.

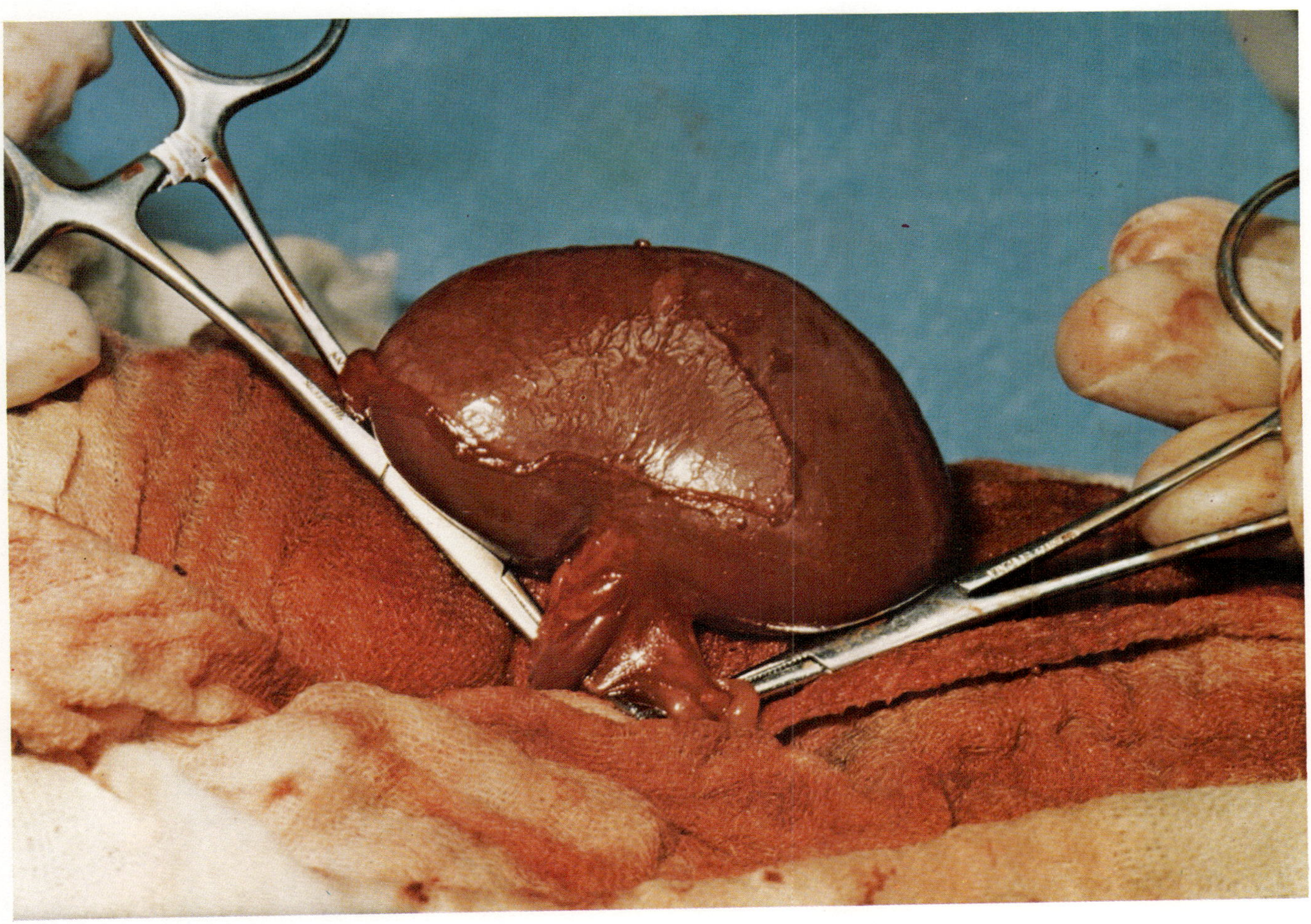

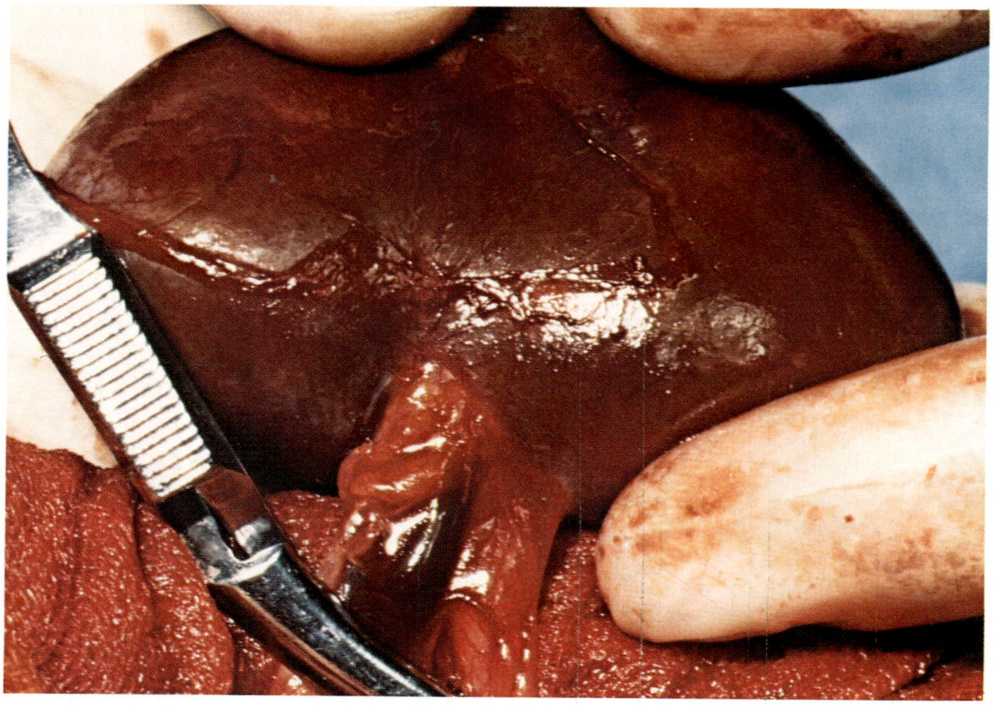

Figure 2—A bulldog vascular clamp is applied to the renal artery and vein.

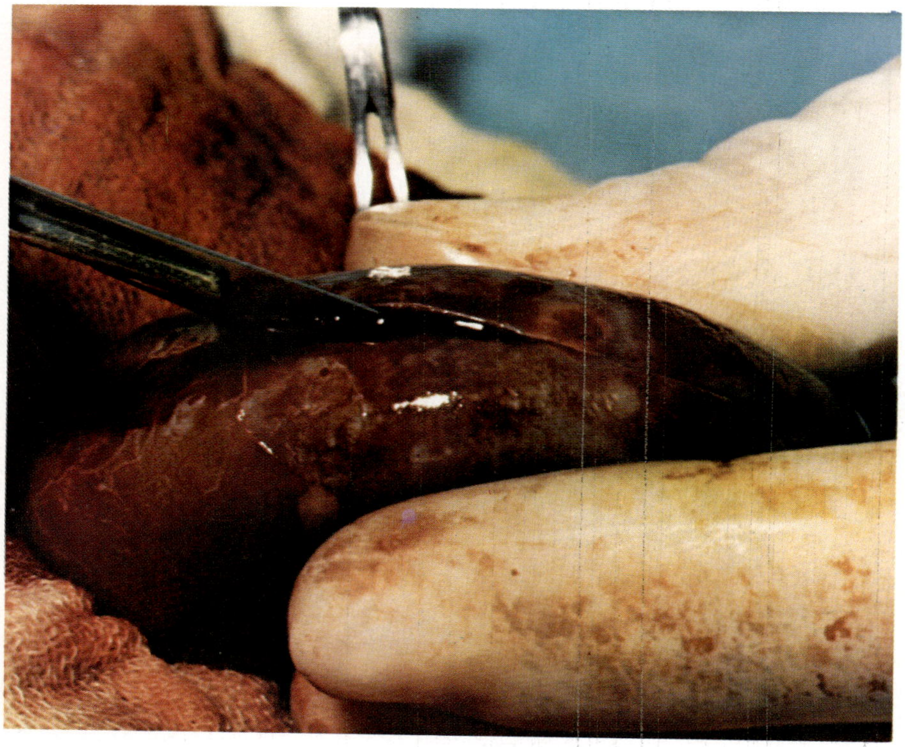

Figure 3

The nephrotomy incision is made on the greater curvature of the kidney.

Figure 4

The renal pelvis is exposed.

Figure 5

(far right)

The halves of the kidneys are gently held together for 5 to 7 minutes after the vascular clamp is removed.

Indications and procedure

Nephrotomy should be considered the treatment of choice for renal uroliths and for infestation of the kidneys by *Dioctophyma renale*, provided that irreversible renal insufficiency has not developed.[1] Standard approaches to the kidney include flank or ventral abdominal incisions.

In the ventral midline approach, the peritoneal cavity is opened. Laparotomy sponges are used to cover both sides of the incision, and the abdominal cavity is exposed using self-retaining retractors. The kidney is exposed by the application of traction on the abdominal viscera. The peritoneum over the kidney is incised and the kidney is elevated from its retroperitoneal location, then packed-off with the laparotomy sponges. Excessive perirenal fat is removed. The renal artery and vein are separated from the ureter (*Figure 1*).

Before an incision is made into the kidney, a bulldog vascular clamp is applied to the renal artery and vein (*Figure 2*). The incision is made on the greater curvature of the kidney. The size of the incision is determined by the degree of exposure required (*Figures 3 & 4*).

The nephrotomy is closed simply by holding the halves of the incised kidney together with the fingers for five to seven minutes. The halves should be as nearly perfectly aligned as is possible (*Figure 5*). The bulldog clamp is released and the time is noted. Some hemorrhage from the incision may be seen initially (*Figure 6*). In our experience, after the halves of the kidney have been held together for five to seven minutes, hemostasis is usually complete. However, in some cases a small amount of

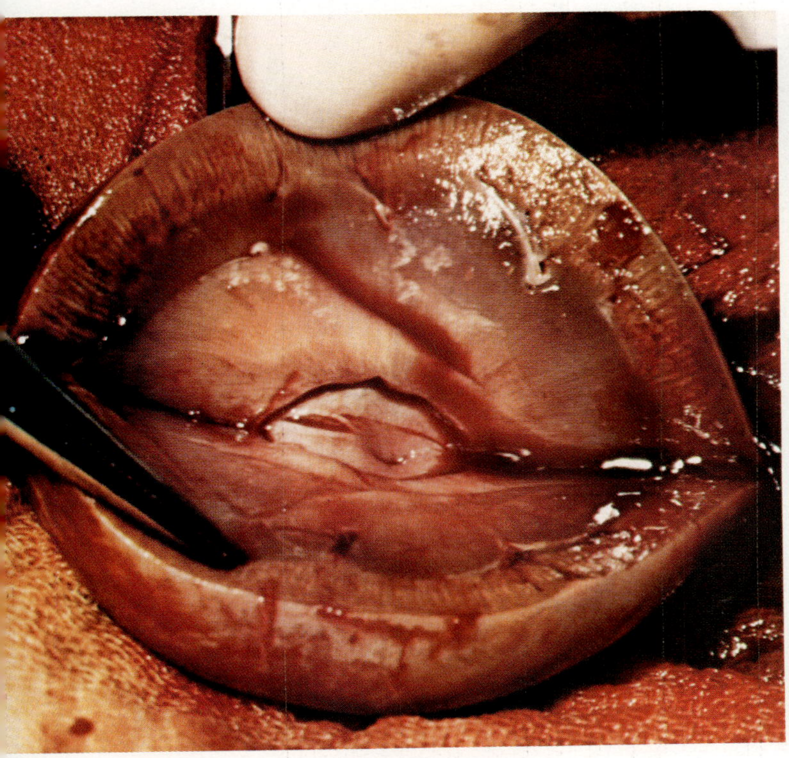

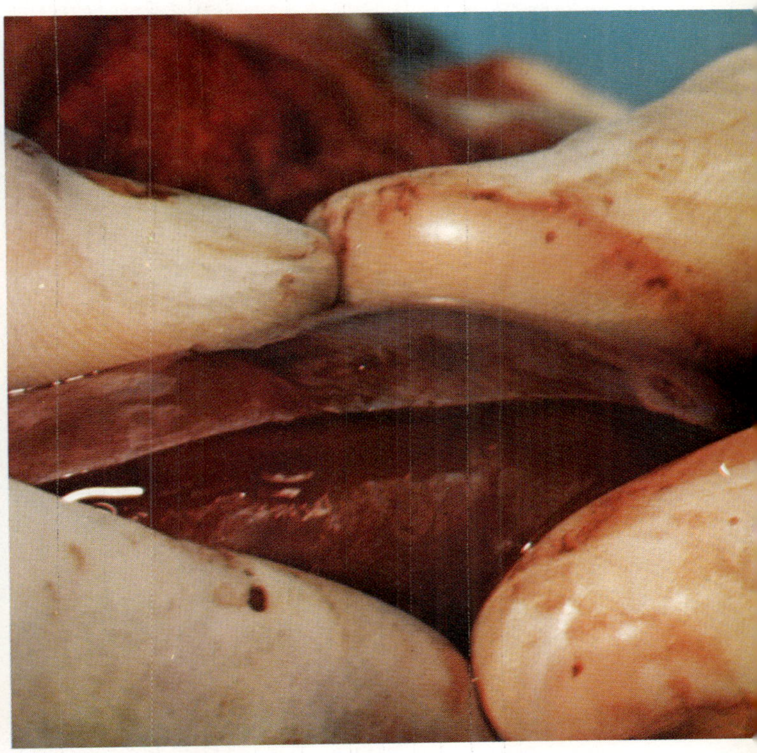

Figure 6—Appearance of the incision after digital compression for five minutes.

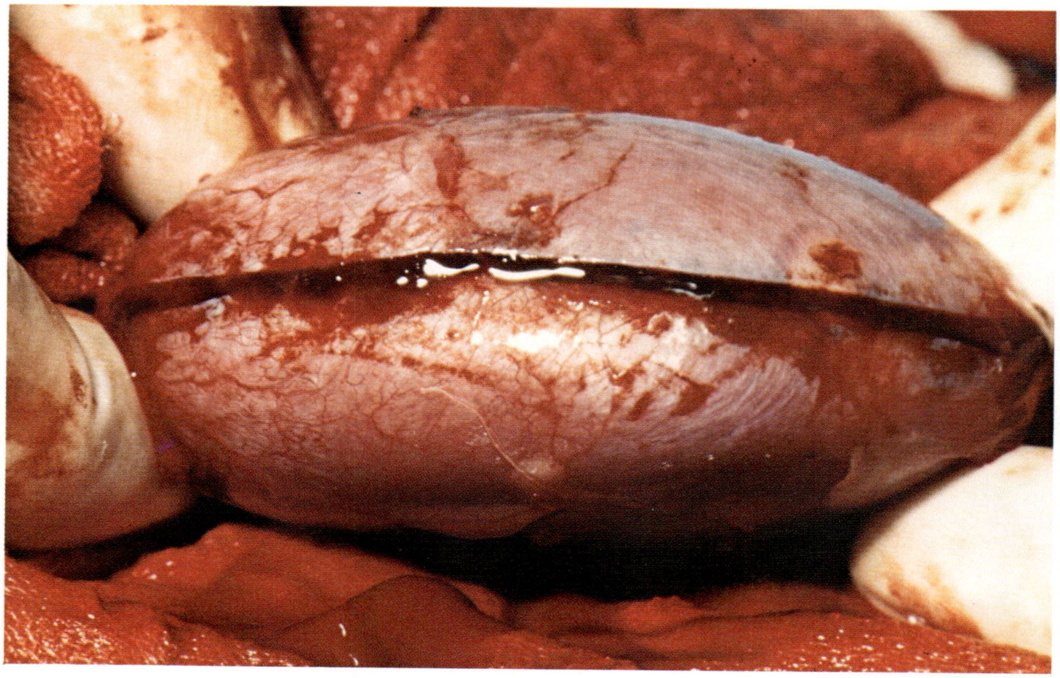

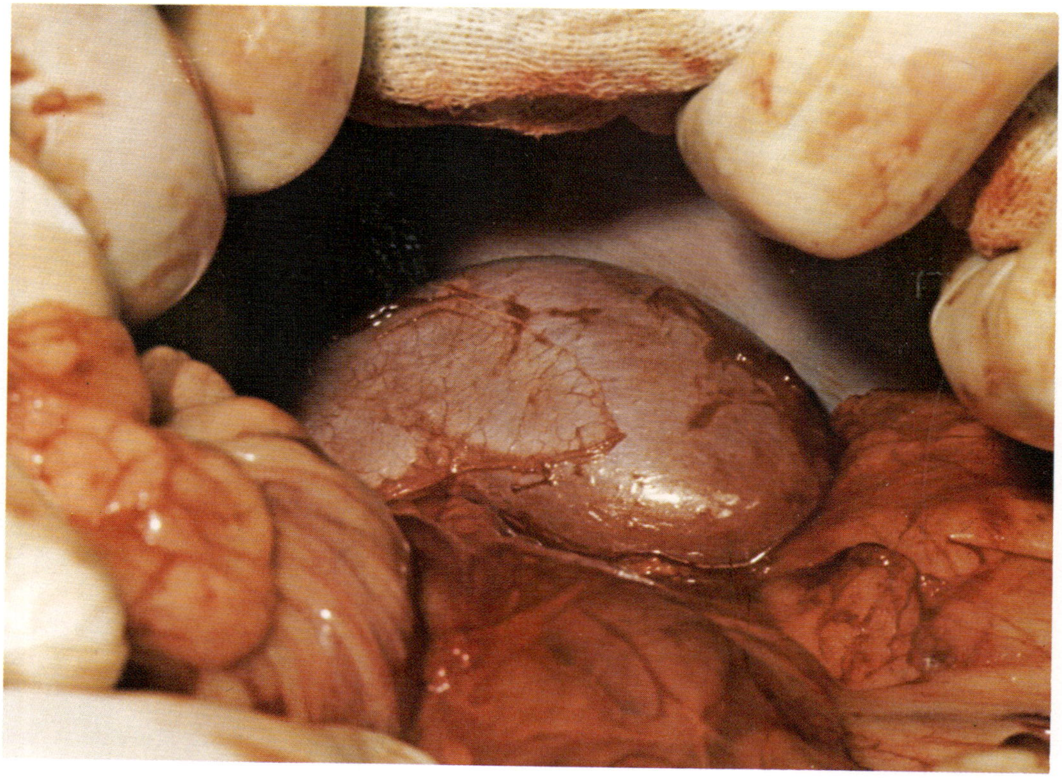

Figure 7—The kidney is returned to the abdominal cavity and observed again for hemorrhage.

bleeding may occur for a few minutes.

At this point digital pressure can be removed. The kidney is then rinsed with warm saline solution. After a final inspection for hemorrhage, the kidney is returned to its normal position (*Figure 7*). The kidney is again inspected for hemorrhage.

The peritoneal cavity is lavaged with warm saline solution. The abdominal and skin incisions are closed routinely.

Discussion

When renal parenchyma is incised, some nephrons are destroyed as a direct result of the incision and indirectly as a result of severed blood vessels.[4] Sutures placed in the renal parenchyma cause further destruction of nephrons and blood vessels. There also exists the possibility of ischemic necrosis from excessive tightness of the sutures. Placement of sutures also leads to permanent reduction of functional renal tissue by subsequent replacement with connective tissue.[5]

Sutureless closure of the nephrotomy has been shown to cause significantly less damage to renal tissue than do closures with sutures.[4] This is especially important in the case of a patient with previously compromised renal function, such as a geriatric animal.

It is especially important to assess the clotting profiles before performing the sutureless nephrotomy.

ACKNOWLEDGMENT

The authors thank Mr. Tom Huffman for photographing the procedure.

REFERENCES

1. Rosin, E.: *Current Techniques in Small Animal Surgery I* (M.J. Bojrab, ed.). Lea & Febiger, Philadelphia, Pa., 1975.
2. Rawlings, C.A.: *Small Animal Surgery: An Atlas of Operative Techniques* (W.E. Wingfield and C.A. Rawlings, eds.). W.B. Saunders, Philadelphia, Pa., 1979.
3. Paramo, P.G. *et al*: Sutureless Nephrotomy. *J. Urology 98*:456-458; Oct. 1967.
4. Gahring, D.R. *et al*: Comparative Renal Function Studies of Nephrotomy Closure With and Without Sutures in Dogs. *JAVMA 171*: 537-541; 1977.
5. Gerlaugh, R.L. *et al*: The Healing of Renal Wounds: II. Surgical Repair of Contusions and Lacerations. *J. Urology 80*:529-534; May 1960.

Small Animal Surgery

NEUROLOGIC

a **RONGEURING TECHNIQUE** for performing thoracolumbar hemilaminectomies

Steven F. Swaim, DVM, MS
Dept. of Small Animal Surgery & Medicine
School of Veterinary Medicine
Auburn University
Auburn, Alabama 36830

A FACTOR that discourages many practitioners from performing spinal surgery (especially hemilaminectomy) is the fear of damaging the spinal cord. Entering the spinal canal by means of trephination entails drilling blindly toward the spinal cord, which can be unnerving if the practitioner is inexperienced and has not developed a feel for using a trephine. A micrometer trephine with a stop has been designed to help prevent over-trephination.[1]

The use of a pneumatic surgical instrument in spinal surgery has been described.[2] As the bone is removed with this instrument, the progress of bone removal can be directly observed. This eliminates guessing as to how close the instrument is to the spinal cord. The technique may be faster, especially for use with large dogs. However, many practitioners do not have pneumatic surgical instruments.

The following is a description of a technique for hemilaminectomy that may help the practitioner who feels uneasy about trephination and who does not have a pneumatic surgical instrument. The technique is best suited to the lumbar vertebrae of smaller-to-medium-sized dogs, but it may also be used on the thoracic vertebrae and in large dogs.

Surgical Procedure

The involved vertebrae are exposed in a routine manner from the tip of the dorsal spinour processes to the heads of the ribs (thoracic vertebrae) or transverse processes (lumbar vertebrae). (*See* Figure 1.)

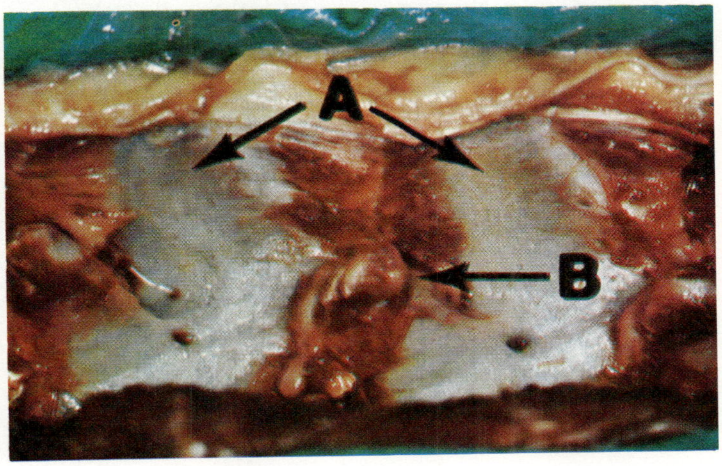

Figure 1—Exposure of L2 and L3 vertebrae. Dorsal spinous processes (A); articular processes (B).

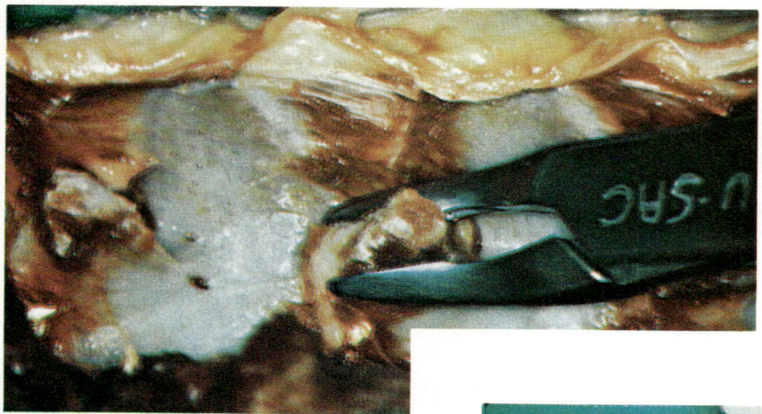

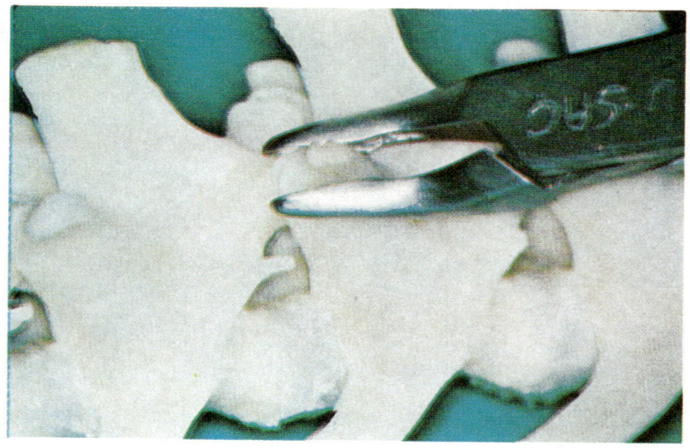

Figures 2A & 2B—The articular processes of L2 and L3 are removed with a rongeur.

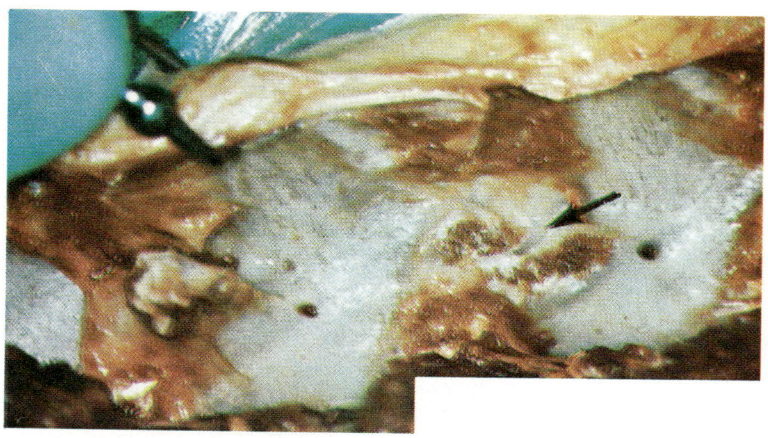

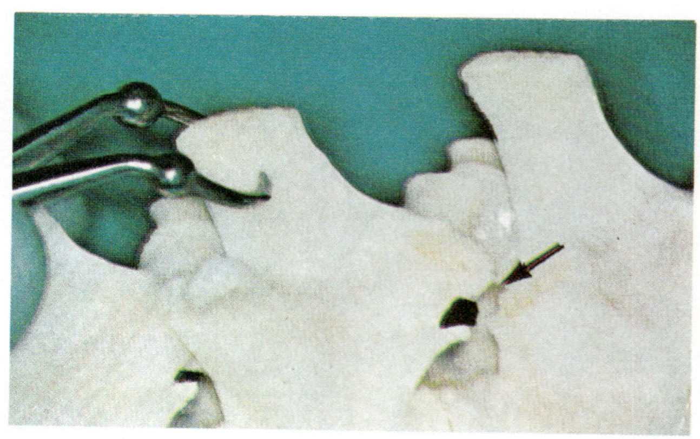

Figures 3A & 3B—A towel forceps is affixed to the dorsal spinous process of L2, applying dorsal traction for opening of the interarcual and articular space (*arrow*).

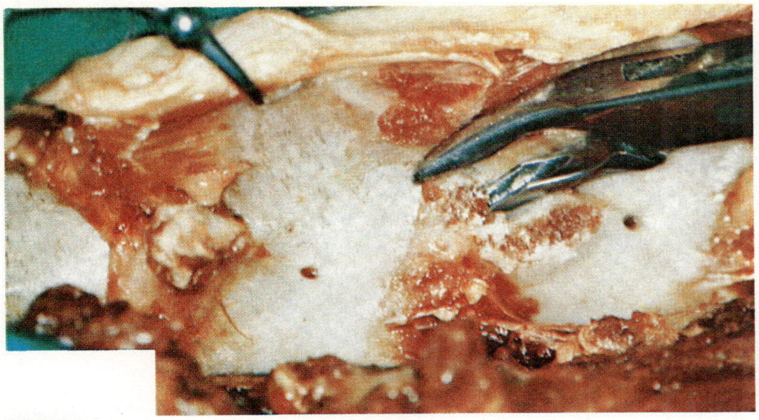

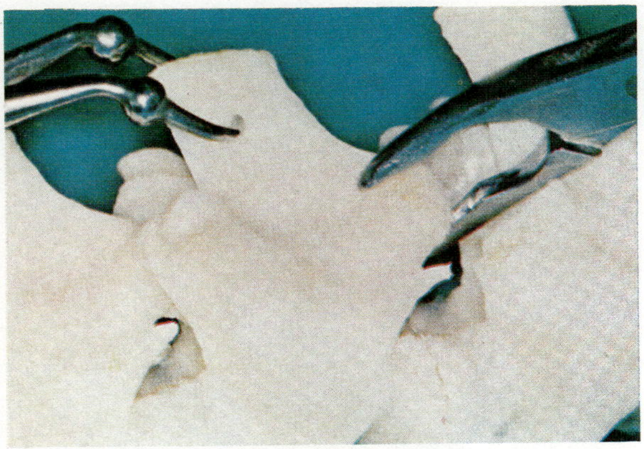

Figures 4A & 4B—One blade of a small rongeur is inserted into the interarcual space between L2 and L3.

A bone rongeur is used to remove the articular processes of the involved vertebrae (*Figures 2A & 2B*). With towel forceps affixed to the dorsal spinous process of the cranial-most involved vertebra, dorsal traction is applied (*Figures 3A & 3B*). By this procedure the interarcual space at the base of the dorsal spinous process is opened sufficiently to allow the introduction of one blade of a small bone rongeur (Lempers Rongeurs—Richards Mfg. Co.). (*See* Figures 4A & 4B).

While dorsal traction is maintained on the cranial-most vertebra, a small amount of bone is removed. This entrance to the spinal canal provides a starting point from which performance of

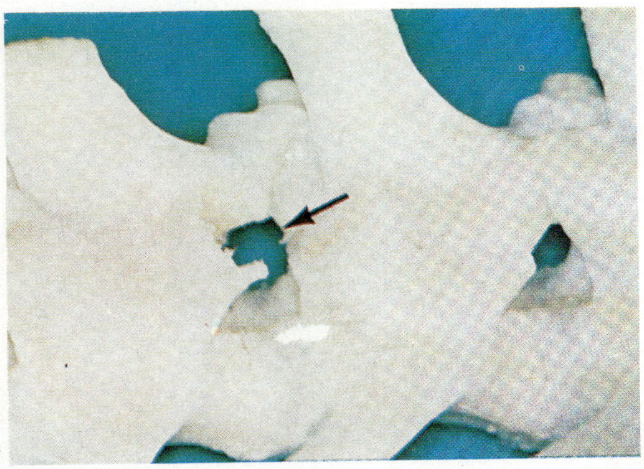

Figures 5A & 5B—A small opening into the spinal canal serves as a starting point for the hemilaminectomy (*arrow*).

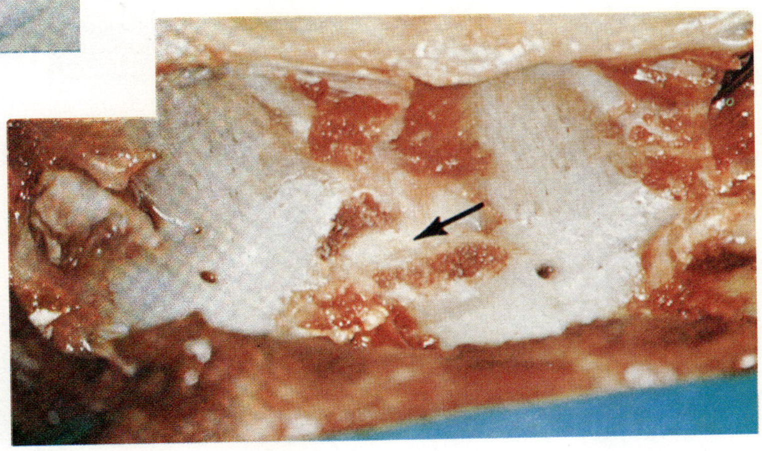

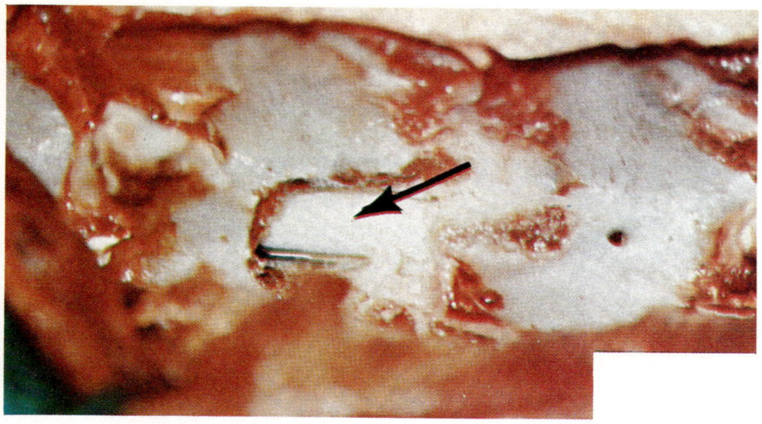

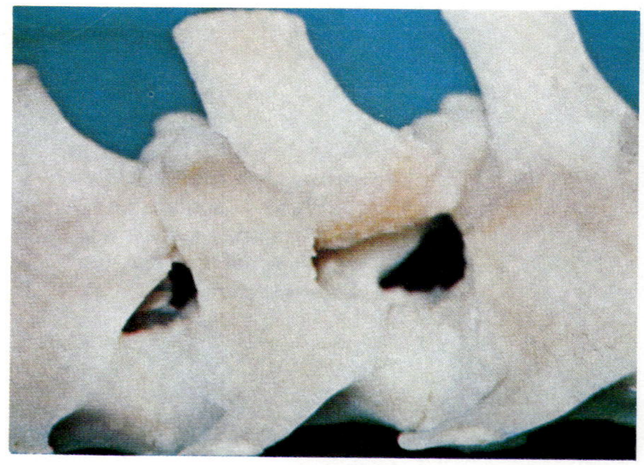

Figures 6A & 6B—The cranial half of the hemilaminectomy has been completed on L2; spinal cord (*arrow*).

the hemilaminectomy can progress (*Figures 5A & 5B*). A small rongeur is then used to remove the bone of the dorsolateral laminae on the cranial-most vertebrae (*Figures 6A & 6B*) and the caudal-most vertebrae (*Figures 7A & 7B*).

REFERENCES

1. Lippincott, C.L.: Use of the Micrometer Trephine in Surgery Treatment of the Intervertebral Disc Syndrome. *VM/SAC 67:* 643-648;1972.
2. Swaim, S.F.: Use of Pneumatic Surgical Instruments in Neurosurgery—Part I: Spinal Surgery. *V/SAC 68*:1275-1280; Nov. 1973.

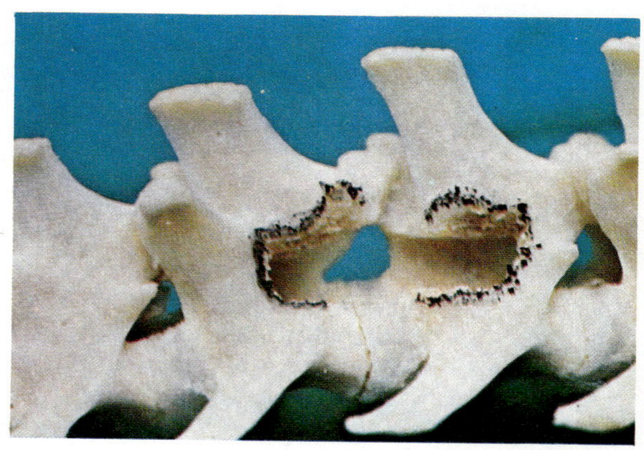

Figures 7A & 7B—The completed hemilaminectomy at L2-L3; spinal cord (*arrow*).

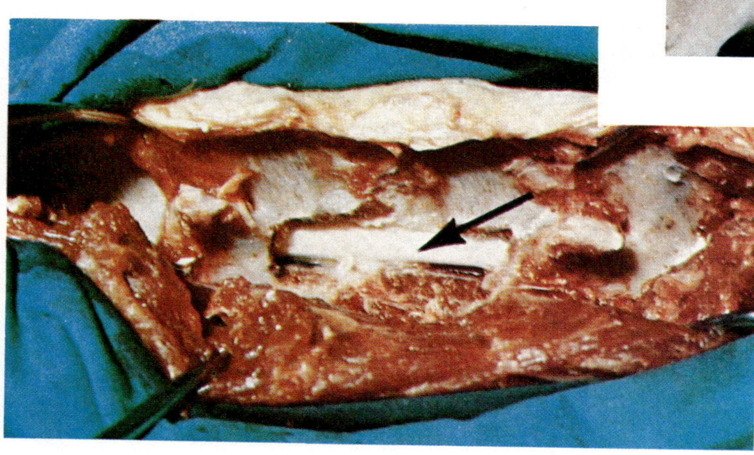

the dorsal approach for CERVICAL LAMINECTOMY in the dog

Vincent W. Chaffee, DVM*
Small Animal Clinics
School of Veterinary Medicine
Purdue University
West Lafayette, Indiana 47907

*Diplomate, American College of Veterinary Surgeons and American College of Laboratory Animal Medicine

CERVICAL LAMINECTOMY is performed in the dog to decompress the spinal cord in an area of intravertebral pressure. In our clinic, it is most commonly used to relieve spinal pressure caused by intervertebral disc extrusion[1] and the structural defects of wobbler syndrome.[2]

Some practitioners avoid the dorsal approach[3] to the cervical region in the dog because of the muscle mass in the area and the possibility of hemorrhage. Complications can usually be avoided by separating the musculature on the exact midline (median raphe),[3] especially through the first superficial muscle layer. If the surgeon deviates from the midline and inadvertently opens the thin muscle bellies of the first superficial muscle layer (platysma, cleidocervicalis, and trapezius), excessive hemorrhage inevitably results.

This thin layer of muscles is richly supplied with branches of the superficial cervical vein and artery.[4] The second superficial muscle layer (rhomboideus, splenius and biventer cervicis) is much thicker. It can be separated on the midline without disruption of the muscle bellies. The nuchal ligament can then be readily exposed and retracted for deeper dissection.

Figures 1-19 illustrate the dorsal approach to a cervical laminectomy. The photographs depict dissection of a live animal.

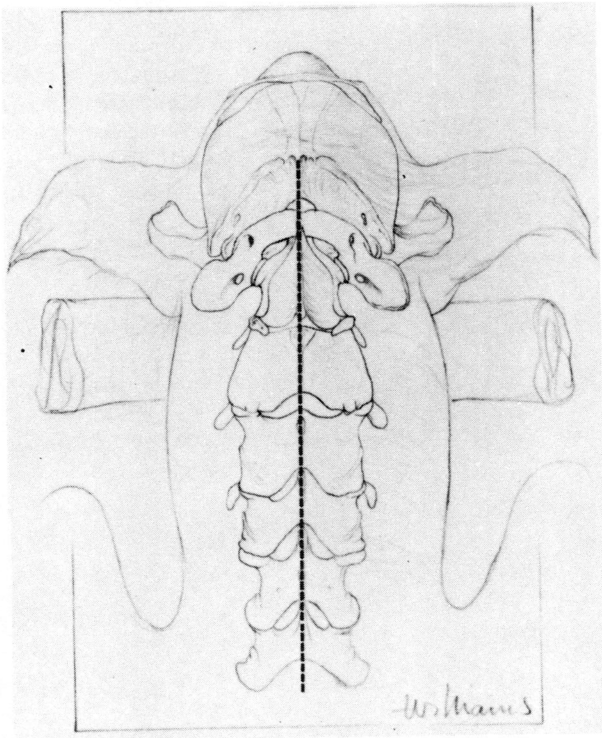

Figure 1—The midline skin incision is started at the occiput and extended to the first thoracic dorsal spine. The dog's nose is at the top.

REFERENCES

1. de Lahunta, A.: Spinal Cord Disease. In *Veterinary Neuroanatomy and Clinical Neurology* (A. de Lahunta, ed.). W.B. Saunders Co., Philadelphia, Pa., 1977; p 192.
2. Dueland, R.: Cervical Spondylolisthesis - Treatment by Fusion and Wiring for Internal Fixation. In *Current Techniques in Small Animal Surgery—I* (M. Bojrab, ed.). Lea & Febiger, Philadelphia, Pa., 1975; p 383.
3. Piermattei, D.L.; Greeley, R.G.: Approach to the Cervical Vertebrae Through a Dorsal Incision. In *An Atlas of Surgical Approaches to the Bones of the Dog and Cat* (Piermattei & Greeley, eds.). W.B. Saunders Co., Philadelphia, Pa.; p 24.
4. Miller, M.E.: The Heart and Arteries. In *Anatomy of the Dog* (M.E. Miller, ed.). W.B. Saunders Co., Philadelphia, Pa., 1964; p 320.

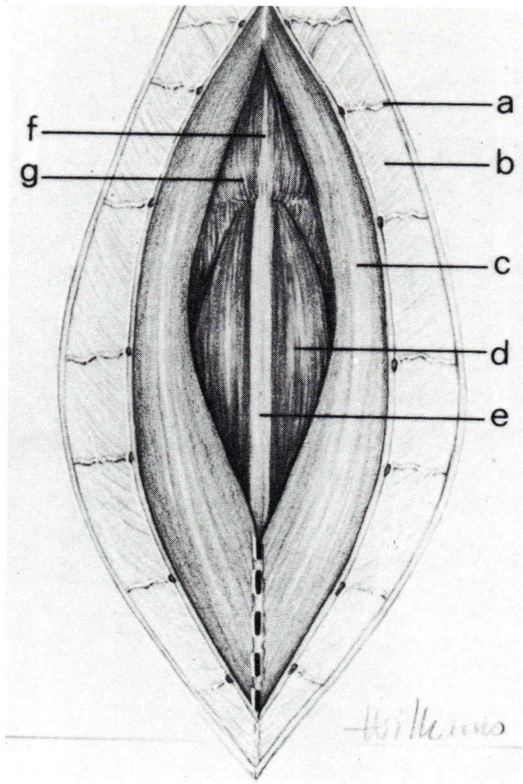

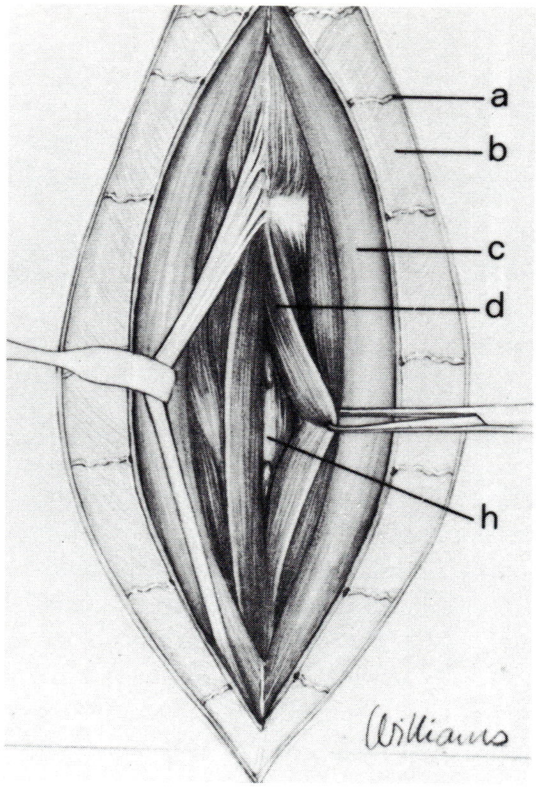

Figure 2—Identification of musculature after the incision on the medial raphe has separated the muscles to the depth of the nuchal ligament: a) cutaneous branch of C_2 spinal nerve; b) thin first superficial muscle layer (platysma overlying the cleidocervicalis and trapezius); c) thick second superficial layer (rhomboideus, splenius, and biventer cervicis); d) deep paired ribbon muscles that sandwich the dorsal cervical spines (spinalis cervicis bordered by multifidus) and lie below the nuchal ligament; e) nuchal ligament; f)dorsal spine of C_2; g) rectur capitis dorsalis major, which covers C_2.

Figure 3(*above*)—The nuchal ligament is retracted. Deep dissection between the ribbon muscles and their retraction (d) exposes the dorsal arch of a cervical vertebra (h).

Figure 6—The skin incision has been completed. The hemostat is on the dorsal spine of C_2. The platysma muscle, which overlies the cleidocervicalis and trapezius, can be seen. The cutaneous branches of segmental cervical nerves approach the median raphe from each side.

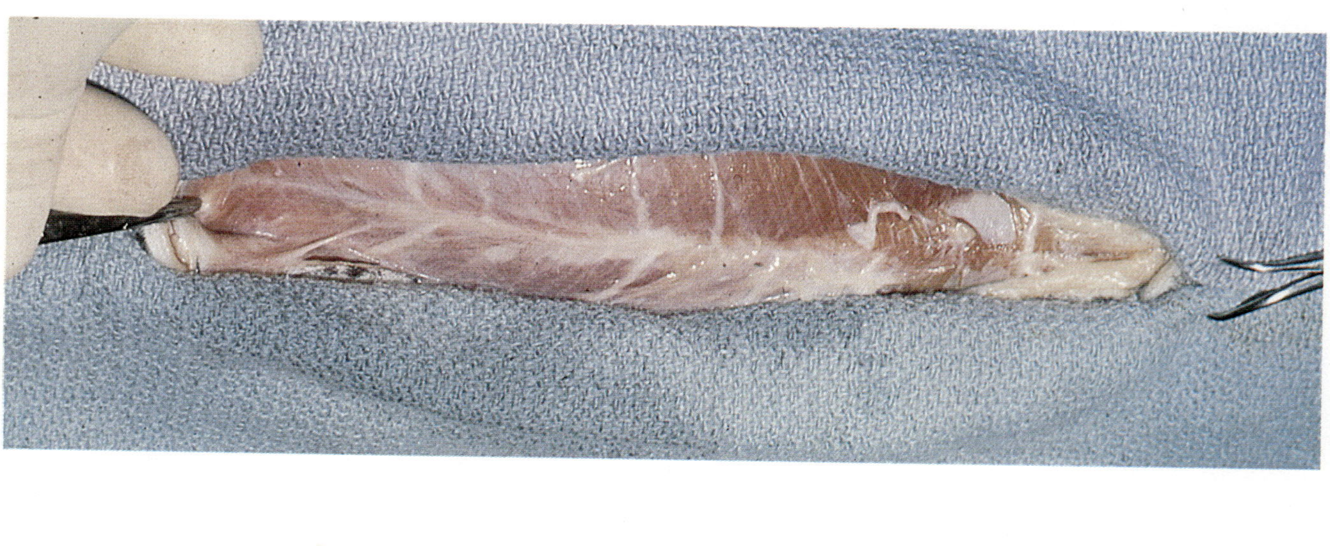

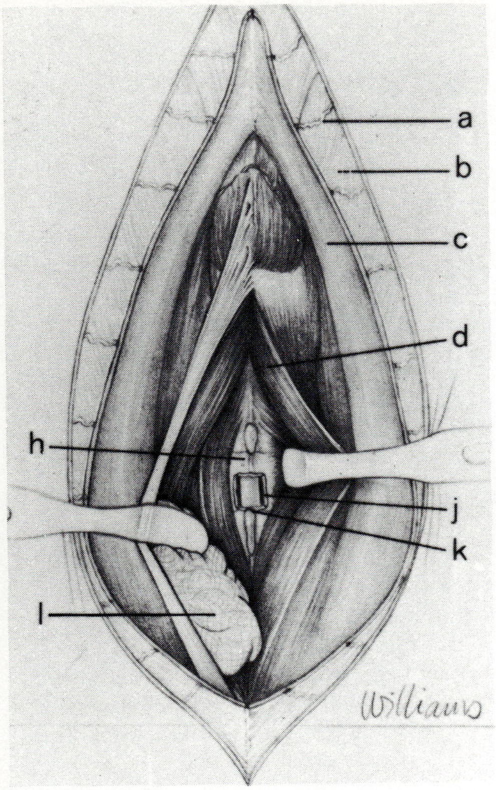

Figure 4—The nuchal ligament and deep ribbon muscles d) are retracted and the small muscle fibers cleared from the dorsal arch of the cervical vertebra for laminectomy; h) dorsal arch of the cervical vertebra; j) site of laminectomy (spinal cord is exposed); k) position of interarcuate ligament cranial to each dorsal spine; l) sponge.

Figure 5—Site of the skin incision. The dog's nose is to the right side on all succeeding photos.

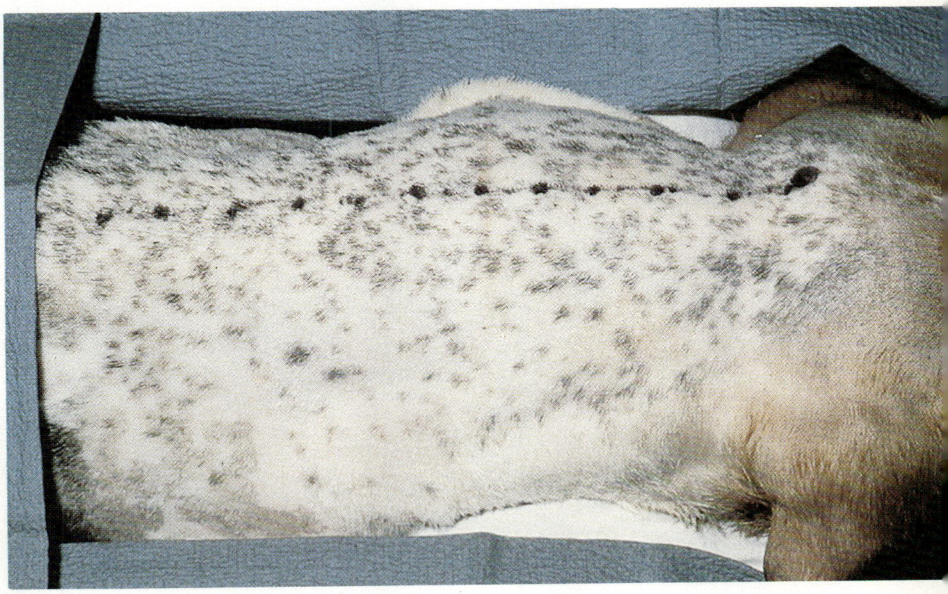

Figure 7—A scalpel incision exposes the thin first superficial muscle layer (platysma overlying the cleidocervicalis and trapezius). The point of the scalpel blade is directly in the center of this layer. When muscle bellies are cut, as often happens, hemorrhage should be controlled. The thick second superficial muscle layer (rhomboideus, splenius and biventer cervicis) can be seen just below the incised muscle bellies of the first superficial layer. The second superficial muscle layer is easily divided on the midline.

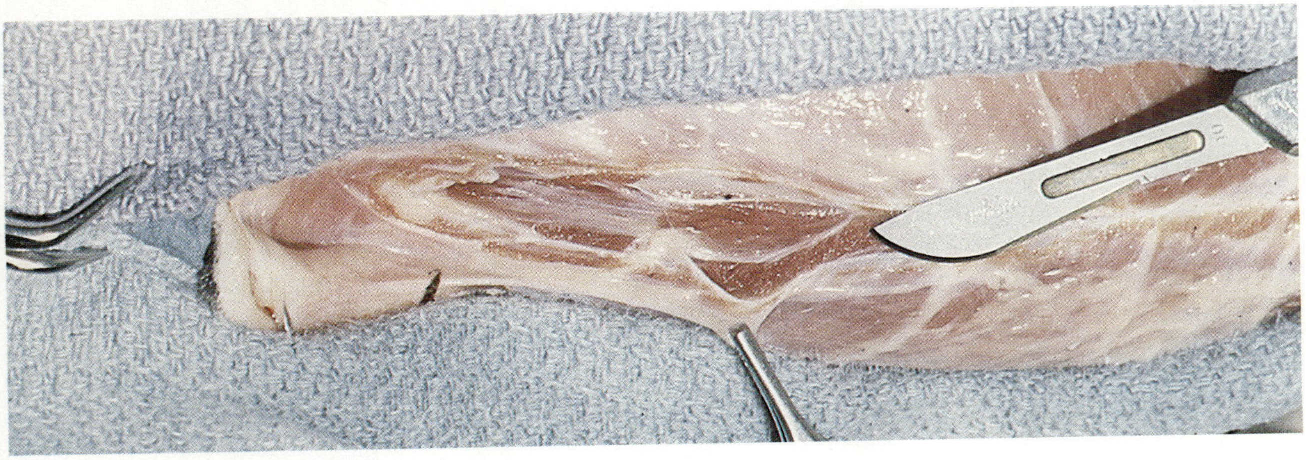

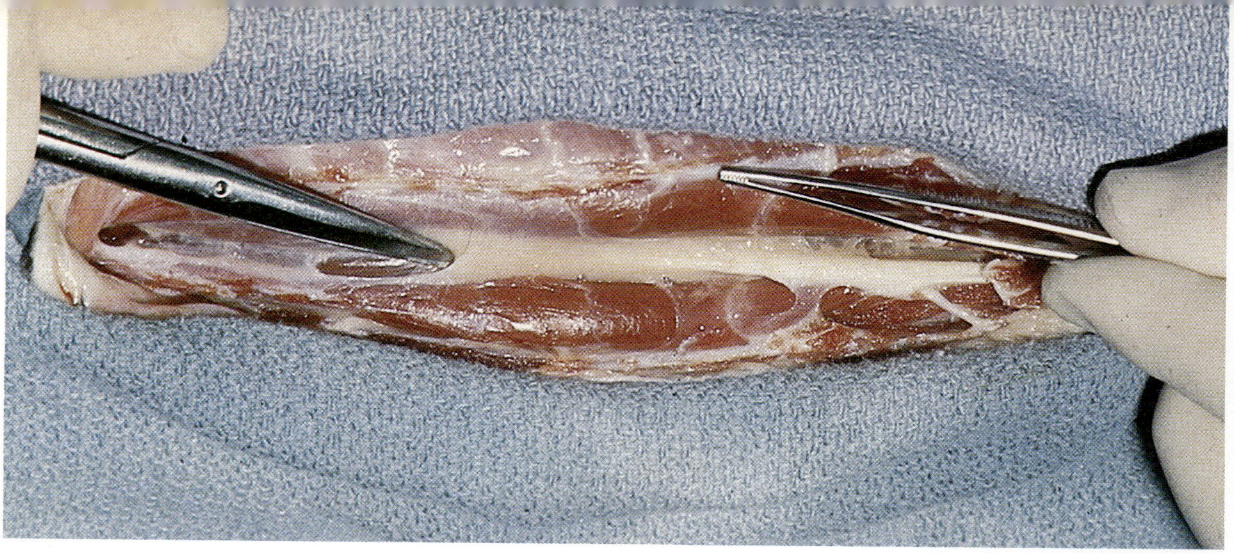

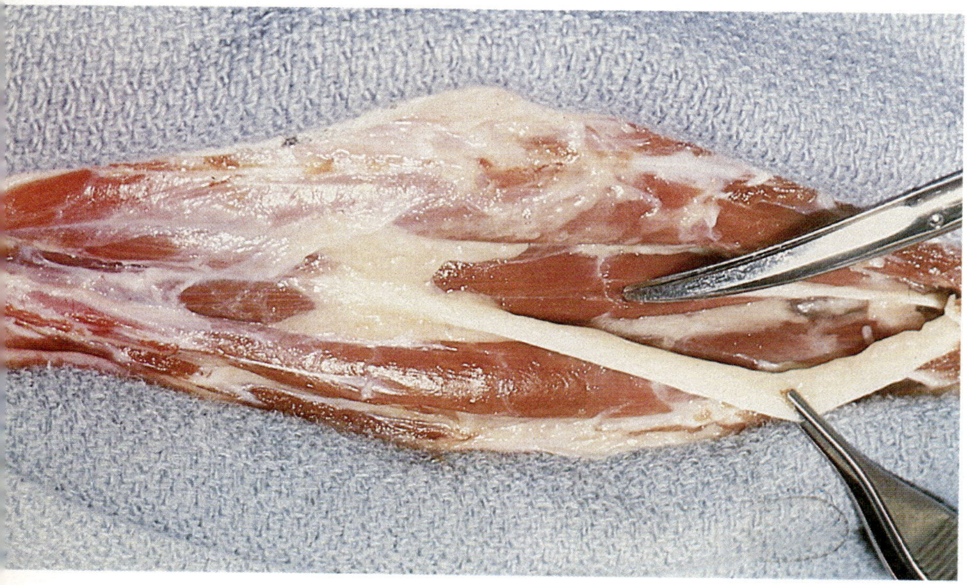

Figure 8—The initial scalpel incision is extended with scissors to the depth of the nuchal ligament. The scissors rest on the dorsal spine of C_2. The thumb forceps rest on the thin first superficial muscle layer which can be very hemorrhagic. The second superficial muscle layer can be seen between the nuchal ligament and first superficial muscle layer.

Figure 9—The anatomy in this photo corresponds to that shown in Figure 2. The scissors rest on the midline of the paired deep ribbon muscles (the spinalis cervicis bordered by the multifidus). The first and second superficial muscle layers are seen above the nuchal ligament.

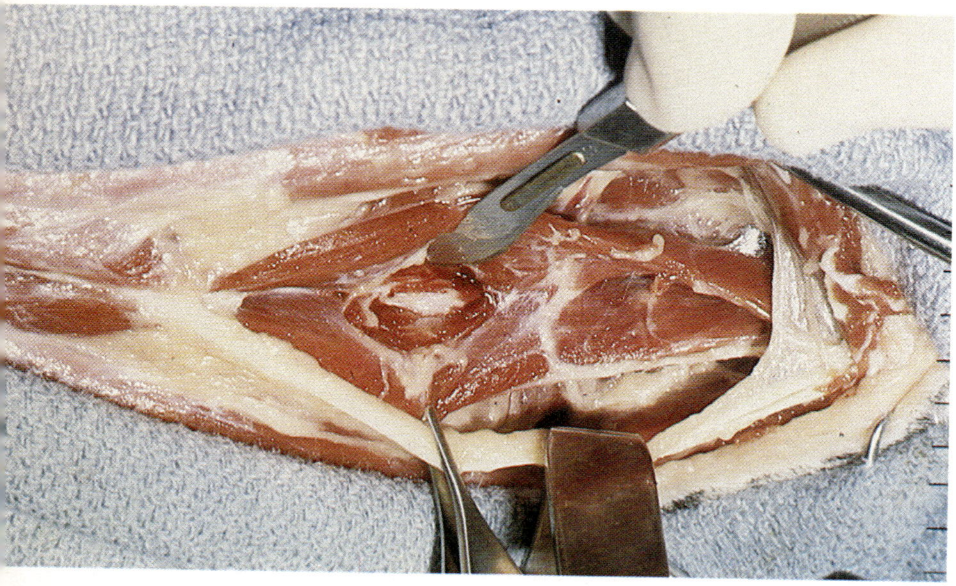

Figure 10—The dorsal spines of the cervical vertebrae can be palpated on the midline. The deep paired ribbon muscles are then retracted, and the short muscle tendons severed from the dorsal spines by sharp dissection. The rectus capitis dorsalis major, overlying C_2, can be seen to the right end of the nuchal ligament.

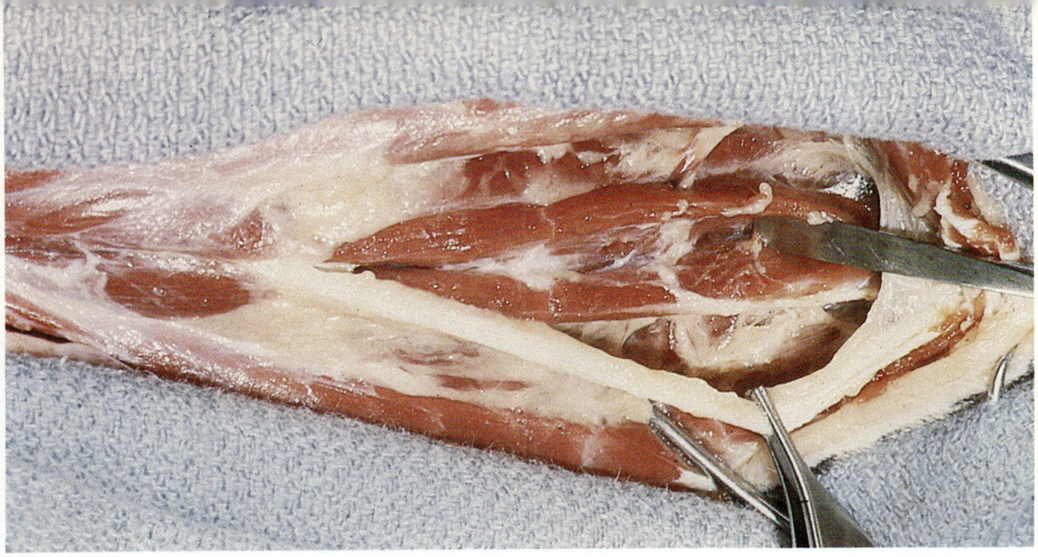

Figure 11—A periosteal elevator is used to clear attached muscle fibers from the dorsal arch of the cervical vertebrae, between the dorsal spines.

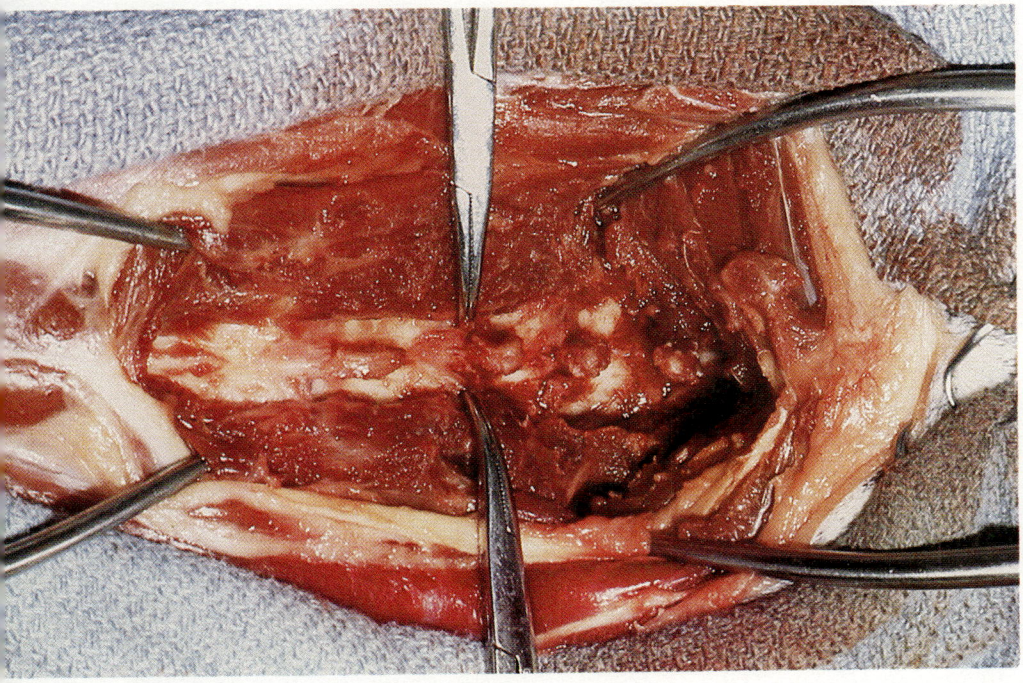

Figure 12—The dorsal portion of the cervical vertebrae is cleared to locate the appropriate interarcuate ligament (between the hemostats). The ligament is just cranial to the dorsal spine of the appropriate cervical vertebra.

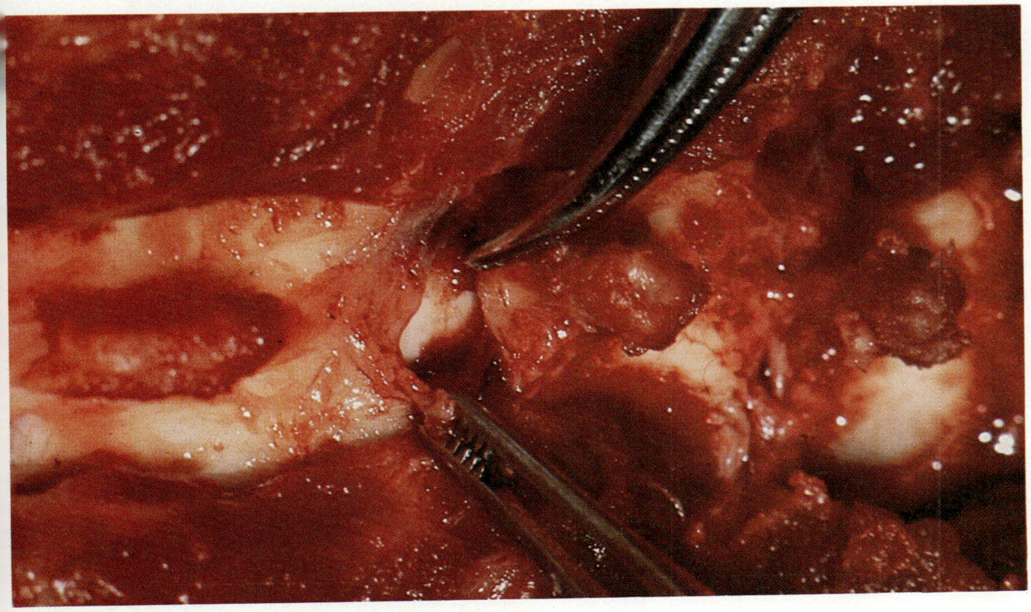

Figure 13—The interarcuate ligament is carefully severed with a No. 15 scalpel blade to expose the underlying spinal cord. Often the spinal cord is immediately next to the interarcuate ligament.

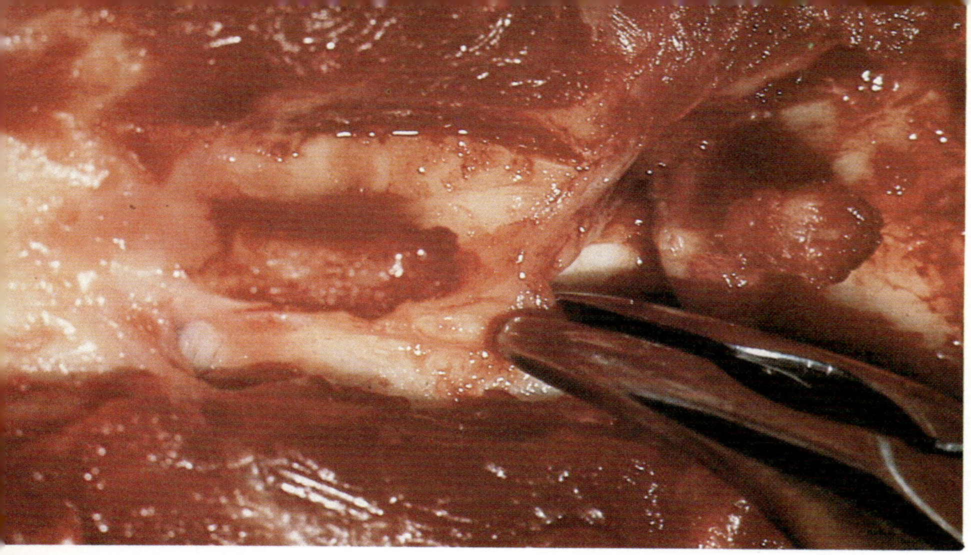

Figure 14
A bone rongeur of appropriate size is used to remove as much of the dorsal vertebral arch as necessary to decompress the bulging spinal cord.

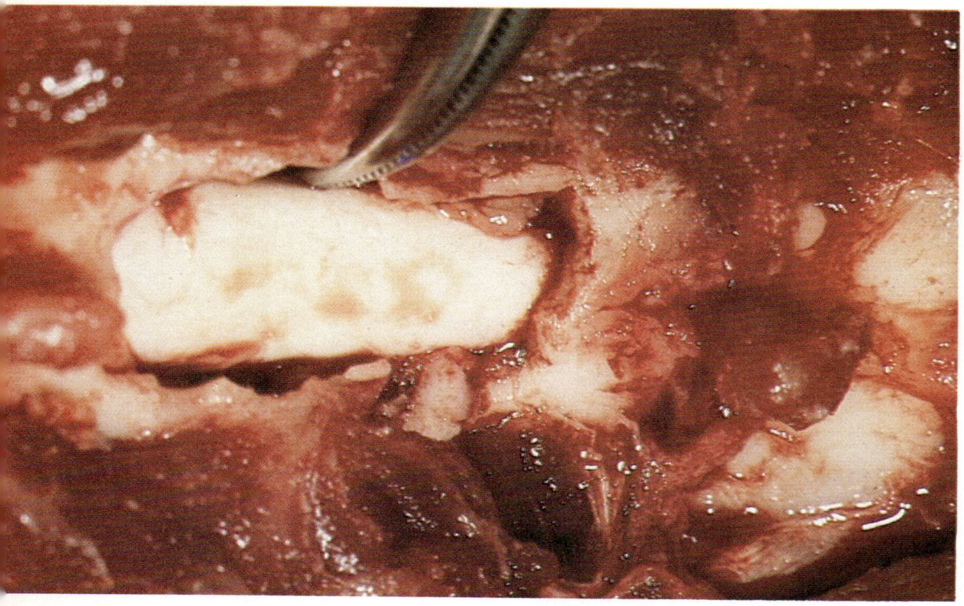

Figure 15
Because the articular facets are left intact, at least two dorsal vertebral arches can be removed without causing instability. In this case, one and one-half vertebral arches have been removed. The hemostat rests in the position of the removed dorsal spine.

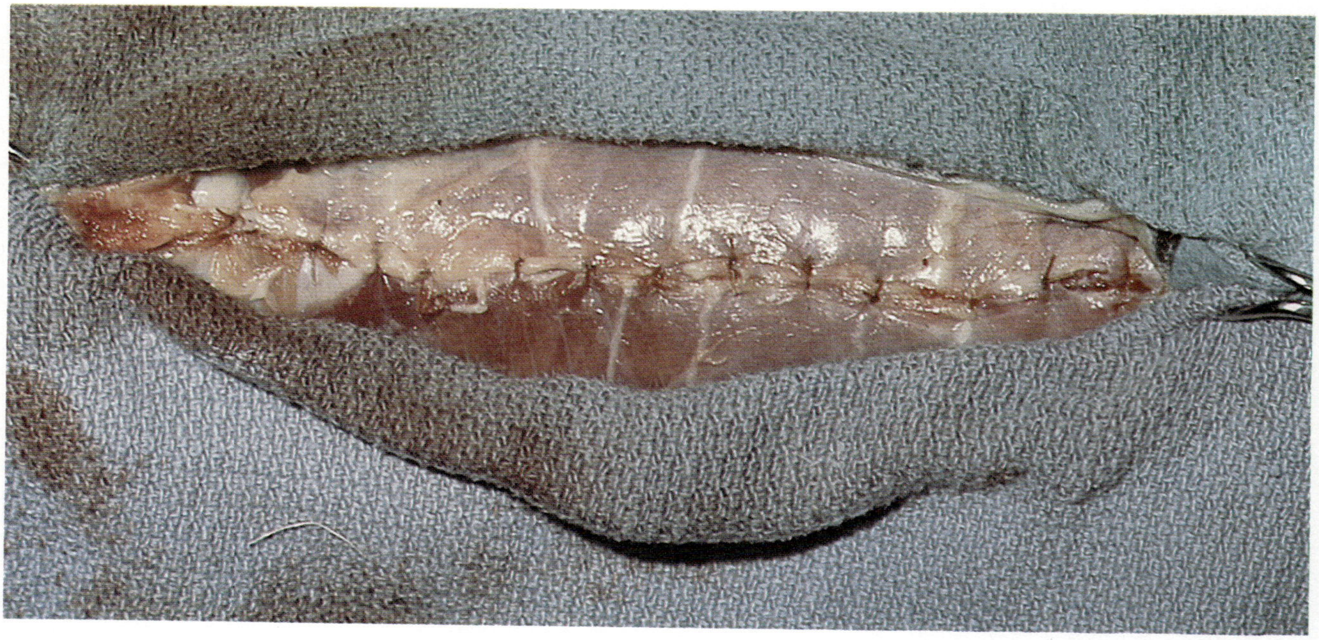

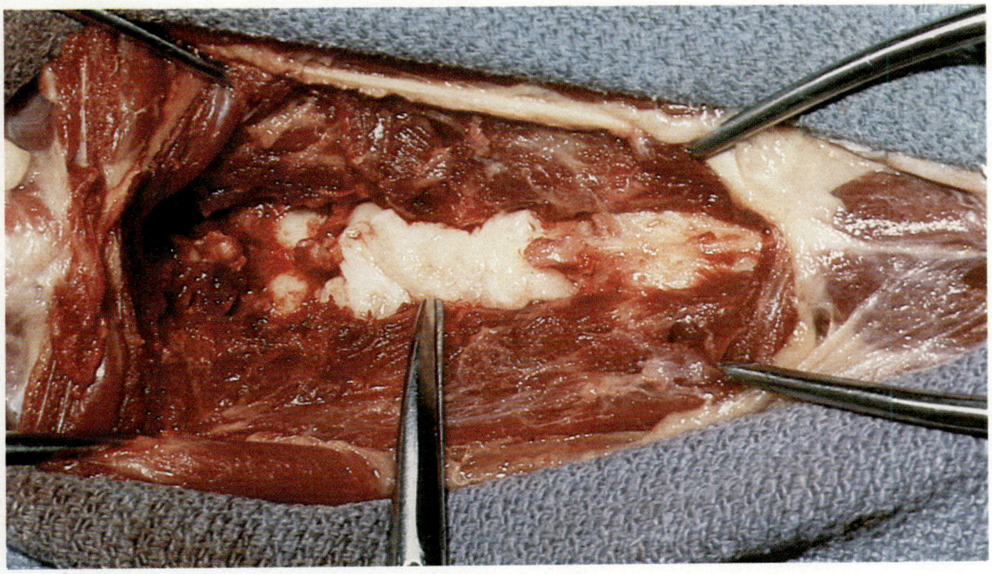

Figure 16
To prevent formation of scars on the dura mater, a fat transplant is used to cover the laminectomy site.

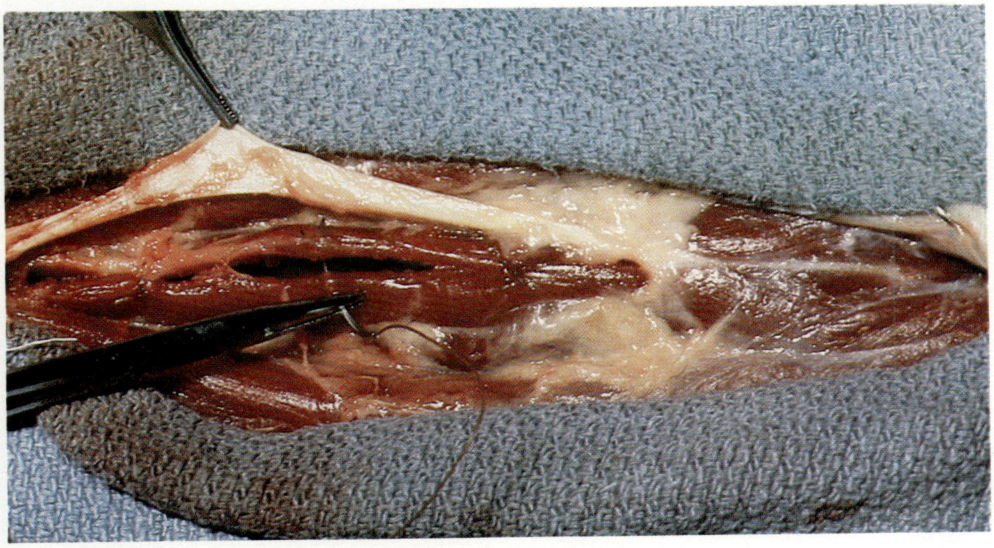

Figure 17
The deep pair of ribbon muscles are apposed with a few chromic sutures in an interrupted pattern.

Figure 18 (*left*)—The fascial layers of the first and second superficial muscle layers are apposed with chromic catgut in a single interrupted pattern.

Figure 19 (*right*)—Closure of the subcutaneous tissue and skin is routine.

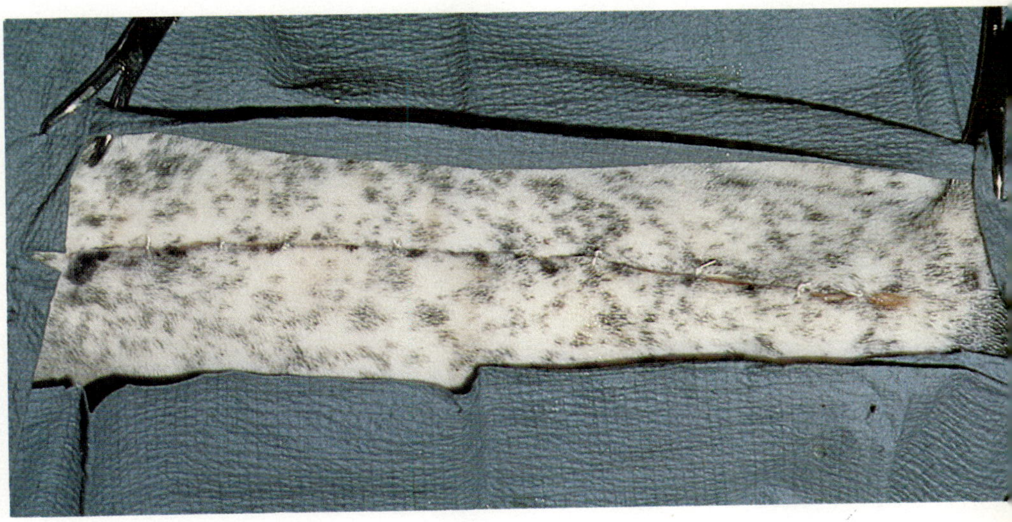

Small Animal Surgery

ORTHOPEDIC

Surgical correction of avulsion of the origin of the long digital extensor muscle in the dog (a case report)

Marvin L. Olmstead, DVM, MS
Hugh C. Butler, DVM, MS
Department of Surgery and Medicine
College of Veterinary Medicine
Kansas State University
Manhattan, Kansas 66506

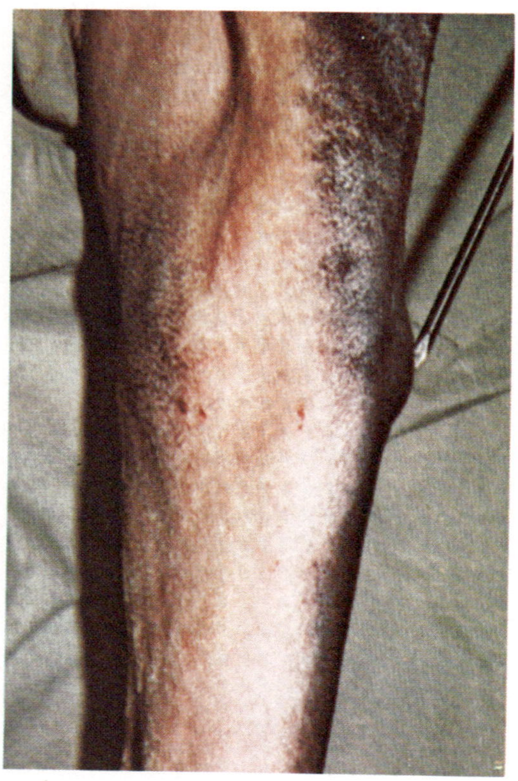

Figure 1—The intramedullary pin indicates the ovoid mass in the stifle joint.

ALTHOUGH most canine lameness related to pathology of the stifle joint involved rupture of the anterior cruciate ligament, arthritis or luxations of the patella, this is not always the case. Presented here is a case where the lameness resulted from an avulsion fracture of the origin of the long digital extensor muscle. The method by which this condition was corrected is described.

Case History

A 45-pound (20.25 kg), 5½-month-old female Doberman Pinscher was presented to Dykstra Veterinary Hospital. The owner noted that an intermittent lameness in the left hind leg had been

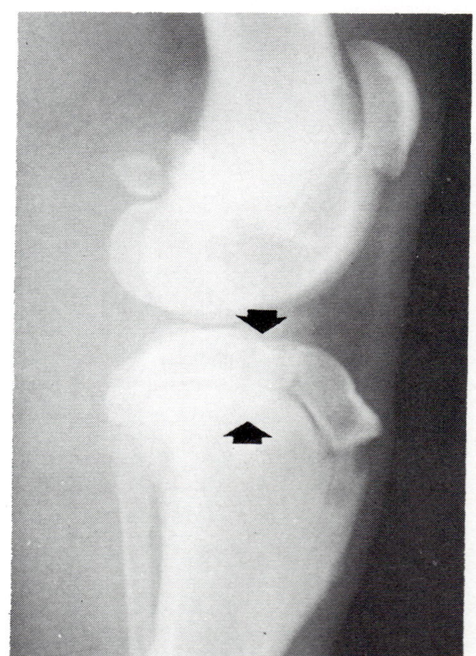

Figure 2—A lateral radiographic view. Arrows indicate the height of the calcified portion of the mass.

present for 11 days. There was no history of known trauma. While the dog would occasionally hold the leg up when walking, the lameness became quite pronounced on exercise.

Physical examination revealed no abnormalities other than those associated with the left stifle joint. Palpation of the left stifle joint revealed a 1.5-cm ovoid mass which seemed to have an elastic attachment distally. The mass could be pushed dorsally but when pressure was released it would return to its position along the lateral side of the tibial crest (*Figure 1*).

Radiographs of the left stifle joint were taken in the following views: anterior to posterior (AP), lateral to medial (FM), and posterior to anterolateral to medial oblique (PALMO). In the LM and PALMO views the mass appeared as a crescent-shaped calcified structure lateral to the tibial tuberosity (*Figures 2 & 3*). The tentative diagnosis of avulsion of the origin of the long digital extensor muscle was made.

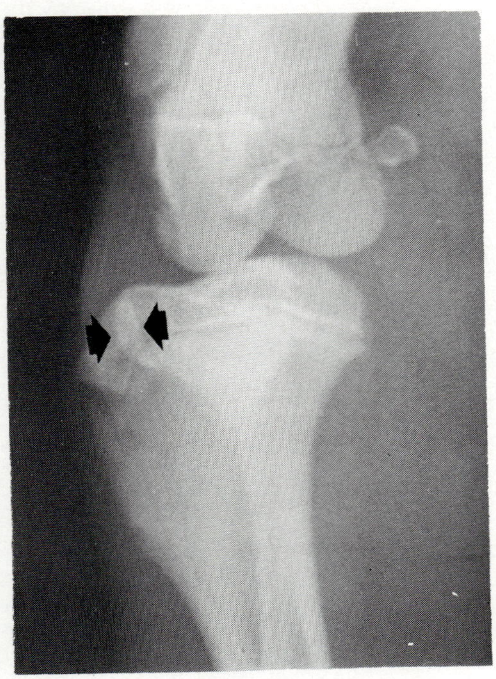

Figure 3—A posterior to anterolateral to medial oblique view. Arrows indicate the width of the calcified portion of the mass.

Surgical Procedure

The dog was anesthetized with inhalant anesthetic and the left stifle joint prepared for surgery. A lateral incision was made over the stifle joint just caudal to the straight patellar ligament from the distal one-third of the femur to a point just below the tibial crest.

An arthrotomy incision was made 1 cm caudal to and parallel with the straight patellar tendon. This exposed a roughened depression along the lateral condyle, as well as the ovoid mass of cartilage and bone to which the long digital extensor

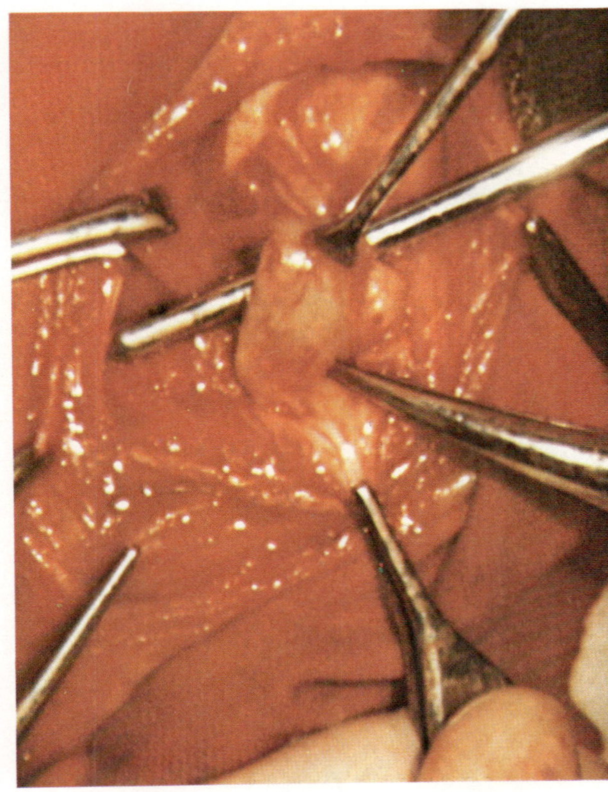

Figure 4—The tip of the Mayo scissors touches the mass of bone and cartilage. The original site of the mass is situated directly under the Allis tissue forceps grasping the mass.

tendon of origin attached along its ventral border (*Figure 4*). The small chip of bone and cartilage was severed from its tendinour attachment.

No further abnormalities were noted in the joint. Closure was carried out in a routine manner.

By histopathologic examination the external surface of the chip was found to be cartilaginous and the center to be made up of bone. The structure appeard to be viable.

Postoperative Course

The progress of this dog was followed for nine months. During that period no recurrences of the preoperative lameness were reported and the only abnormality noted in the dog's gait was a slight tendency to rotate the leg outward when walking.

Discussion

During the course of surgery consideration was given to lagging the bone chip to its original site; however, this idea was rejected for several reasons. Since the object seen radiographically was a small crescent-shaped calfified bone chip and the structure which was seen at the surgical site was larger and more ovoid, it was felt that most of this structure was made up of cartilagenous material rather than bone. This would decrease the ability of the structure to hold a screw.

The structure would be further weakened by the debridement necessary to achieve a freshened edge that would result in proper healing.

The traume that would result from creating a bed in the femur could not be justified in view of the minimal benefits that would be gained from reattaching the long digital extensor at its original site.

It was felt that by removing the bone chip, normal locomotion would result and the patient would be exposed to minimal trauma and anesthetic time. The results were quite satisfactory in the opinion of the authors and the owner.

medial approach to bone plating in REPAIR OF HUMERAL-SHAFT FRACTURES

Ira M. Zaslow, AB, DVM
Paula L. Hanssen, MT
Morrisey Animal Hospital, Inc.
255 Freeport Street
Dorchester, Massachusetts 02122

IN REPAIRING fractures of the humeral shaft during the past few years we have routinely applied the neutralization or compression plate to the medial surface of the bone. The medial approach affords greater exposure of the bone, is easier and thus less time-consuming than the more commonly employed lateral approach. The configuration of the canine humerous makes the medial surface ideal for application of a plate. In all of our cases, some followed for as long as three years, normal function of the leg has been restored without postoperative complications.

Case History

On May 28, 1974, a male Irish Setter weighing 48 lb (21.6 kg) was presented because of severe lameness of the left foreleg. The owner reported that the dog had disappeared for two days and was lame when it returned.

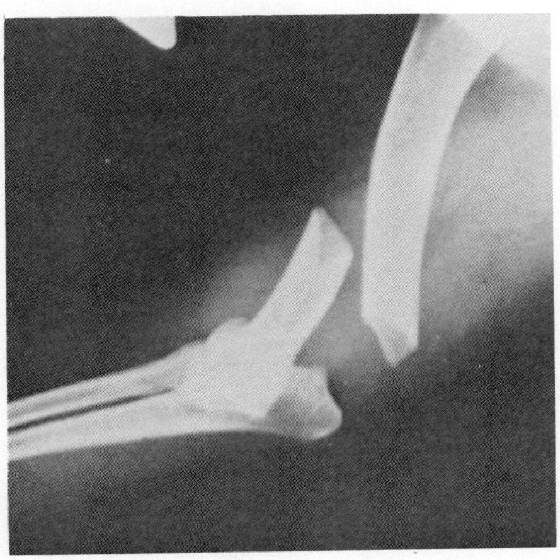

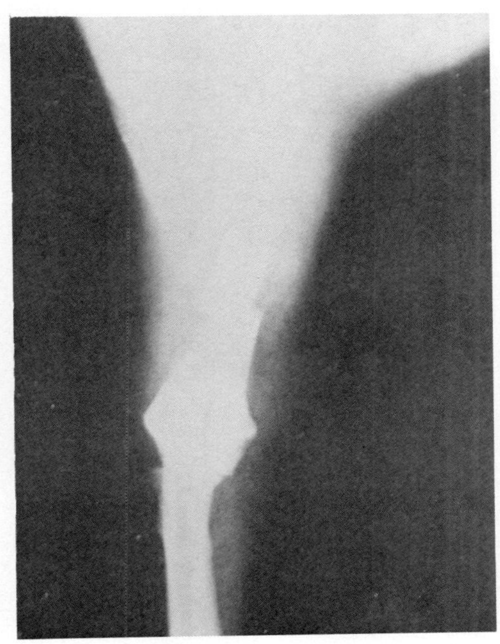

Figure 1A & 1B—Lateral and anteroposterior radiographs showing an oblique fracture at the distal one-third of the humerus.

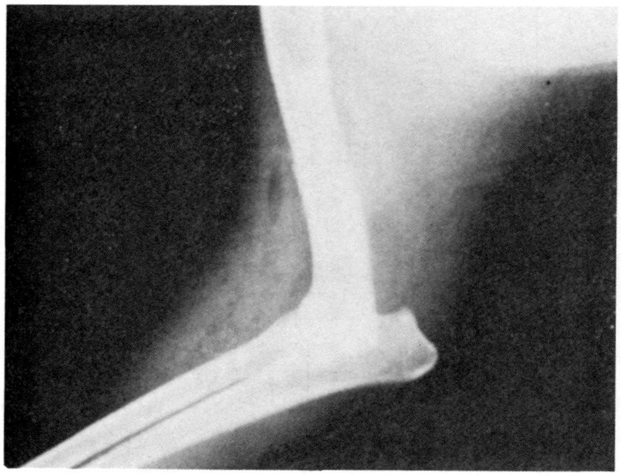

Figure 2—Lateral radiograph taken after application of the compression plate to the medial surface of the humerus. *(See Figure 1A.)*

Figure 3A—Medial aspect of the humerus. The skin incision for the medial approach is started at the proximal two-thirds point on the humerus and extended distally to the medial epicondyle. The biceps muscle is reflected cranially, and the medial head of the triceps muscle and associated vessels and nerves are reflected caudally.

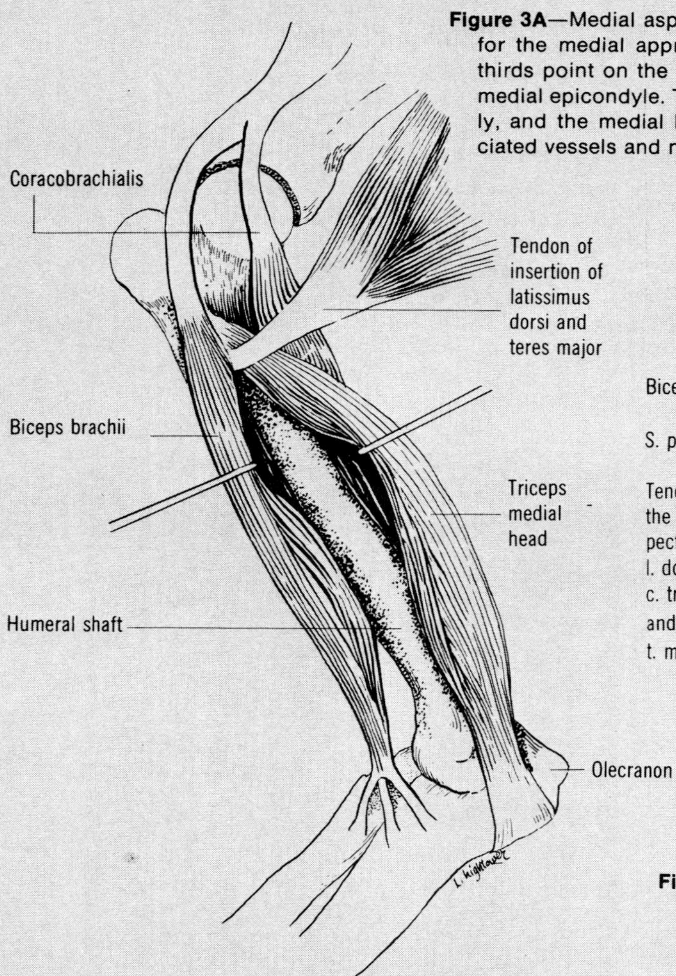

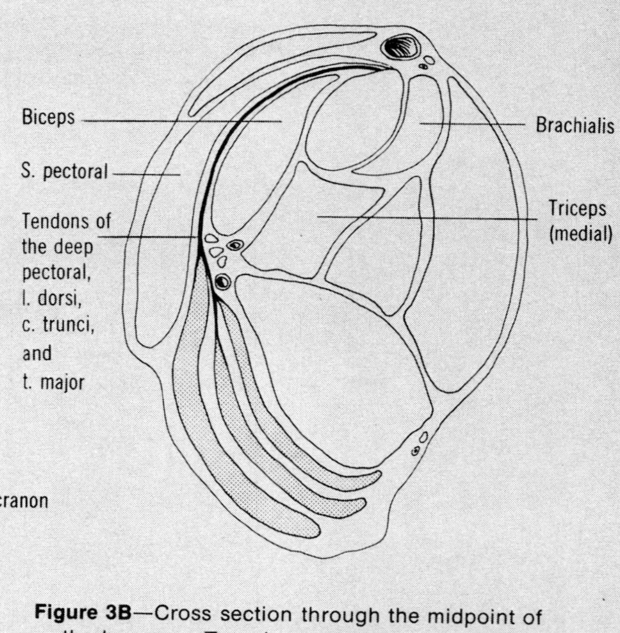

Figure 3B—Cross section through the midpoint of the humerus. To gain access to the upper one-third of the humerus, the tendons of insertion of the teres major, latissimus dorsi, cutaneous trunci, and superficial and deep pectoral muscles are reflected proximally.

The dog was bright and alert and all vital signs were within normal limits. The affected leg was swollen and tender. Blood was drawn for hematologic examination and analysis of blood chemistry. Radiographs showed an oblique fracture at the distal one-third of the humeroud (*Figures 1A & 1B*).

The day after presentation the dog was prepared routinely for surgery. Anesthesia was induced with Surital® (Parke-Davis) and maintained with Fluothane® (Ayerst) administered via a bird® small animal anesthesia machine.

The dog was laid on a circulating hot-water blanket (Gorman-Rupp Industries) and its body temperature was monitored with a battery-powered rectal thermometer (Tele-Thermometer—Yellow Springs Instrument Co.). Arterial and venous blood samples were drawn before, during, and after surgery. Blood gases were closely monitored. During surgery and for a short time thereafter, lactated Ringer's solution was given via the cephalic vein. Crystalline penicillin was introduced at the fracture site.

The fracture was exposed using the medial approach (description of procedure follows), and a narrow, four-hole compression plate (Synthes) was applied (*Figure 2*). No external fixation was employed. Recovery was uneventful.

This patient has been followed with periodic physical and radiologic examinations for two years. Function of the leg is normal and the dog appears healthy in all respects.

The Medial Approach

A skin incision is started at the proximal two-thirds point of the humerus and extended distally to the level of the epicondyle, paralleling the cranial border of the humerus. After the skin and subcutaneous tissues have been freed, skin towels are affixed with Michel clamps.

The brachial artery and vein, their branches, and the median and ulnar nerves are identified. This entire group is reflected caudally with the medial head of the triceps muscle. The biceps muscle is reflected cranially, to complete the exposure of the middle and distal parts of the humeral shaft.

To gain additional exposure, the tendons of insertion of the teres major, latissimus dorsi, cutaneous trunci, and superficial and deep pectoral muscles are reflected proximally (*Figures 3A & 3B*).

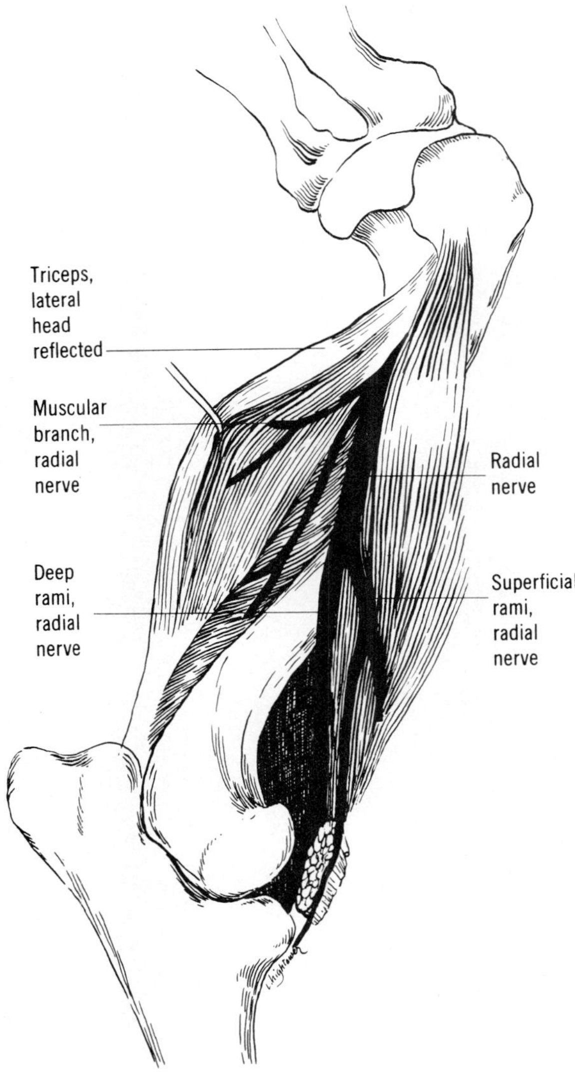

Figure 4—Lateral aspect. In the lateral approach, the lateral head of the triceps muscle is reflected to expose the radial nerve and its branches and rami. Excess stress when the muscles surrounding the radial nerve are retracted can damage the nerve. The superficial and deep rami of the radial nerve must be identified and carefully protected at the distal end of the incision.

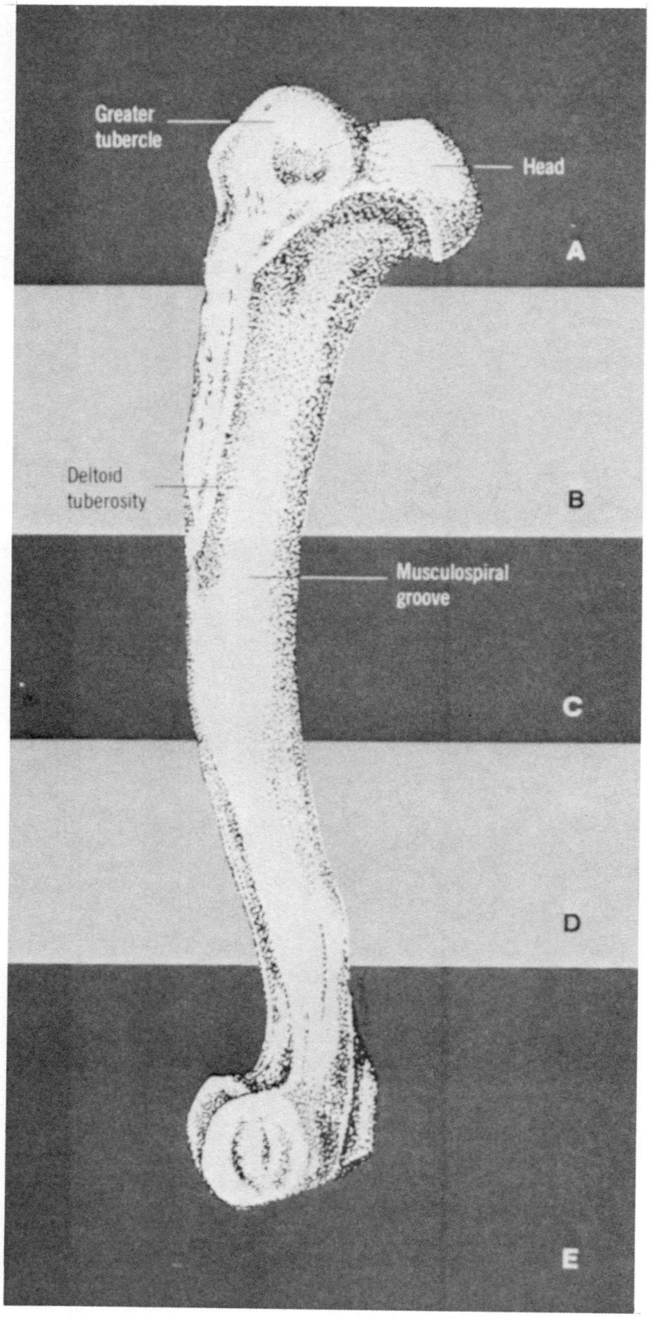

Figure 5—Lateral aspect of the left humerus. Note the sigmoid curvature of the anterior surface. When the lateral approach is made, the bone plate must conform to this configuration. *(See Figures 7A-7E for explanation of the lettered transverse segments.)*

Figure 6—Cranial aspect of the left humerus. Note that the medial surface is relatively straight. The anterior surface tends to blend into the lateral surface at the level of the musculospiral groove.

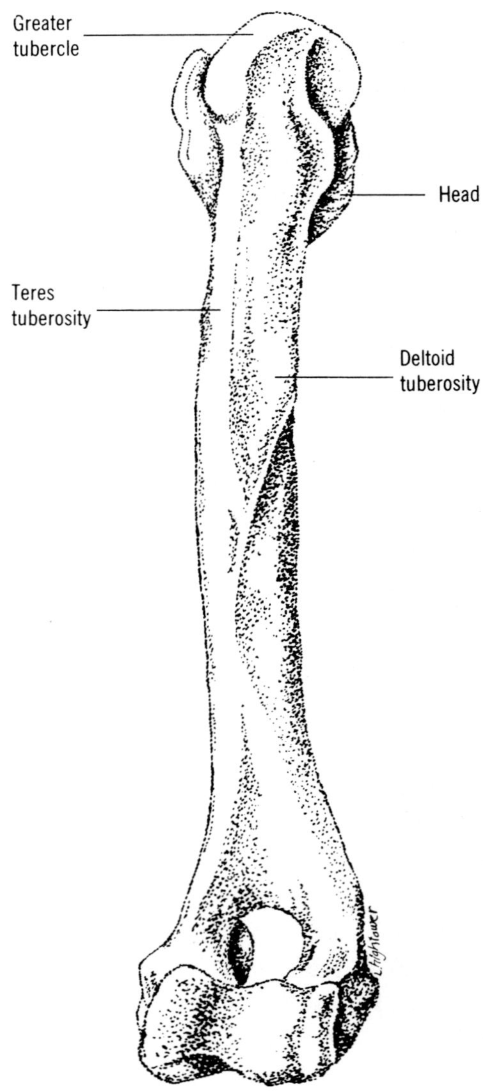

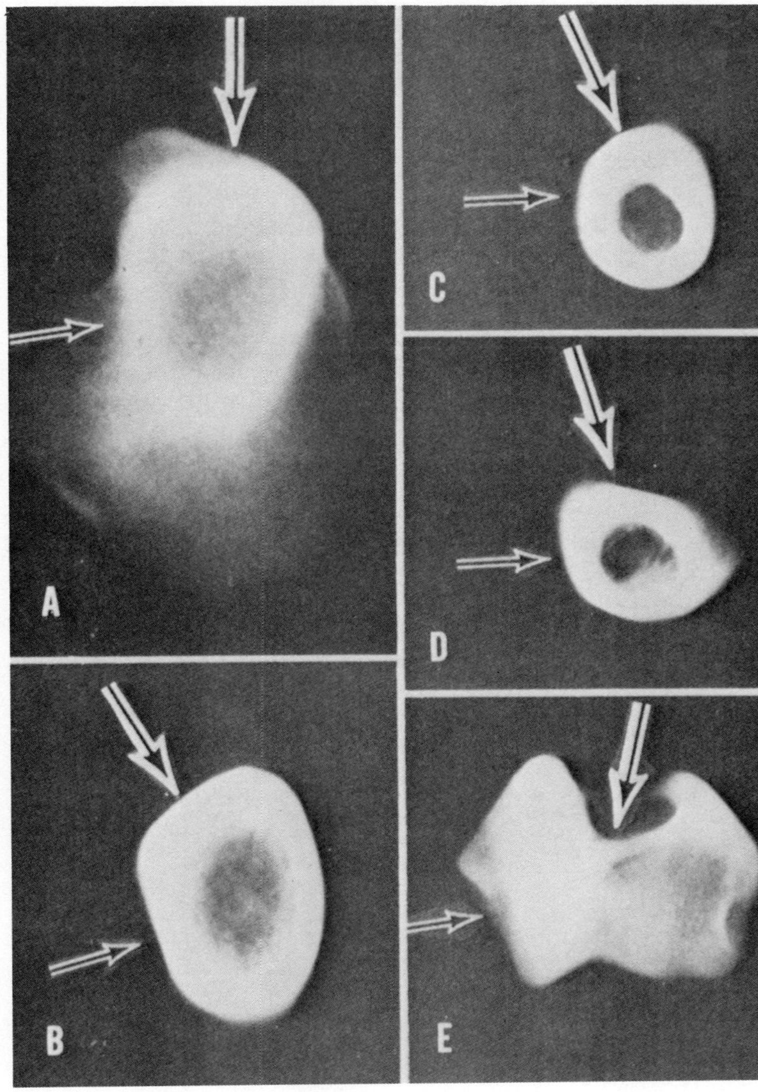

Figures 7A - 7E—The cross sections shown here correspond to the segments indicated by letters A through E in Figure 5. The central ray was directed through the center of the marrow cavity in a proximal-to-distal direction. Large arrows indicate the medial surface. Small arrows indicate the anterior surface. Throughout the length of the humeral shaft, the medial surface maintains relatively uniform size, shape, and thickness of cortex. The anterior surface not only varies in size and shape; it also tends to lose identity as it blends into the lateral surface at the level of the musculospiral groove (*Figures 7C & 7D*).

At this time the entire medial aspect of the shaft is visible and an appropriate plate can be applied with ease.

Discussion

The described medial approach offers a number of advantages over the lateral approach. With the lateral approach, the muscles that must be retracted for adequate exposure of the humeral shaft are large and cumbersome to manipulate. The lateral head of the triceps muscle and the brachialis muscle must be retracted caudally, while the superficial pectoral and brachiocephalicus muscles are reflected cranially. The large bellies of these muscles make adequate manipulation of the fracture fragments awkard and time-consuming. Due to the muscle masses and the contours of the humeral shaft we have seldom been able to apply a bone clamp for temporary stabilization of the fracture.

The radial nerve further complicates the lateral approach. This nerve crosses the musculospiral groove and is closely associated with the brachialis muscle. We have noticed that when the brachialis muscle or the lateral head of the triceps muscle is retracted, undue stress is often exerted on the radial nerve and its deep and superficial rami which arise in the distal third of the shaft (*Figure 4*). With the lateral approach, the radial nerve and rami must be identified and carefully protected at the distal end of the incision.

Application of a bone plate through a lateral incision must be made on the anterior surface (so-called tension side) of the humeral shaft. This surface follows a sigmoid curve (*Figure* 5), and the proximal half is convex while the distal half is concave. Thus, the plate must be bend to conform to this configuration, with the proximal segment of a mid-shaft fracture under tension and the distal segment under compression. In addition, the proximal part of the anterior surface is wide and curves laterally while the distal surface narrows and enjoins the musculospiral groove. Thus, with the lateral approach the surgeon must content with a surface that is both curved and tapering-not an optimally desirable configuration for satisfactory application of a bone plate.

In contrast to the anterior surface of the humeral shaft, the medial surface has less curvature than any other aspect of the shaft (*Figure* 6). The medial surface is rounded throughout the length of the shaft (*Figures* 7A-7E). This facilitates inital reduction of the fracture and permits application of a plate with minimal bending of the plate. Application of a compression device can be accomplished with relative ease.

Comment

Our experience indicates that the medial surface of the humeral shaft is the most acceptable site for application of a bone plate. The medial aspect of the humerus is relatively uniform in structure throughout the length of the bone, and is slightly convex rather than concave. Thus, a bone plate at this site seems to be subjected to less stress from bending and fracture fatigue.

Biomechanical studies would be of great value in demonstrating the relative merits of the medial and lateral approaches.

indications for stabilization of SACROILIAC LUXATIONS in the dog and cat

Joe Hauptman, BS, DVM
Dykstra Veterinary Hospital
College of Veterinary Medicine
Kansas State University
Manhattan, Kansas 66506

Don Hulse, BS, DVM
John Chitwood, BS, DVM
Department of Medicine and Surgery
College of Veterinary Medicine
Oklahoma State University
Stillwater, Oklahoma 74074

TWENTY to 25% of all fractures are fractures of the pelvis.[1,2] Frequently, when pelvic trauma is sustained the sacroiliac joint is luxated. The luxation is usually craniodorsal[2] and can be either bilateral or unilateral. If unilateral, the luxation is always accompanied by one or more pelvic fractures on the same side, the opposite side, or both sides.

Sacroiliac luxation may be treated surgically or nonsurgically. We believe definite indications exist for surgical stabilization; our method of choice is to fasten a compression screw into the wing of the sacrum.[1-3]

Other methods of treatment for sacroiliac luxations have been reported. In many cases, cage rest is the simple, effective treatment of choice.[1-4] For surgical correction, intramedullary pins have been advocated. A pin may be driven transversely through the opposite iliac crest, caudal to the spinous process of L-7, and through the dorsal edge of the luxated illium.[5,6] Or, the pin may be driven similarly through the wings of the ilia, but also through the dorsal spinous process of L-7.[4] Pins may also be placed through the wing of the ilium into the sacrum or last lumbar vertebra.[2]

Anatomy[7]

The sacroiliac joint is partly synovial and partly cartilaginous, with the crescent-shaped diarthrotic joint caudoventral to the synchondrotic joint of fibrocartilage (*Figure 1*). This fibrocartilaginous joint is rough and has irregular projections and depressions that tend to interlock.

Three sets of ligaments lend support to the sacroiliac joint: 1) the ventral sacroiliac ligament, 2) the more formidable dorsal sacroiliac ligaments, and 3) the sacrotuberous ligament, which extends from the sacrum to the ischiatic tuberosity.

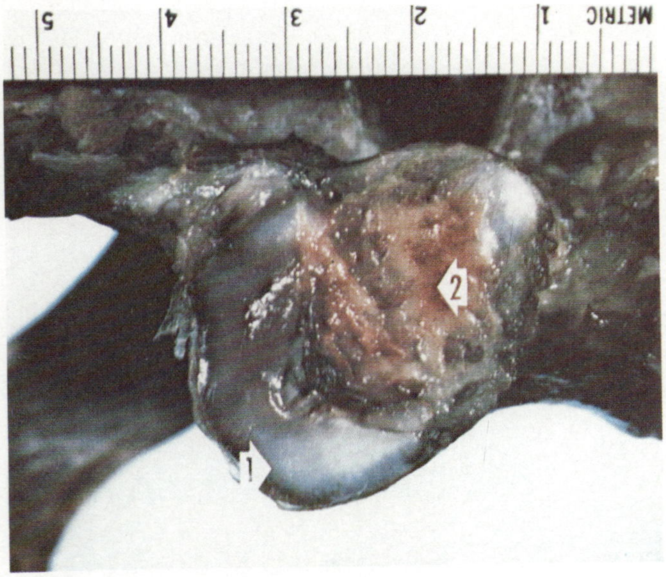

Figure 1—A gross specimen showing the synovial (1) and fibrocartilaginous (2) joints that make up the sacroiliac joint.

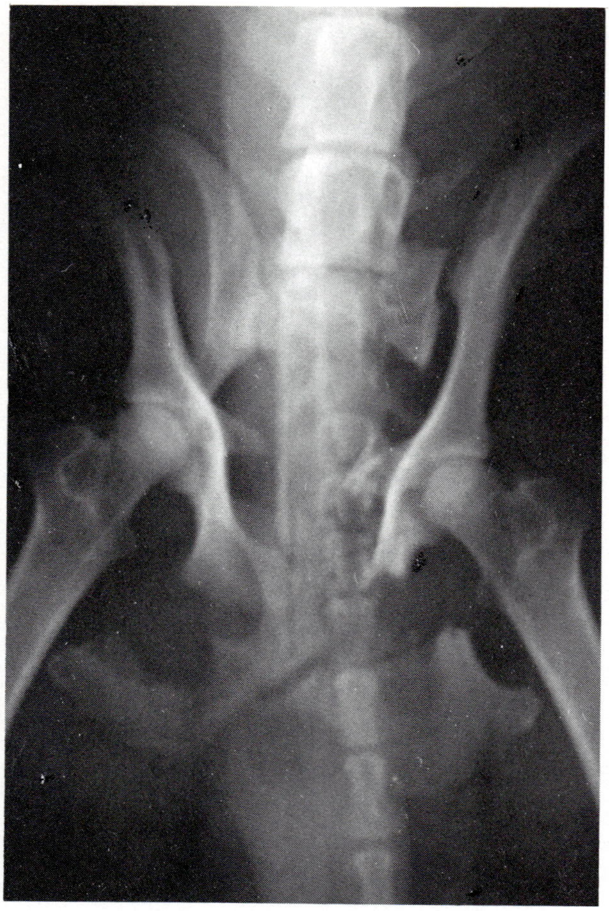

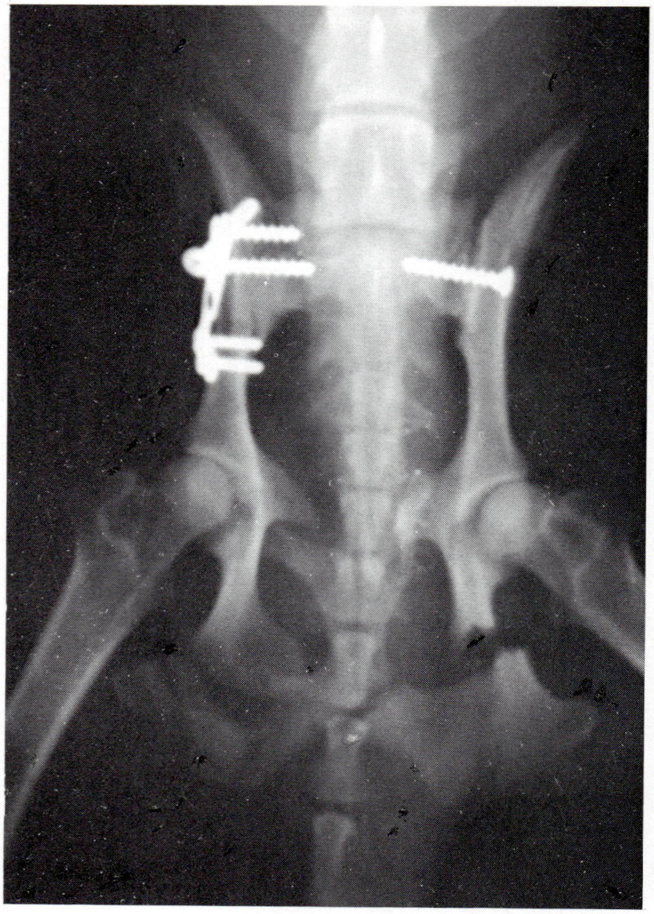

Figures 2A & 2B—Pre- and postoperative ventrodorsal radiographs of a sacroiliac luxation contributing to obstruction of the pelvic outlet.

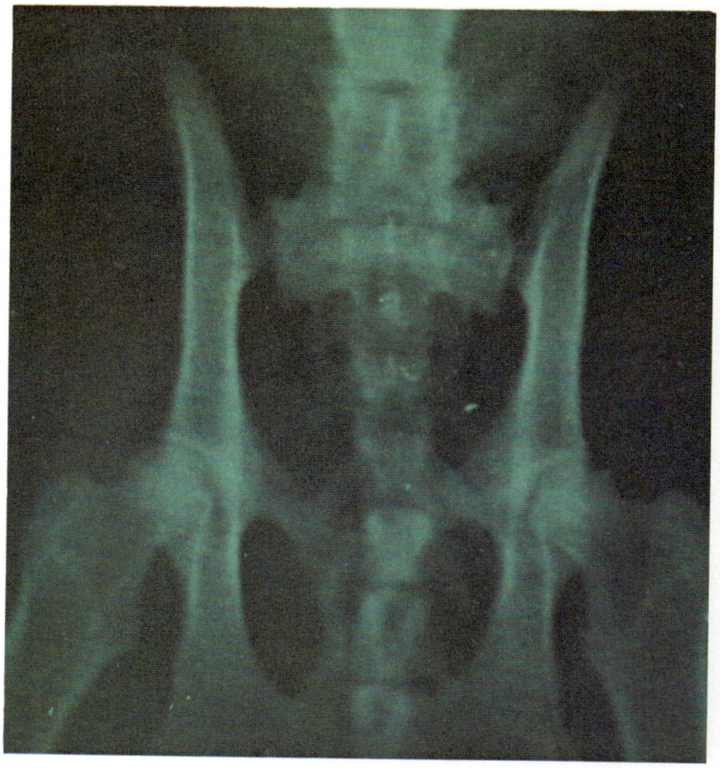

Figures 3A & 3B—Pre- and postoperative ventrodorsal radiographs of a bilateral sacroiliac luxation.

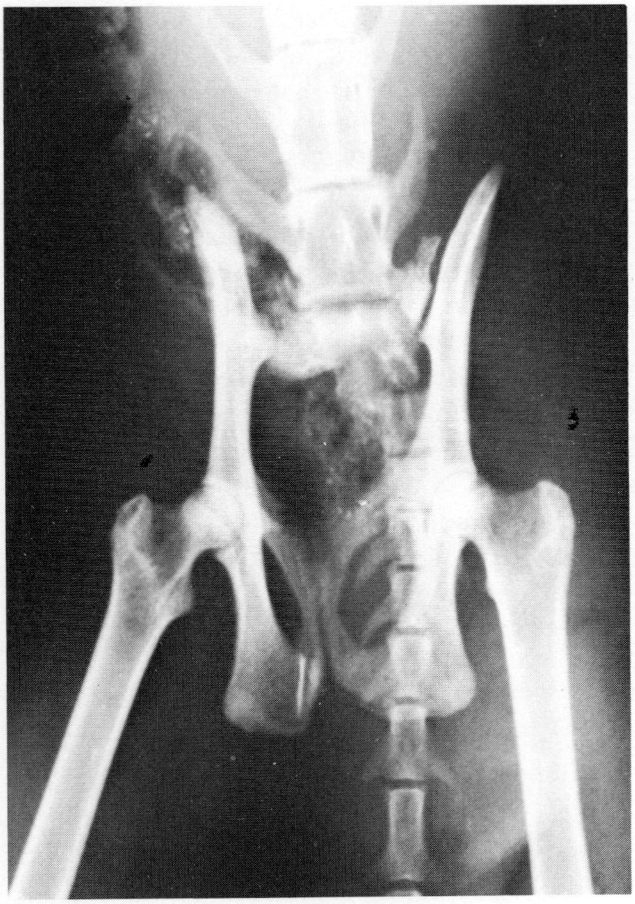

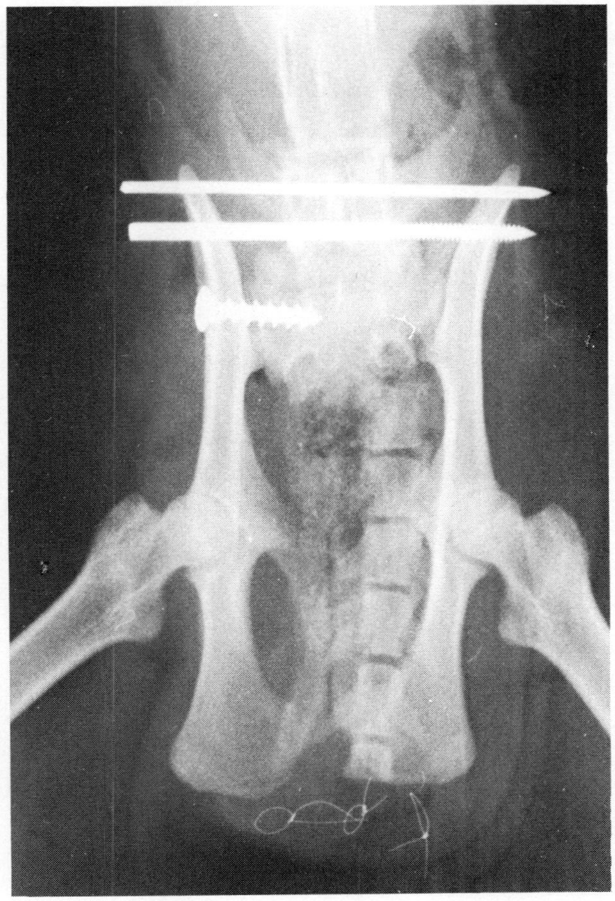

Figures 4A & 4B—Pre- and postoperative ventrodorsal radiographs of a sacroiliac luxation on one side and a fracture through the wing of the sacrum on the other.

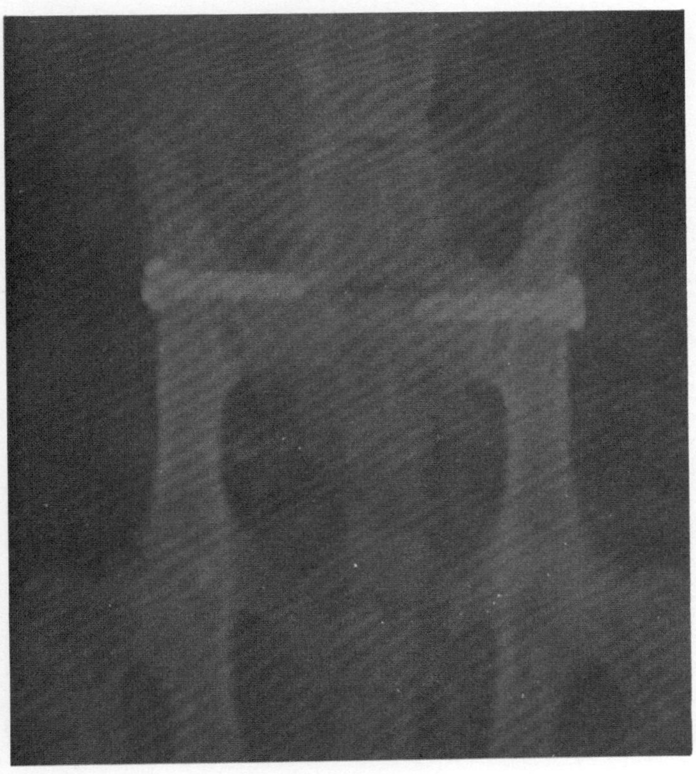

Indications for repair

The primary indication for stabilization of sacroiliac luxations is pain, which is manifest by the degree to which the animal is unwilling to use or support weight with the rear legs. Even without pain, however, obstruction of the pelvic outlet is an indication for stabilization (*Figures 2A & B*). Pain may be associated with 1) bilateral sacroiliac luxation (*Figures 3A & B*), with or without concurrent pelvic fractures; 2) unilateral luxation and pelvic fracture on either or both sides (*Figures 2A & B*); or 3) a sacral fracture on the opposite side (*Figures 4A & B*).

Surgical treatment of sacroiliac luxation reduces or abolishes pain and helps restore anatomic continuity to the pelvis. These are important factors in restoring normal limb function and the ability to bear weight. Surgical treatment shortens hospitalization time and lessens the likelihood that the animal will develop decubitus ulcers or will soil itself with feces or urine. Reduction and stabilization of the sacroiliac luxation also aids in the correction of other pelvic fractures (such as an ischial fracture on the same side) or it alleviates the need for correction.

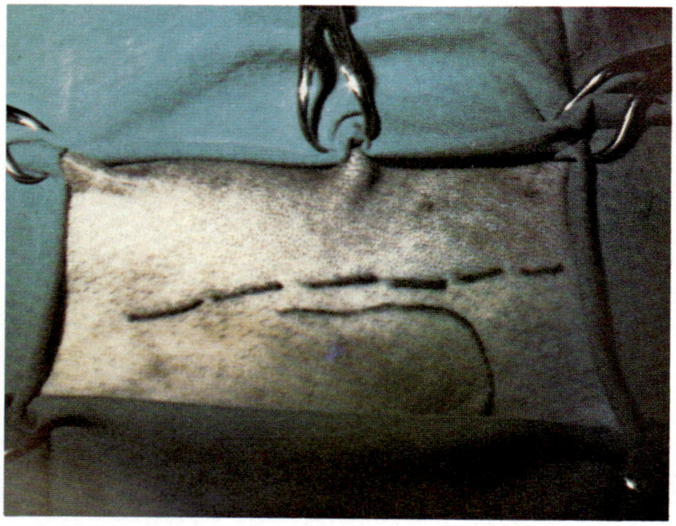

Figure 5—The broken line indicates the line of incision in relation to the wing of the ilium (*curved line*).

Surgical technique

The patient is anesthetized and routinely prepared for aseptic surgery. With the patient in ventral recumbency, the rear quarters are elevated with a sandbag. The sacroiliac luxation is exposed by a described technique (*Figures 5-9*).[1,8]

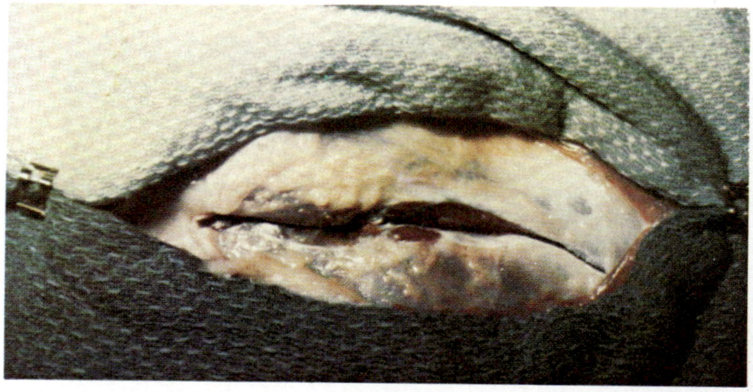

Figure 6—An incision is made through the deep gluteal fascia separating the middle gluteal and dorsal lateral sacrococcygeal muscles.

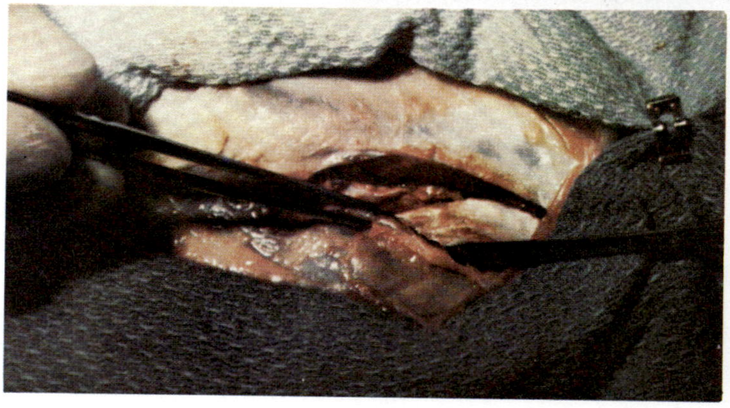

Figure 7—The middle gluteal muscle is reflected off the wing of the ilium with a periosteal elevator.

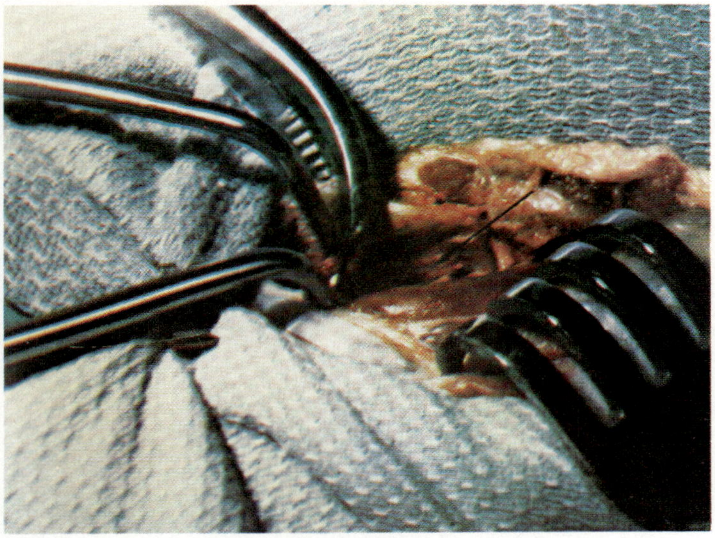

Figure 8—The exposed luxation. The arrow indicates the fibrocartilaginous articular surface of the ilium.

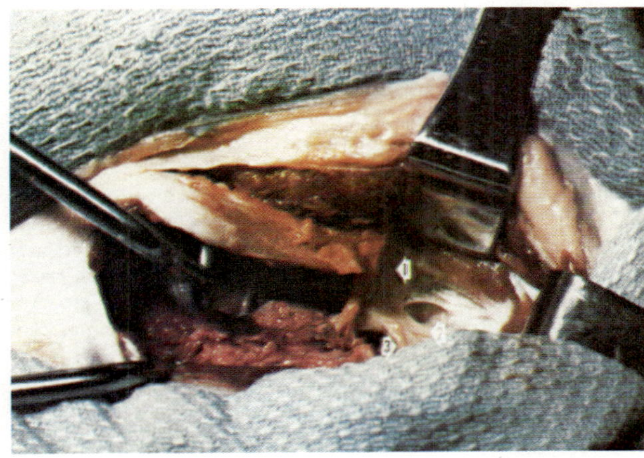

Figure 9—The cranial gluteal artery, vein, and nerve (1), sciatic nerve (2), and first sacral nerve (3). These structures need not be exposed during surgery, but the surgeon must be aware of their presence in relation to the sacrum.

With the luxation exposed, bone-holding forceps are placed on the wing of the ilium to aid in the reduction. Because of contracture of the longissimus dorsi, iliocostalis lumborum, and quadratus lumborum muscles, anatomic reduction may be difficult if more than 48 hours have passed since the trauma was sustained. Contraction of these muscles, however, may be overcome with gradual reduction.

When reduction has been achieved, a compression screw is inserted through the wing of the ilium into the wing of the sacrum for stabilization. Compression can be accomplished with a cortical screw and overdrilling of the wing with the proper bit (*Figures 10 & 11*). Compression can also be achieved with a cancellous bone screw of proper total length and thread length.

Whether or not a cortical screw of a cancellous bone screw is used, proper screw length is important to prevent damage to the sacral nerves coursing in the spinal canal (*Figures 12—14*). Proper screw length is determined by measuring the width of the wing of the ilium and wing of the sacrum on the preoperative ventrodorsal radiograph.

When stabilization has been accomplished (*Figure 15*), the surgical site is flushed with sterile saline solution and the wound closed in a routine manner.

Postoperative care requires the administration of antibiotics for five days. The animal should be kept inside for five weeks, with exercise limited to walks on a leash.

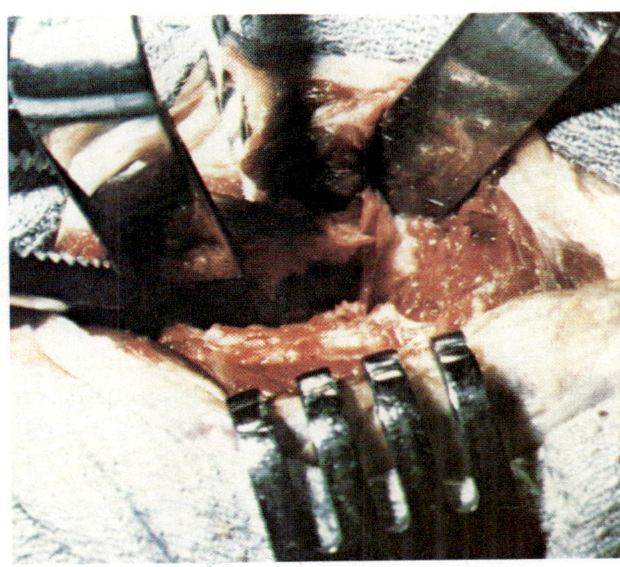

Figure 10—The wing of the ilium is overdrilled through the fibrocartilaginous joint surface.

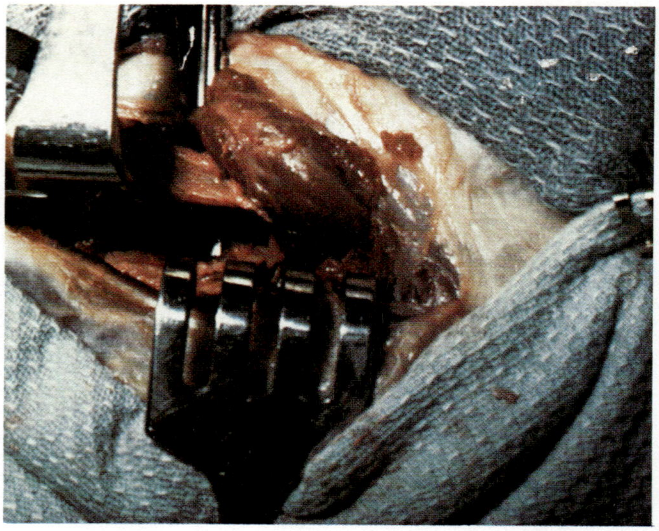

Figure 11
The wing of the sacrum is drilled at the level of the fibrocartilaginous joint surface.

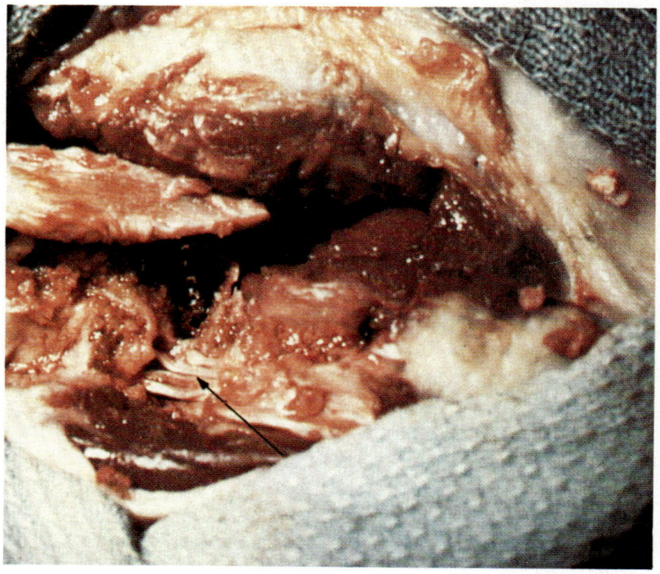

Figure 12
Dissected specimen with the dorsal wing of the sacrum removed to show the relation of the screw to the sacral nerves (*arrow*) coursing in the spinal canal.

Discussion

We routinely use this technique to repair sacroiliac luxations. Although others use two or more compression screws,[1-3] we invariably use only one. In our experience, one screw has been satisfactory. Multiple screws would certainly be advantageous if an ischial fracture were present in a large dog whose stability depended upon fixation of the sacroiliac luxation. Aided by the anatomy of the joint and pelvis and by the surrounding heavy musculature, the one-screw technique often stabilizes satisfactorily.

This technique is reasonably fast, effective, and safe. When it is used with the proper indications, results are satisfactory.

REFERENCES

1. Bojrab, M.J.: *Current Techniques in Small Animal Surgery.* Lea & Febiger, Philadelphia, Pa., 1975; pp 414, 415, 424-426.
2. Archibald, J., ed: *Canine Surgery*, 2nd ed. American Veterinary Publications, Inc., Santa Barbara, Calif., 1974; pp 987-988, 1067-1069.
3. Singleton, W.B.: Limb Fractures in the Dog and Cat. V-Fractures of the Hind Limb. *J. Small Anim. Pract.* 7:163-168; 1966.
4. Whittick, W.G.: *Canine Orthopedics.* Lea & Febiger, Philadelphia, Pa., 1974; Chapter 18.
5. Leighton, R.L.: Surgical Treatment of Some Pelvic Fractures. *JAVMA 153*:1739-1741; Dec. 15, 1968.
6. Rudy, R.L.: In *Scientific Presentations of the 42nd Annual Meeting AAHA*, vol. 1: p 378; 1975.
7. Miller, M.E. *et al: Anatomy of the Dog.* W.B. Saunders Co., Philadelphia, Pa., 1964; p 119.
8. Piermattei, D.L.; Greeley, R.G.: *An Atlas of Surgical Approaches to the Bones of the Dog and Cat.* W.B. Saunders Co., Philadelphia, Pa., 1966; p 76.

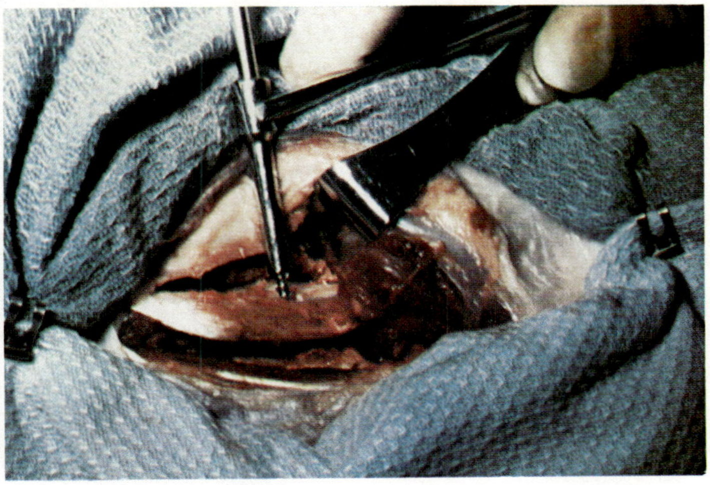

Figure 13
The hole drilled into the wing of the sacrum is tapped.

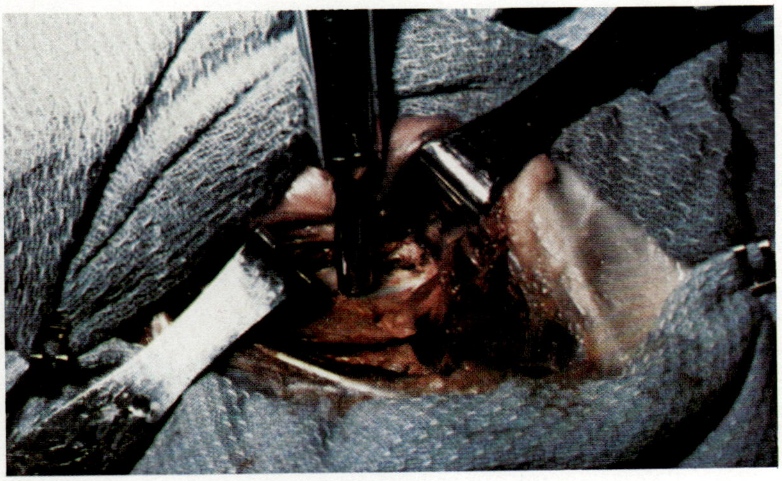

Figure 14
A depth gauge is used to determine the proper length of the screw to be inserted

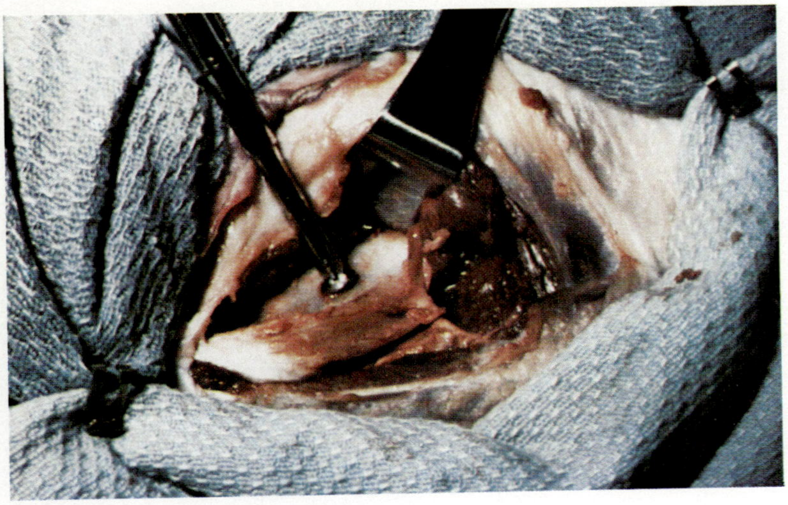

Figure 15
A screw of proper length is inserted to achieve compression.

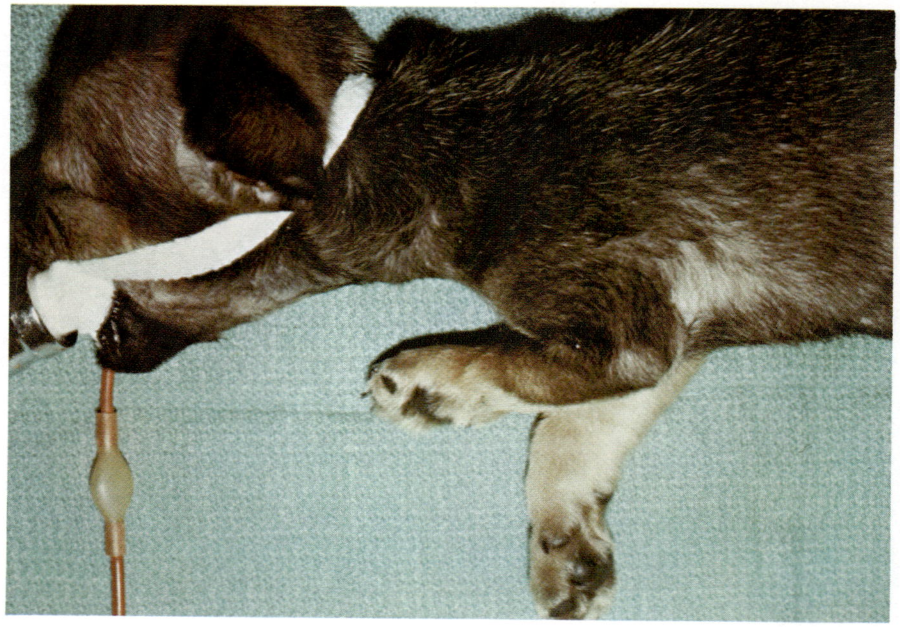

Figure 1—Appearance of the affected left foreleg before surgery. Note the marked inward rotation of the leg.

management of a congenital elbow luxation by

Temporary Transarticular Pinning

Stephen J. Withrow, DVM
Dept. of Veterinary Clinical Studies
Western College of Veterinary Medicine
University of Saskatchewan
Saskatoon, Canada S7N OWO

Percutaneous transarticular pinning was used successfully to stabilize a reduced elbow luxation in a 6-week-old puppy. Although this treatment violates several principles of orthopedics, the potential benefit was thought to outweigh the possible disadvantages. Recovery was uneventful and the patient regained normal use of the elbow. No degenerative joint disease or epiphyseal abnormality was detected 16 months after surgery.

NEITHER congenital nor early acquired luxation of the elbow is common in small animals.[1] The prognosis is usually very guarded, regardless of therapy.[1-3] Proposed management has included open reduction (often involving several surgeries),[1] and nonintervention which permits formation of a false joint.[2] Unlike acute elbow luxations in adult dogs, closed reduction and extension coaptation is rarely feasible in the young animal.

In this paper I describe a technique of closed reduction and percutaneous transarticular pinning that led to successful recovery of elbow function in a 6-week-old puppy. The technique is simple and rapid to perform. Possibly, the procedure could be used to treat other traumatic or congenital luxations.

Case History

A 6-week-old female terrier-cross was presented to the Western College of Veterinary Medicine for evaluation of an abnormal left front leg. The owner stated that the dam had delivered a normal litter without apparent difficulty. The problem with this puppy was first noted when the animal was 1 week old. The owner also reported that the puppy was only half as large as its littermates. It had been weaned one week before presentation and reportedly had a good appetite.

The puppy weighed only 0.7 kg but was in excellent physical condition except for the left front leg (*Figure 1*). Little weight could be borne on the affected leg, but the foot was put on the ground with each step. Muscle atrophy of the entire leg was apparent, most noticeable from the elbow distally. A bulge could be palpated on the lateral aspect of the elbow. Neither crepitus nor pain was noted when the leg was flexed or extended. Marked internal rotation at the carpus caused the medial aspect of the paw to bear most of the weight.

A tentative diagnosis of an early acquired or congenital lateral elbow luxation was confirmed radiographically (*Figure 2*).

The owners were consulted as to their wishes, and we decided to attempt closed reduction and percutaneous transarticular pinning. The prognosis for return of the leg's normal function was guarded.

Surgical Technique

General anesthesia was induced via mask and inhalation of 2.5% halothane. The puppy was intubated and maintained on halothane and oxygen, using a non-rebreathing system.

Palpation of the elbow revealed that the luxation could be reduced with the elbow in flexion but that it reluxated with any movement of the leg.

The posterior aspect of the elbow and olecranon was clipped and surgically prepared for insertion of a pin. While the elbow was held reduced in a functional position (135°), a small Kirschner wire (0.045 in.) was inserted from 1 cm distal to the point of the olecranon, through the semilunar notch of the ulna, and seated 2 cm into the distal humerus (*Figure 3*). The pin was cut off flush with the skin.

Figure 2—Preoperative radiograph of the leg giving an anteroposterior view of the humerus and a lateral view of the radius and ulna.

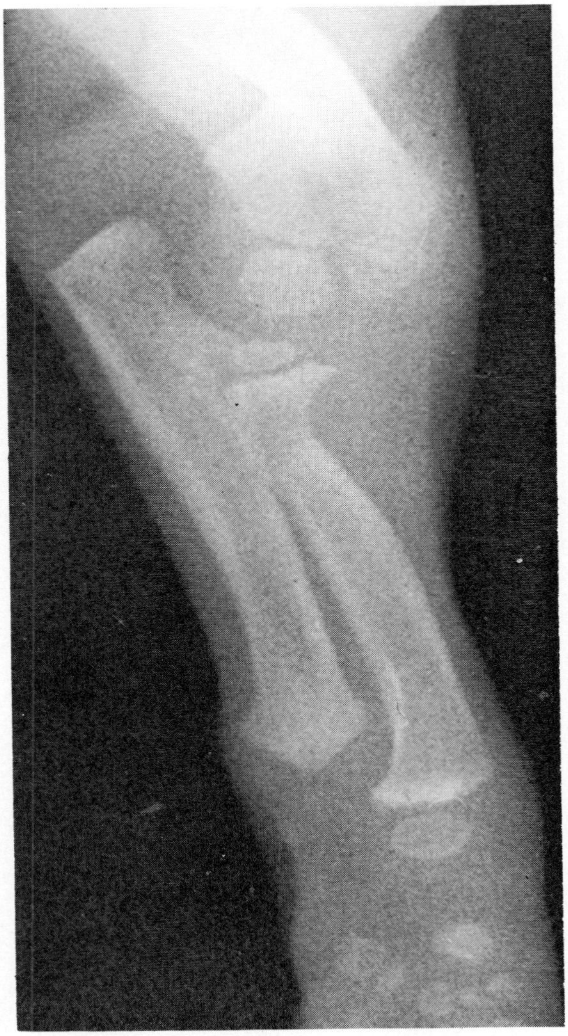

Postoperative radiograph showed good reduction of the luxation (*Figure 4*). Perfect reduction could not be confirmed due to lack of ossification and the small size of the bones.

The patient was discharged the next day with instructions to the client to restrict the puppy's activity and return it in 10 days for removal of the pin. When released from the hospital the puppy was bearing more weight on the injured leg than before surgery.

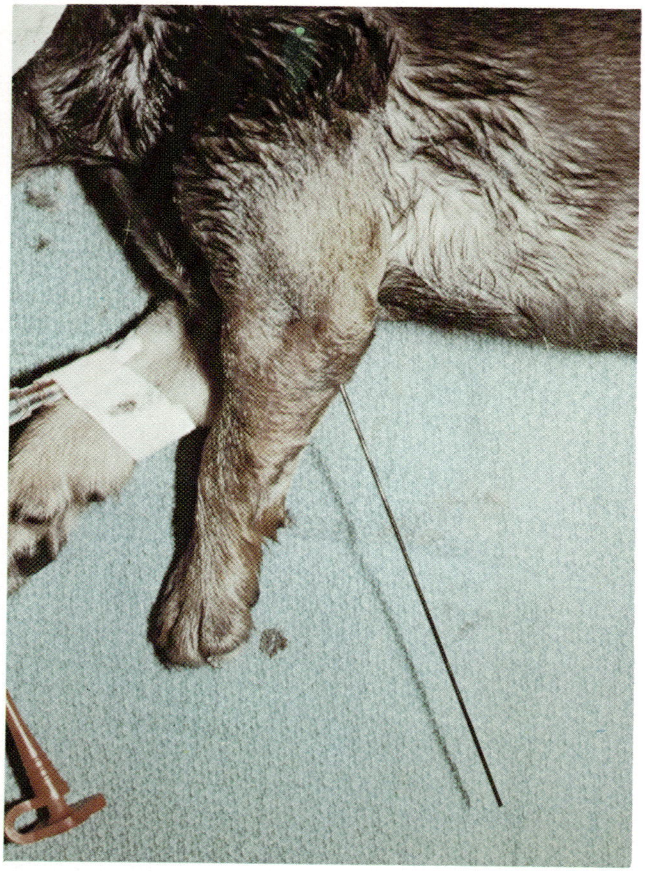

Figure 3—Appearance of the reduced elbow joint before the pin was cut off flush with the skin. Note the proper functional angle of the joint.

Figure 4—Postoperative radiograph showing the relative realignment achieved by insertion of the pin.

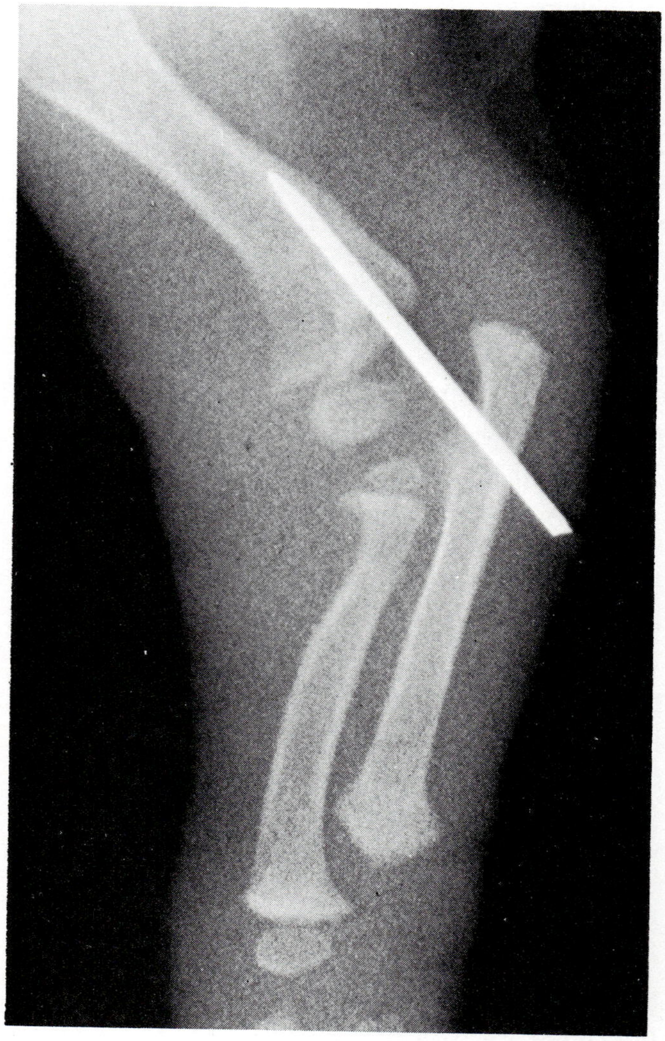

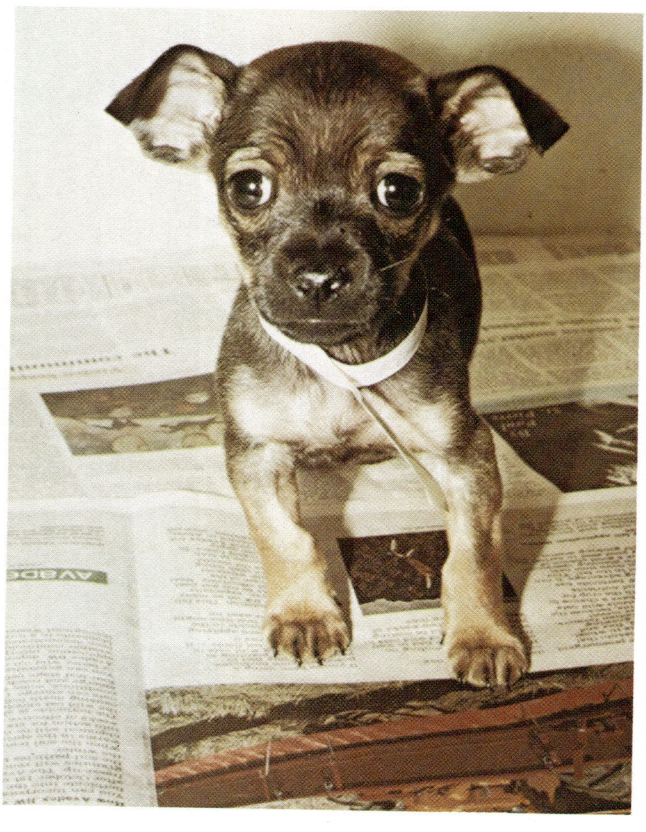

Figure 5—The puppy 10 days postoperatively. Muscle atrophy is minimal and alignment is good.

Follow-Up

Nine days after surgery the owner presented the dog after noticing that the pin had fallen out. The dog was walking on the leg most of the time without difficulty. Range of motion was reduced only minimally. No crepitus was noted and there was no evidence of pain in the joint. Except for minimal muscle atrophy, the positioning of both front legs was the same (*Figure 5*). Radiographs revealed a well-reduced elbow joint with only slightly greater than normal distance between the ulna and the humeral condyles (*Figure 6*).

Figure 6—This lateral radiograph, taken 10 days postoperatively, shows good reduction of the luxated elbow. Pin tracts are slightly visible in the proximal ulna and distal humerus.

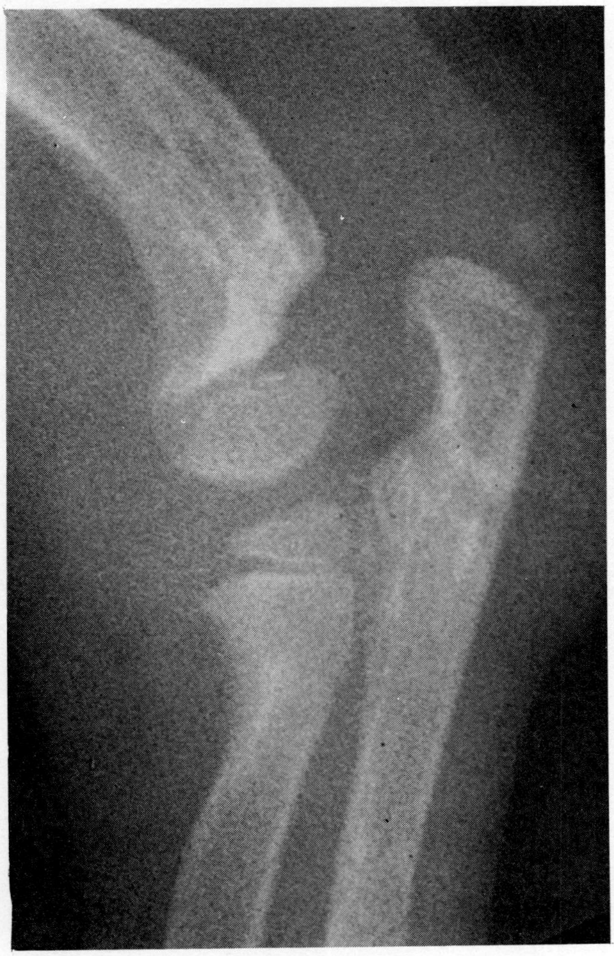

The owners were instructed to avoid strenuously exercising the puppy and to return it in one month for further evaluation. At the five-week check-up the dog was found to be 100% sound and free of pain. The length and position of the leg appeared normal and no muscle atrophy was noted. No abnormalities were seen on radiographs. The animal was released with no restrictions on activity.

When the dog was 8 months old, it was presented for an ovariohysterectomy, affording an additional opportunity for follow-up. The owner reported that the dog was active and exhibited no lameness or signs of pain even after considerable exercising. Full range of motion was present, no evidence of pain could be elicited, and full muscle size was evident. Radiographs revealed a normal elbow with no evidence of a degenerative joint disease.

At the last follow-up, 16 months postoperatively, the dog was clinically normal in all respects. Radiographs again showed a normal elbow and front legs of equal length (*Figures 7A & B*).

Discussion

Congenital or early acquired elbow luxations in small animals have carried a grave prognosis regardless of whether or not open reduction is employed. Problems encountered may include atrophy as a result of disuse; internal rotation from the elbow distally; bone deformity secondary to lack of normal stress and strain of growing bones (*i.e.* distal humerus, radius, and ulna); poor radiographic definition due to lack of bone density in the ossification centers of the elbow; the need for general anesthesia; and extremely small size of structures for operative reconstruction.

Several aspects of transarticular pinning are theoretically not ideal. The first problem is that the procedure violates the principle of not crossing a joint surface with an implant. Long-standing fixation will lead to contracture of the joint capsule and surrounding structures so that the elbow's range of motion may be limited. Early removal of the pin (seven to 10 days) should prevent permanent irreversible joint stiffness. It is important that

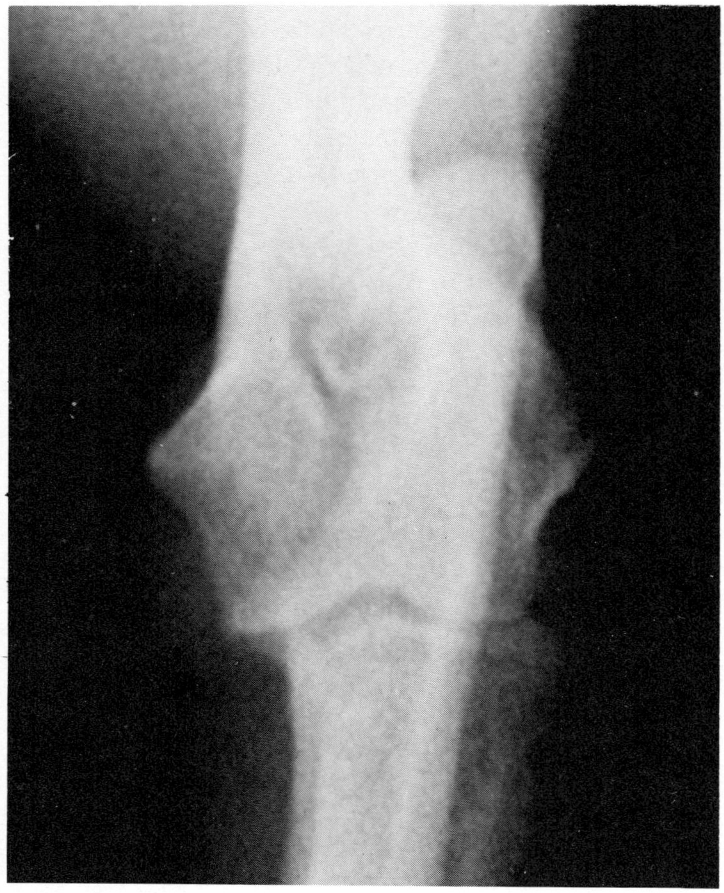

Figures 7A & B
Anteroposterior *(left)* and lateral *(below)* radiographs taken 15 months after surgery. No degenerative joint disease was apparent at this time.

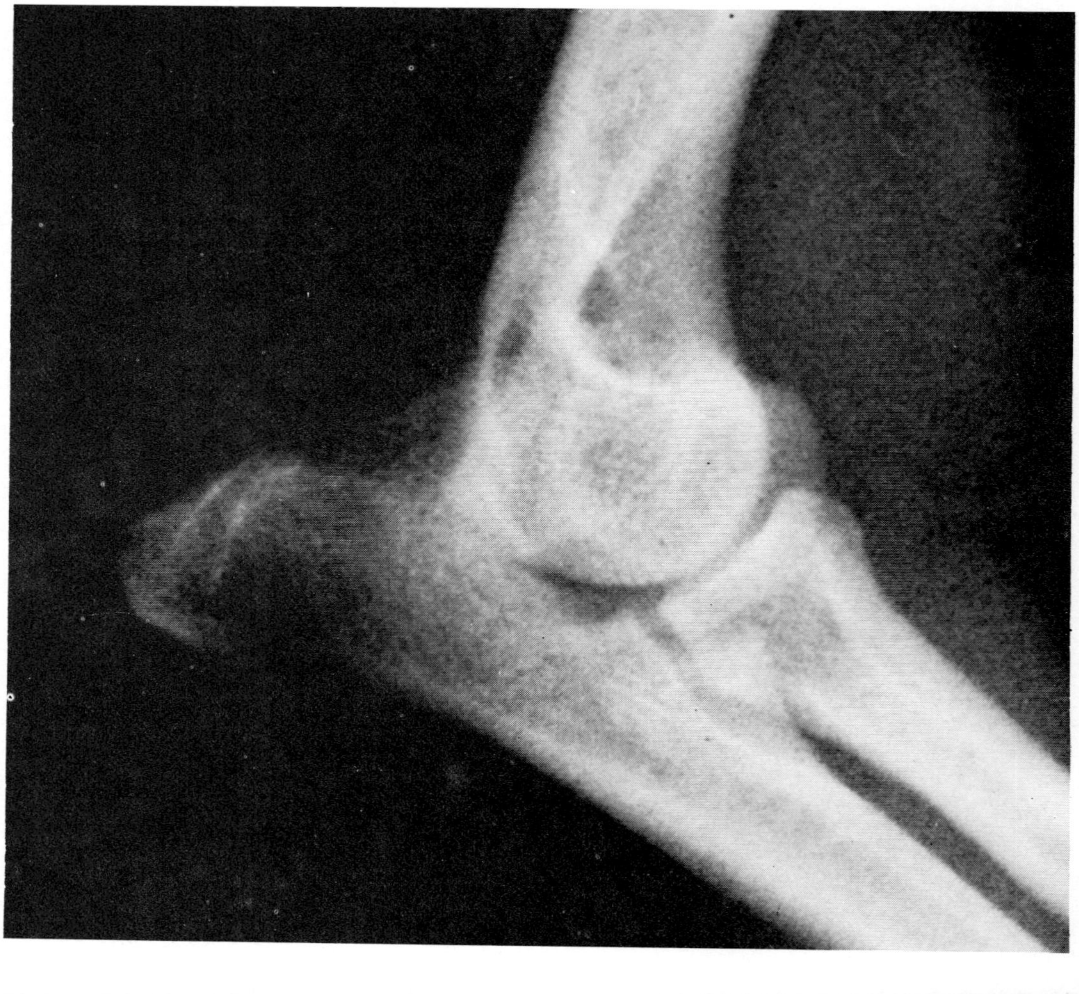

the elbow be held in a functional position so that the leg has maximal ability to break out of the contractions when it is either flexed or extended.

Transarticular pinning also damages some joint cartilage, which may contribute to degenerative changes in the elbow. If degenerate joint disease did ensue, however, the cause could be the trauma of the luxation and/or a reduction rather than the pinning. In the case reported here, no degenerative changes were noted more than one year after surgery.

The last potential problem with this technique is the possiblity of closing or altering epiphyseal growth of the pinned bones. Unless a very large pin or threaded pins have been used, this possibility is unlikely.[4] Small, straight-shafted pins allow the epiphyses to grow around the pin and maintain proper length. Even if arrested for seven to 10 days, growth may start again after the pin has been removed.

The use of temporary transarticular pinning can be expanded to include any unstable joint that must be immobilized for any of a variety of reasons (postoperative collateral ligament repair, deranged stifles, shearing wounds, hip luxations, etc.). If used judiciously, the procedure allows a joint to be "put at rest" as treatment for various lesions. Except in small puppies, care must be taken to prevent excessive weight-bearing on the operated leg. Continual cycling of the metal will eventually cause sufficient stress fatigue to break the pin within the joint. The pin in large or mature animals should be protected with external coaptation or slings.

REFERENCES

1. Stoyac, J.M.: The Elbow: Dislocation of the Elbow In *Current Techniques in Small Animal Surgery.* Lea & Febiger, Philadelphia, Pa., 1975; pp 523-526.
2 .Flipo, J.: Joints of the Pectoral Limb: Dislocation. In *Canine Surgery, 1st Archibald ed.* American Veterinary Publications, Inc., Santa Barbara, Calif., 1965; pp 930-933.
3. Campbell, J.R.: Nonfracture Injuries of the Canine Elbow. *JAVMA 155*(5);735-744; Sept. 1, 1969.
4. Campbell, C.J. *et al:* The Effects Produced in the Cartilagenous Epiphyseal Plate of Immature Dogs by Experimental Surgical Trauma. *J. Bone & Joint Surg. 41-A*(7): 1221-1242; Oct. 1959.

treatment of CANINE OSTEOSARCOMA for limb preservation using osteotomy, adjuvant radiotherapy and chemotherapy (a case report)

G. H. Theilen, DVM
Robert Leighton, VMD
Department of Surgery
Section of Clinical Oncology
Roy Pool, DVM, PhD
Department of Pathology
School of Veterinary Medicine
University of California
Davis, California 95616
R. D. Park, DVM, PhD
Dept. of Radiology & Radiation Biology
School of Veterinary Medicine
Colorado State University
Fort Collins, Colorado 80521

On March 23, 1975, a 10-year-old spayed Doberman Pinscher was referred to the Veterinary Medical Teaching Hospital with radiographic evidence of a primary bone tumor of the right distal ulna. There was no radiographic evidence of metastasis to the lungs. Three years earlier the animal had undergone surgery for removal of the axillary mammary glands. Grossly, the glands were tumorous at that time, but a histologic examination was not done. The dog was spayed two weeks after the mammary gland surgery.

As acute lameness of the right foreleg developed two weeks previous to the initial examination and four weeks before the dog was admitted to the Veterinary Medical Teaching Hospital. Although the leg was not noticeable swollen, it was hot to touch and apparently painful. The dog was in good physical condition, and no other physical abnormalities were found.

Clinical Findings

Complete blood counts, alkaline phosphatase, blood urea nitrogen, serum glutamic pyruvate and glutamic oxyloacetic transaminase levels were within normal range. Plasma proteins were slightly below normal range with an albumin:globulin ration of 0.7:1. Serum copper was 75 mcg/dL and zinc was 120 mcg/dL, both elevated above normal limits.

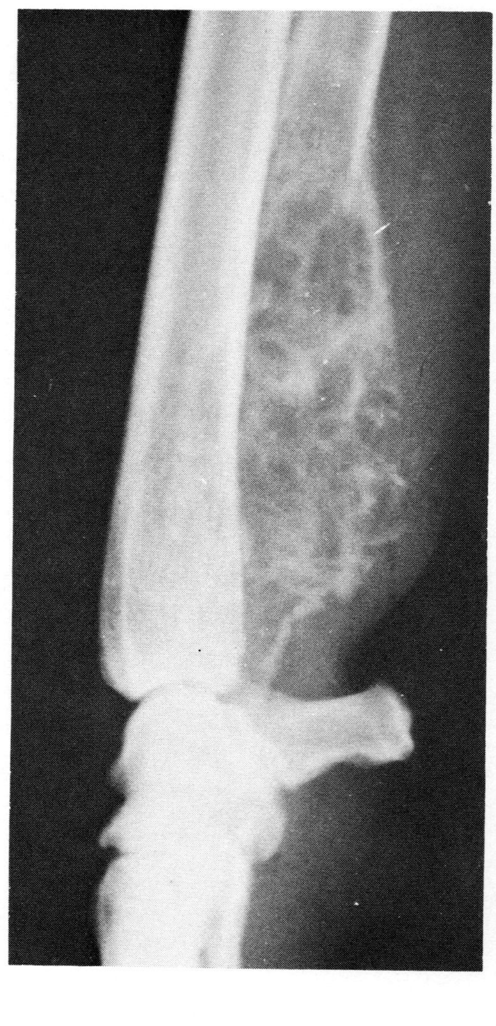

Figure 1—Radiograph of the distal radius and ulna taken when the dog was first hospitalized. Osteosarcoma had resulted in severe osteolysis and soft-tissue swelling.

Initial radiographs revealed a highly destructive malignant bone tumor of the distal ulna (*Figure 1*). Lung fields were normal for a 10-year-old dog. Osteotomy of the involved distal ulna was performed; thus saving the affected limb. This approach was used because we have tried in the past to maintain the affected limb by various treatments, but never before had tried surgical removal of the involved bone.

Histologically the neoplasm was identified as a primary telangiectatic osteosarcoma (*Figure 2*).

Treatment

The osteotomy, performed two days after the dog was admitted to the hospital, consisted of removing a 10-cm length of the distal right ulna. All signs of lameness disappeared approximately 10 to 14 days after surgery and never recurred.

Two weeks after surgery, radiation therapy was begun on the distal right foreleg in an area extending from the carpus to mid-diaphysis. Radiation was administered from a distance of 50 cm with a Westinghouse Orthovoltage-250 Quadricondex machine operated at 15 mA and 250 kVp. The half-layer value was 1.58 mm of copper equivalent, and the added filters were 0.5 mm of copper and 1.0

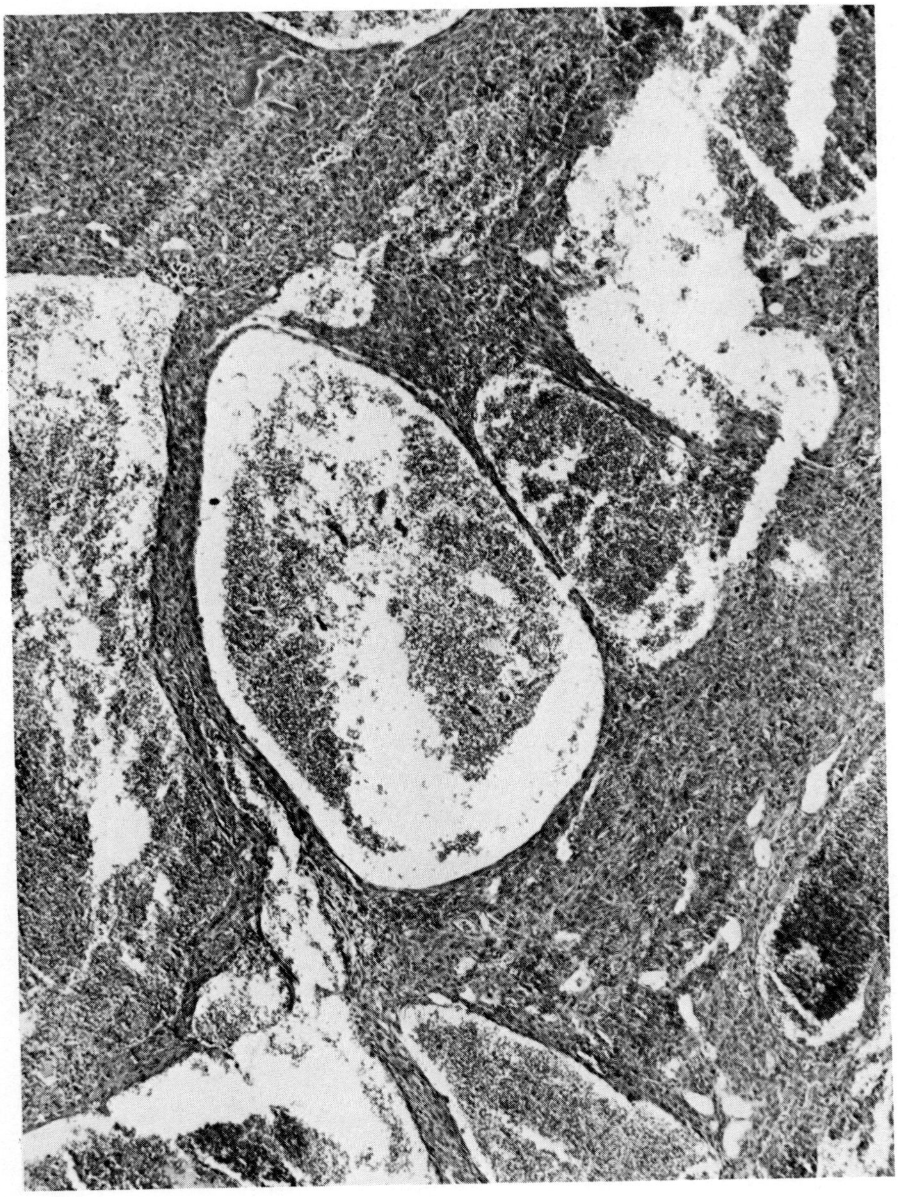

Figure 2
Photomicrograph of a telangiectatic osteosarcoma arising in the distal ulna. Blood-filled spaces of irregular caliber have developed within a field of anaplastic cells having low osteoplastic potential (H&E x200).

mm of aluminum. Total dosage for treatment of the osteotomy site was 5,000 rads to 2 cm depth. This was applied over a field of 5 x 10 cm divided into 10 equal doses of 500 rads. Three treatments were given each week, with the direction of the beam being alternated 90° from lateral to medial and posterior to anterior.

When radiotherapy was completed, eight weeks after the initial diagnosis was made, adjuvant chemotherapy began. The therapeutic regimen consisted of Adriamycin (Doxorubicin® —Adria Labs) and cyclophosphamide (Cytoxan® Mead Johnson). Adriamycin was given intravenously at the rate of 50 mg/M^2 daily for four days each week when Adriamycin was not given. Chemotherapy continued for 23 weeks.

A slight moist dermatitis with loss of hair occurred at the irradiation site about three weeks after radiotherapy began. The skin reaction healed in 60 days with care (keeping the lesion clean with cool water and preventing the animal from licking the affected sites). Alopecia was persistent. There was little evidence of drug toxicity, with the exception that 2½ months after treatment began, blood platelet counts were below normal, and 2% red blood cells found in peripheral blood were nucleated. Thrombocytopenia was a transient finding.

One month after surgery, the lateral cortex of the right radius was rough and a periosteal reaction was evident at the stump of the amputated ulna. The lungs remained free of radiographically visible metastatic foci. Two months after surgery there was still no evidence of local recurrence; however, there was a small nodule in the lung that later proved to be a metastatic lesion.

One month after surgery, the lateral cortex of the right radius was rough and a periosteal reaction was evident at the stump of the amputated ulna. The lungs remained free of radiographically visible metastatic foci. Two months after surgery there was still no evidence of local recurrence; however, there was a small nodule in the lung that later proved to be a metastatic lesion.

Five months after surgery and three months after initation of chemotherapy a small definitive metastatic focus, measuring 0.5 cm in diameter, was present in the lung.

Despite continuation of chemotherapy, this focus enlarged to 1.2 cm in diameter during the next month. The right radius and remaining portion of the ulna were free of tumor and the periosteum of the radius appeared normal (*Figure 3*). The dog continued to use the leg normally.

One month after completion of adjuvant therapy (nearly eight months after diagnosis) the dog suddenly developed signs of extreme dyspnea, became comatose, and was euthanatized.

Pathology

At necropsy there was no evidence of locally recurrent osteosarcoma at the primary site. The tissue had healed normally after the osteotomy (*Figure 4*). Postmortem radiographs, however, showed multiple osteolytic lesions in the distal radius and in the stump of the ulna. These lesions resulted from the

Figure 3—Radiograph of the distal radius at the site of the osteotomy performed five months earlier.

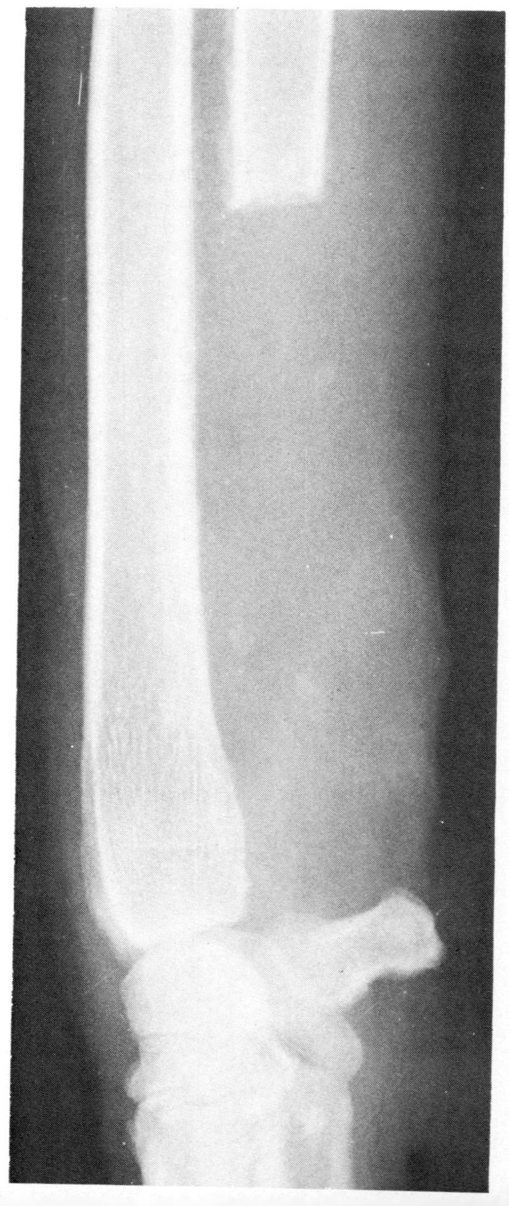

radiation therapy (*Figure 5*). Histologic examination of the radius and ulna revealed cortical bone reorption followed by fibrous rather than osseous repair, peritabecular fibrosis, and myelofibrosis.

The largest of five cystic, bloody, tumor nodules in the lung had eroded through the visceral pleura, leading to extensive hemothorax that produced the sudden terminal signs (*Figure 6*). Each metastatic nodule resembled the primary tumor. Blood-filled spaces of irregular caliber developed within a field of anaplastic cells. This gave both the gross and microscopic structures of the osteosarcoma a characteristic telangiectatic appearance.

The osteolytic character of the lesion seen radiographically in the distal ulna was due to the fact that only a small percentage of the tumor cells produced osteoid that mineralized to form tumorous bone.

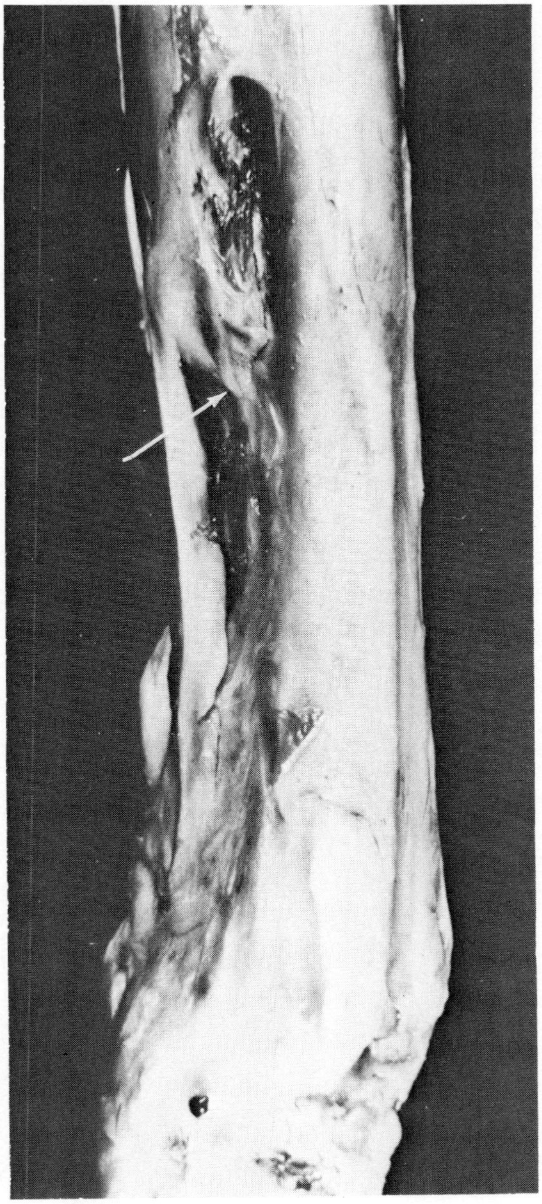

Figure 4—Photograph of the leg at necropsy showing the stump of the ulna (*arrow*). There was no gross or microscopic evidence of primary osteosarcoma.

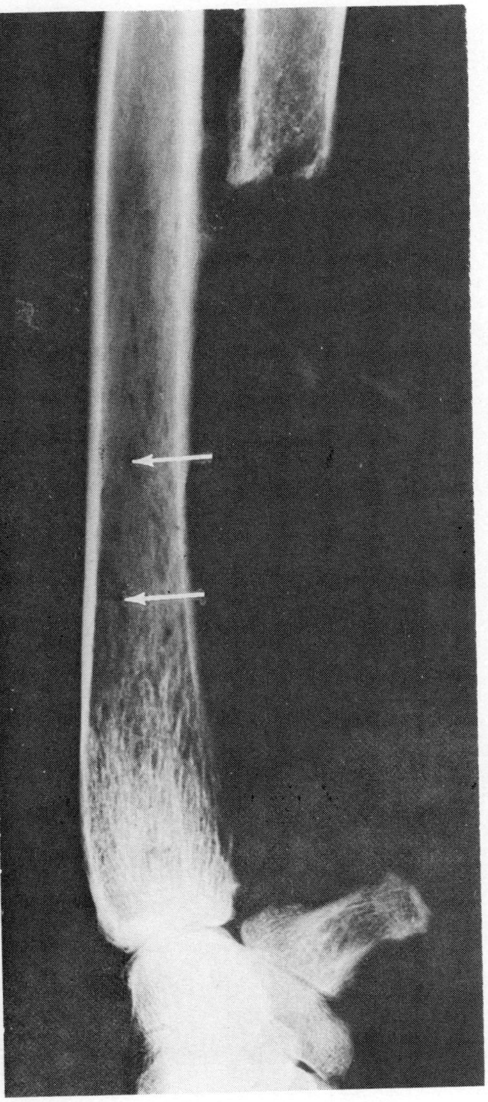

Figure 5—Postmortem radiograph showing the multiple osteolytic lesions (*arrows*) caused by radiation therapy.

Discussion

This report presents for the first time, to our knowledge, a case of canine osteosarcoma in which the neoplasm was surgically removed and the limb was preserved without a local recurrence of the tumor.

Telangietatic osteosarcoma is an uncommon type of canine osteosarcoma which must be differentiated from primary and secondary henamgiosarcomas as well as from other highly anaplastic sarcomas of bone.[1,2] Radiographically, these tumors form lytic, highly destructive lesions with little or no radiodense tumor matrix. In man, the telangiectatic pattern was found in 40 of 1,000 cases of osteosarcoma and was associated with a worse prognosis than were conventional osteosarcomas.[3]

Treatment of canine osteosarcoma had been primarily surgical extirpation.[4,5] In one study, 85% of the dogs showed radiographic evidence of metastasis within eight months after amputation.[6] It is evident, therefore, that surgical removal of the primary tumor seldom results in a cure.

In a previous report, attempts were made to save the involved legs of dogs by combining radiotherapy or the primary tumor with adjuvant chemotherapy or by using adjuvant chemotherapy alone.[7] Survival was longer when the dogs were treated with adjuvant chemotherapy after amputation.[7]

Despite terminal metastasis in the dog in our case, maintaining the leg and preventing metastasis and recurrence at the primary site may prove to be technically feasible. In this vein, we are currently treating another animal with adjuvant chemotherapy after osteotomy. That animal has been free of tumor for eight months.

We anticipate that block dissections, followed with allogenic bone grafts and adequate adjuvant drug therapy, may some day lead to a cure for canine osteosarcoma. Perhaps this technique will become routine for treating osteosarcome in both man and animals.

REFERENCES

1. Ling, G.W. *et al:* Primary Bone Tumors in the Dog: A Combined Clinical Radiographic, and Histologic Approach to Early Diagnosis. *JAVMA 165*:55-67; 1974.
2. Pool, R.R.: Tumors of the Skeleton, In *Tumors in Domestic Animals*, 2nd ed. (J.E. Moulton, ed.). Univ. of Calif. Press, Berkeley, Calif. (In press.)
3. Matsuno, T. *et al:* Telangiectatic Osteosarcoma. Abstracts of Papers, 65th Ann. Mtg. International Academy of Pathology. *Lab. Invest. 34*:325; 1976.
4. Brodey, R.S.: Surgical Treatment of Canine Osteosarcoma. *JAVMA 142*:729-735; 1965.
5. Owen, L.N.: Stevenson, D.E.: Observation on Canine Osteosarcomata. *Res. Vet. Sci. 2*:117-129; 1961.
6. Brodey, R.S.; Riser, W.H.: Canine Osteosarcoma: A Clinicopathologic Study of 194 Cases. *Clin. Orth. 62*:54-64; 1969.
7. Henness, A.H. *et al:* Combination Therapy for Canine Osteosarcoma. *JAVMA*. (In press.)

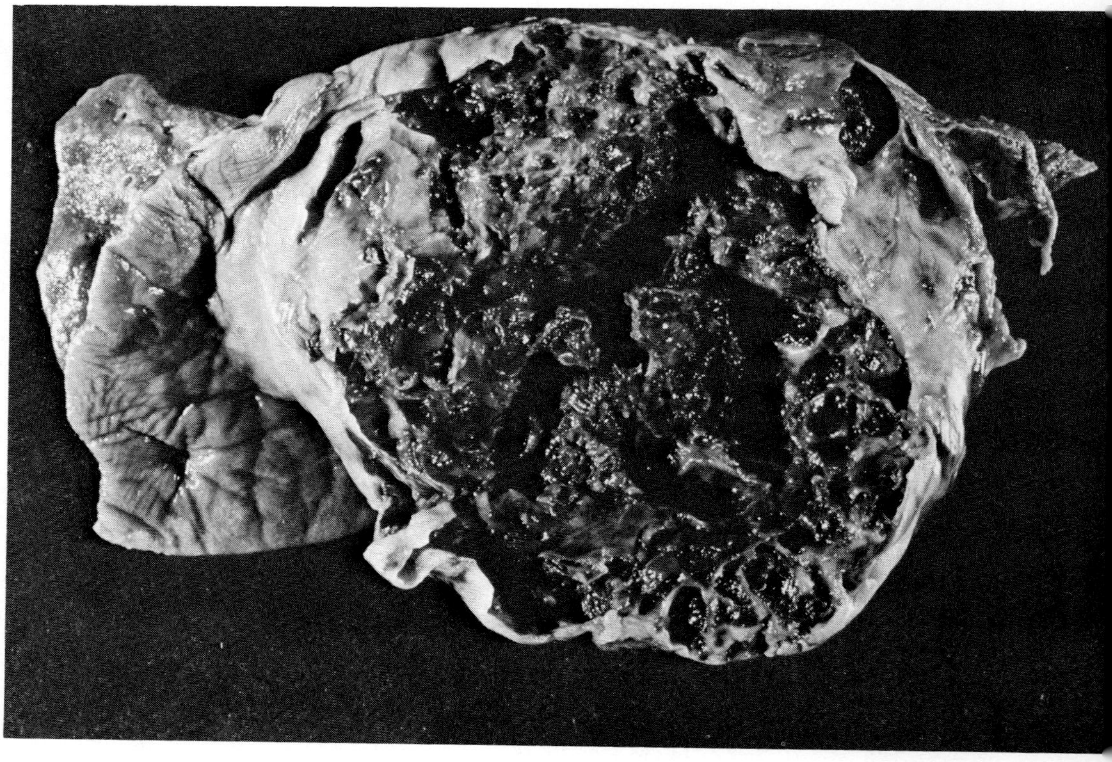

Figure 6 *(right)*—Photograph of the lung showing the large metastatic tumor. The tumor has been incised to demonstrate the blood-filled, cystic character of a telangiectatic osteosarcoma.

Osteochondritis Dissecans of the Elbow in a Dog

R. L. Leighton, VMD
School of Veterinary Medicine
University of California
Davis, California 95616

Diagnosis of osteochondritis dissecans of the elbow is sometimes difficult and may be overlooked as a cause of elbow lameness. By excellent radiographic technique the lesion can be demonstrated. Surgical treatment results in better healing and greater freedom from lameness than conservative measures. The surgical procedure is described and illustrated.

THE OCCURRENCE of osteochondritis dissecans of the canine humeral head with resulting shoulder lameness is well documented and the surgical repair well described.[1-17]

The knee, elbow, hip, and hock are also affected.[18-21] The basic treatment is arthrotomy with removal of the loose fragment(s) and curettage of the lesion. In the less common locations diagnosis is often difficult or may be missed.

In the elbow, the lesion develops in the medial condylar surface. With good techniques it can be shown radiographically *(Figures 1 & 2)*.

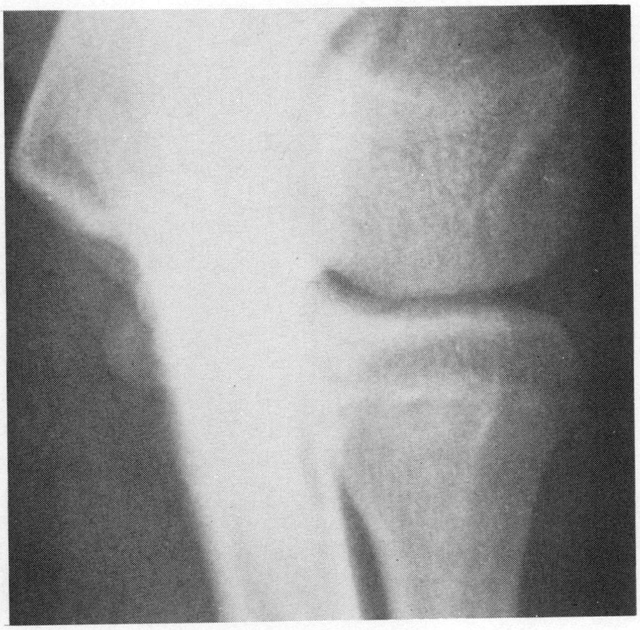

Figure 1—Oblique radiographic view of the normal canine elbow.

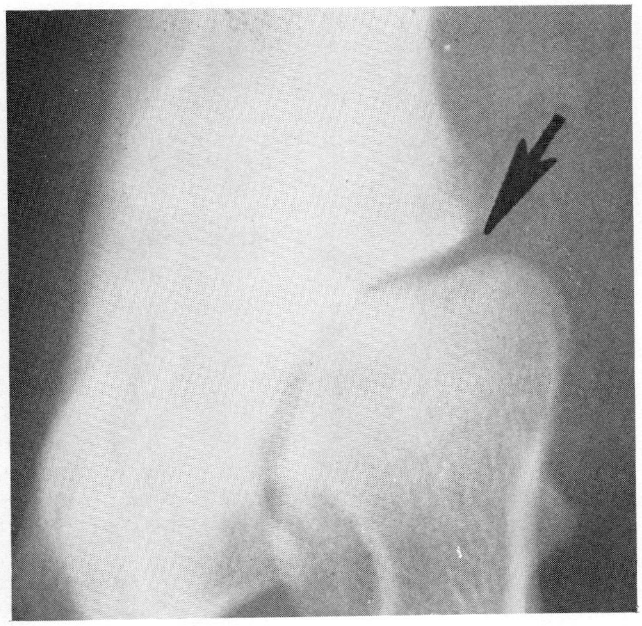

Figure 2—Radiograph showing osteochondritis dissecans of the medial humeral condyle *(arrow)*.

Case History

On August 17, 1977, a 7-month-old male Golden Retriever was presented at the small animal clinic of the Veterinary Medical Teaching Hospital, School of Veterinary Medicine, University of California. The history included limping on left front leg for more than two months. The dog would bear weight on the leg, but often held it up when standing. No external abnormalities were present, nor could pain be elicited on movement or palpation. The entire leg had been radiographed elsewhere with negative findings. Empirical treatment for osteomyelitis had not been beneficial. When most of the causes of foreleg lameness in young dogs were eliminated, a tentative diagnosis of osteochondritis dissecans of the elbow or fragmented coronoid process was made. Evidence of osteochondritis dissecans was shown radiographically.

Surgery was performed on August 22. The dog responded well to halothane and nitrous oxide anesthesia after premedication with acepromazine maleate (Ayerst) and atropine, and induction of anesthesia with Surital® (Parke-Davis).

The postoperative course in the hospital was without incident. Some swelling was noted. On August 25 the dog was discharged. At this time the animal was beginning to touch the paw to the ground. The dog made good progress and the owner was pleased with results of the surgery until October 4, when the dog again became lame in the same leg.

When examined on October 20, the dog was lively and active and only slightly favored the left front leg.

Figure 3—The sterile stockinette is cut over the site of the proposed incision on the caudomedial aspect of the elbow.

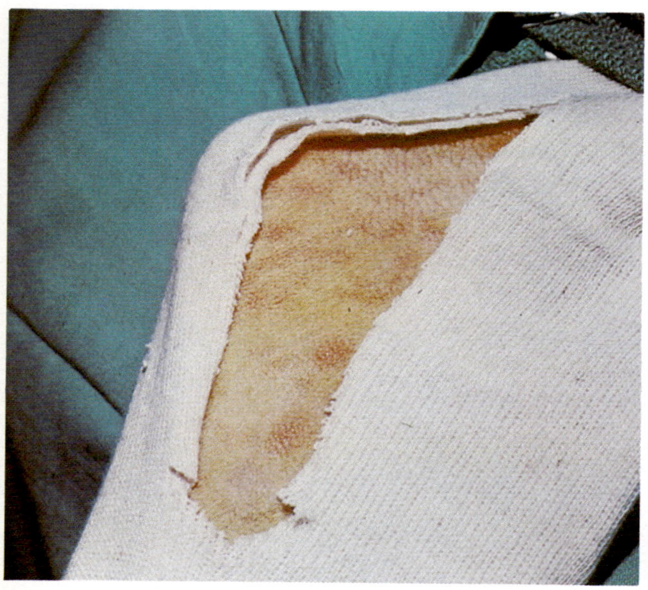

Figure 4—After the skin and subcutaneous tissue have been incised, the edges of the incision are secured to the stockinette with Autoclips® (Clay Adams).

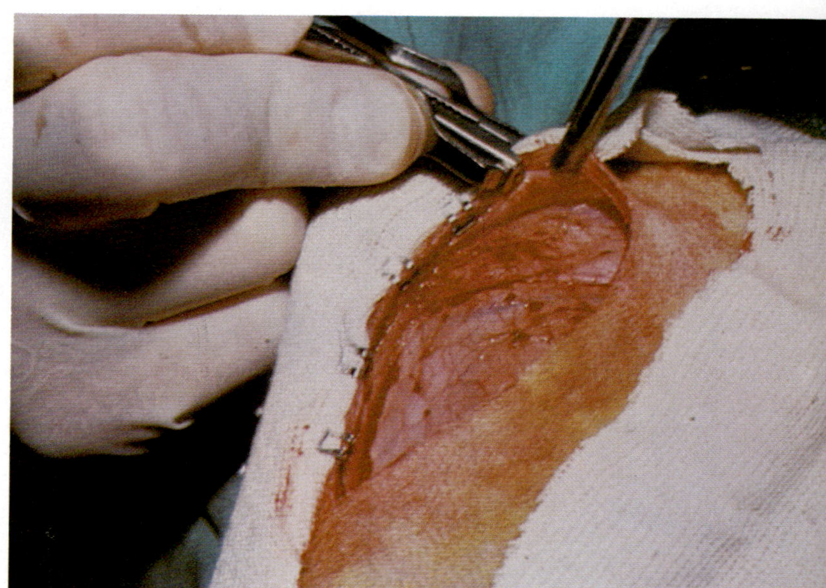

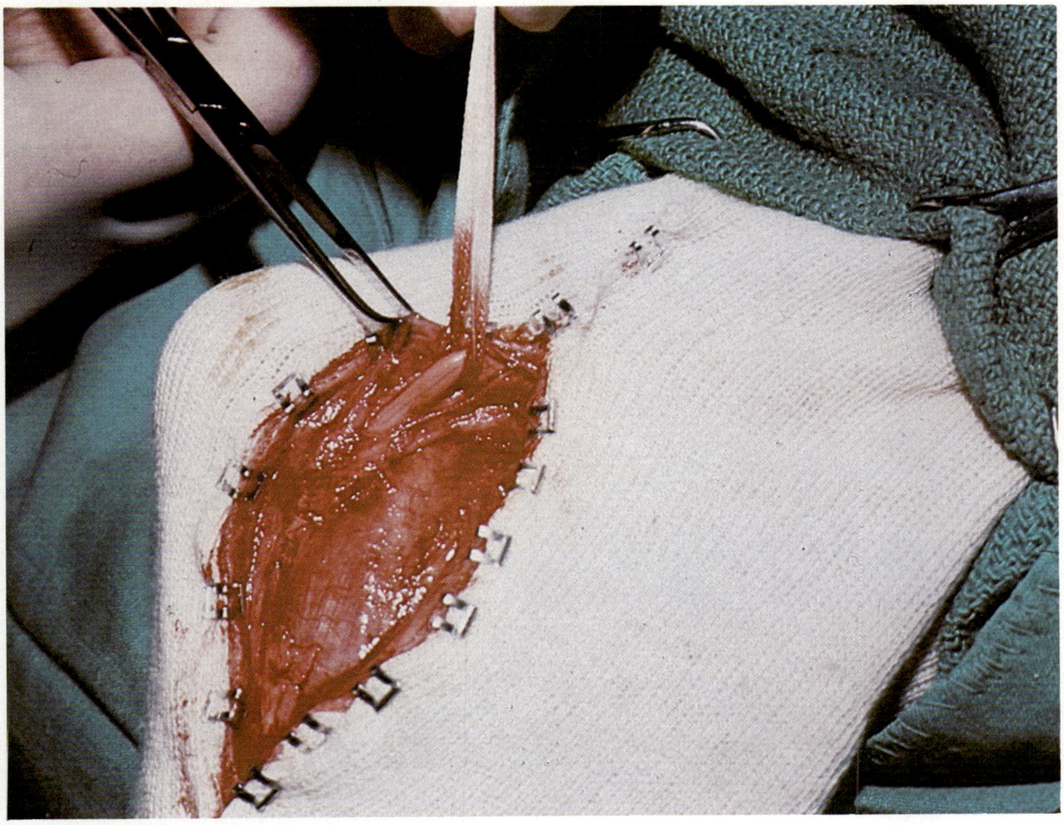

Figure 5
The ulnar nerve is isolated and retracted with umbilical tape.

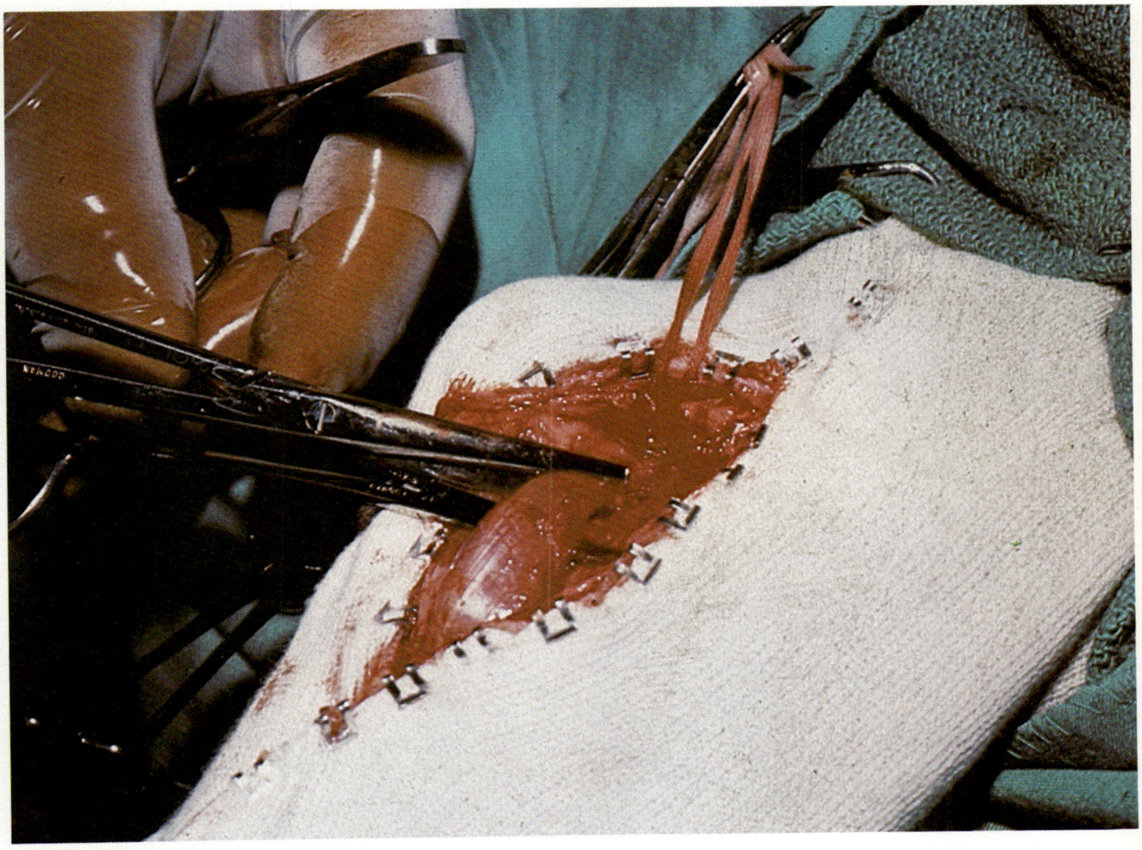

Figure 6
After the overlying fascia has been incised, the origin of the superficial digital flexor is isolated and transected.

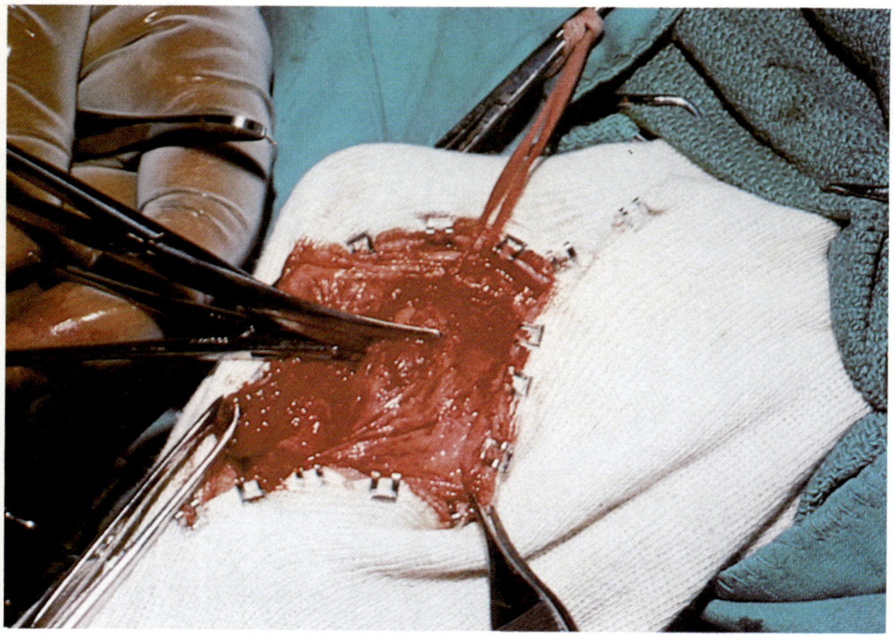

Figure 7 *(left)*—The deep digital flexor is transected at its origin.

Figure 8 *(below)*—When the joint capsule and radial collateral ligament have been incised, the joint is spread apart and the loose cartilage (shown in the mosquito forceps) is removed.

Figure 9 *(right)*—The underlying lesion on the caudal aspect of the medial humeral condyle is exposed.

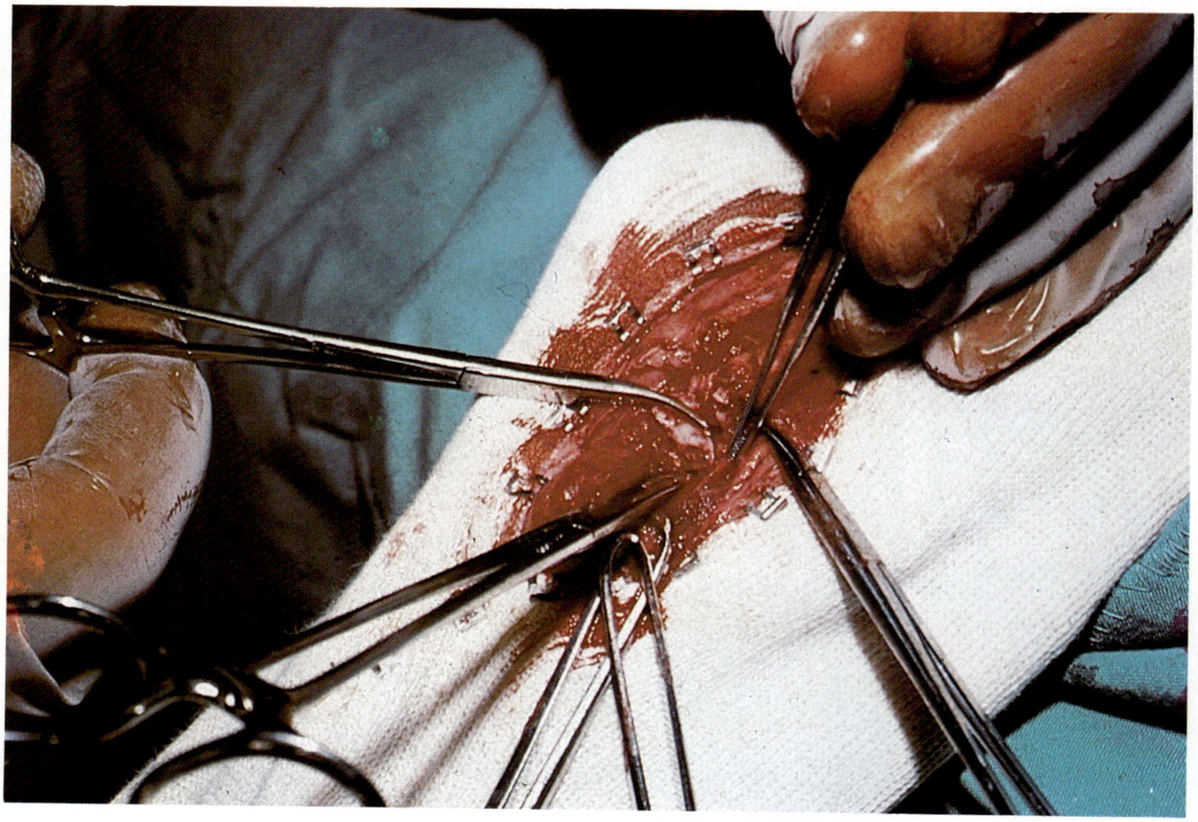

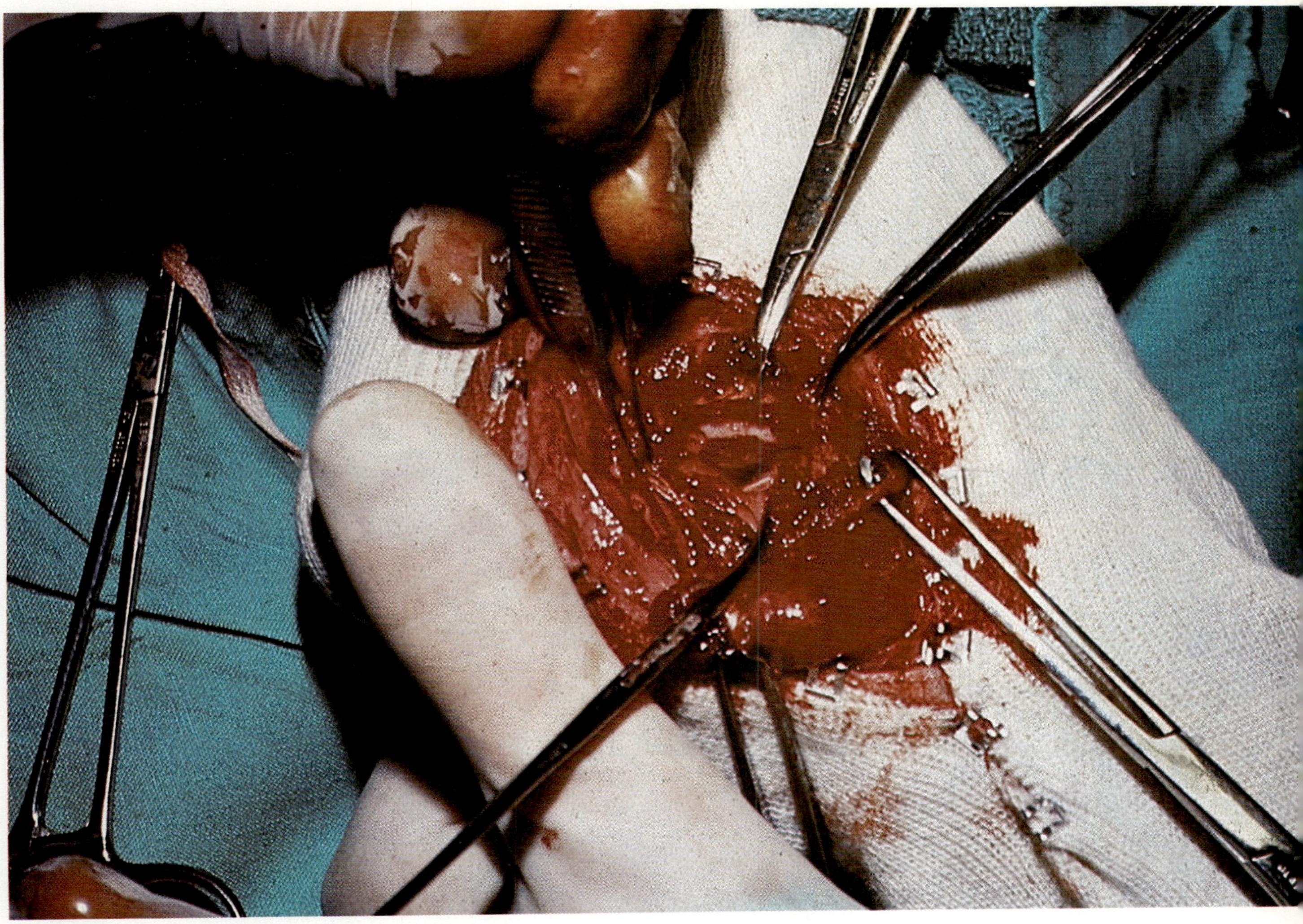

Surgical Procedure

A medial approach to the elbow joint was used. With the dog in the left lateral recumbency the area of the elbow was shaved, surgically prepared, and blocked off with four towels. The leg was covered with stockinette and inserted through a fenestrated drape, thus presenting the medial aspect to the surgeon.

The stockinette was cut with scissors at the proposed line of incision *(Figure 3)*. With the scalpel over the caudomedial aspect of the elbow, an incision was made through the skin and subcutaneous tissue. The stockinette was attached to the skin with Autoclips® (Clay Adams) *(Figure 4)*.

By palpation and sharp and blunt dissection the ulnar nerve was isolated and retracted with moistened umbilical tape *(Figure 5)*. After the overlying fascia had been incised, the origin of the superficial digital flexor was isolated and sectioned with Metzenbaum scissors *(Figure 6)*. The origin of the deep digital flexor was isolated and transected *(Figure 7)*.

The joint capsule and adjacent radial collateral ligament were severed with a scalpel and the joint entered. By distraction of the joint, the caudal aspect of the medial condyle was exposed. When the loose cartilage flap had been removed *(Figure 8)*, the underlying lesion was clearly visible *(Figure 9)*. The lesion was curetted with a 2-mm curette *(Figure 10)*.

After flushing, the joint was closed with 2-0 chromic catgut placed in the joint capsule and the radial collateral ligament *(Figure 11)*. The deep digital flexor head was replaced *(Figure 12)*, followed by the transected origin of the superficial digital flexor *(Figure 13)*. After removal of the tape from the ulnar nerve, the fascia was closed *(Figure 14)*. When the subcutaneous fascia was closed, the Autoclips were removed and a

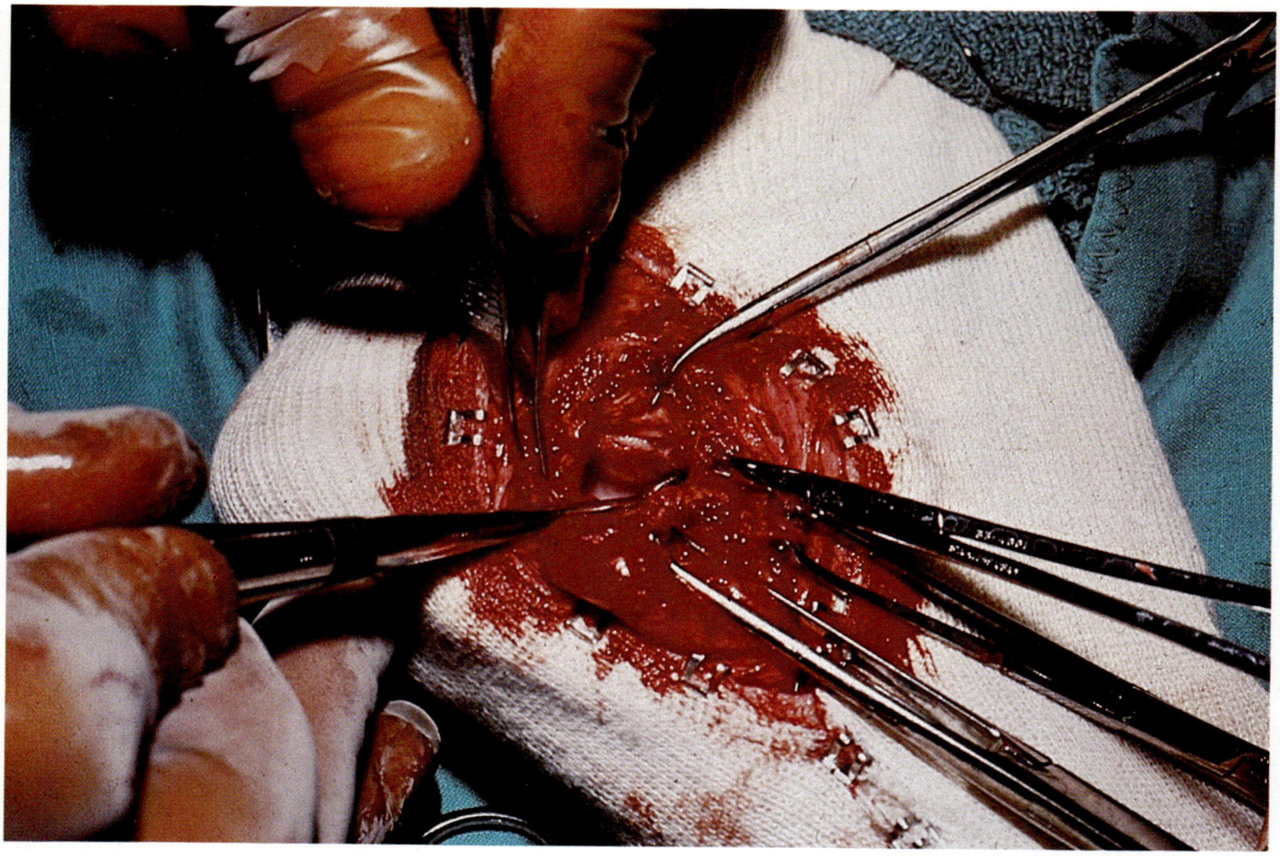

Figure 10
The lesion of osteochondritis dissecans is curetted with a 2-mm curette.

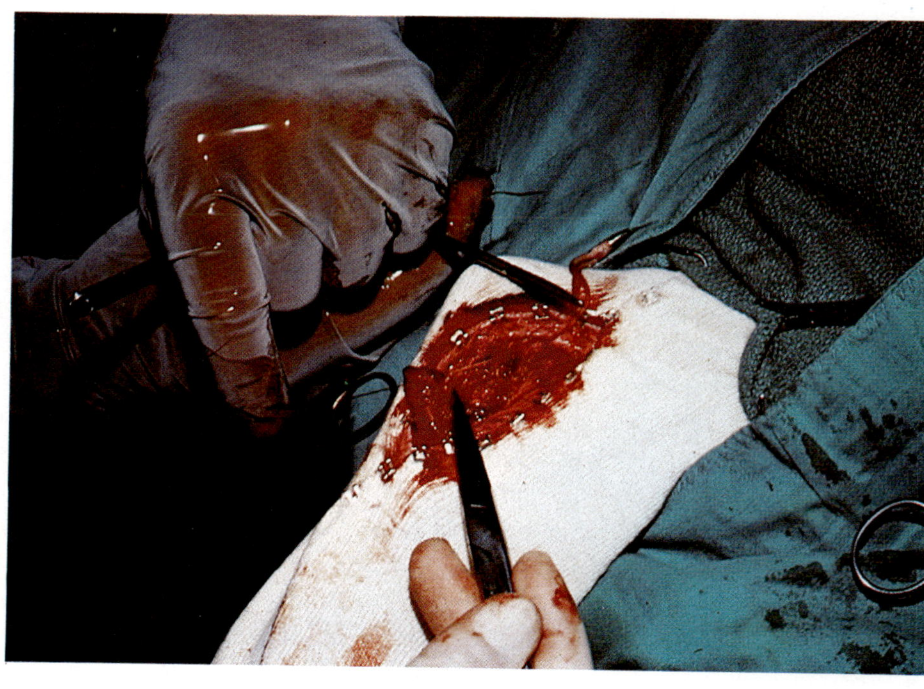

Figure 11
Closure of the joint capsule and radial collateral ligament is made with 2-0 chromic catgut.

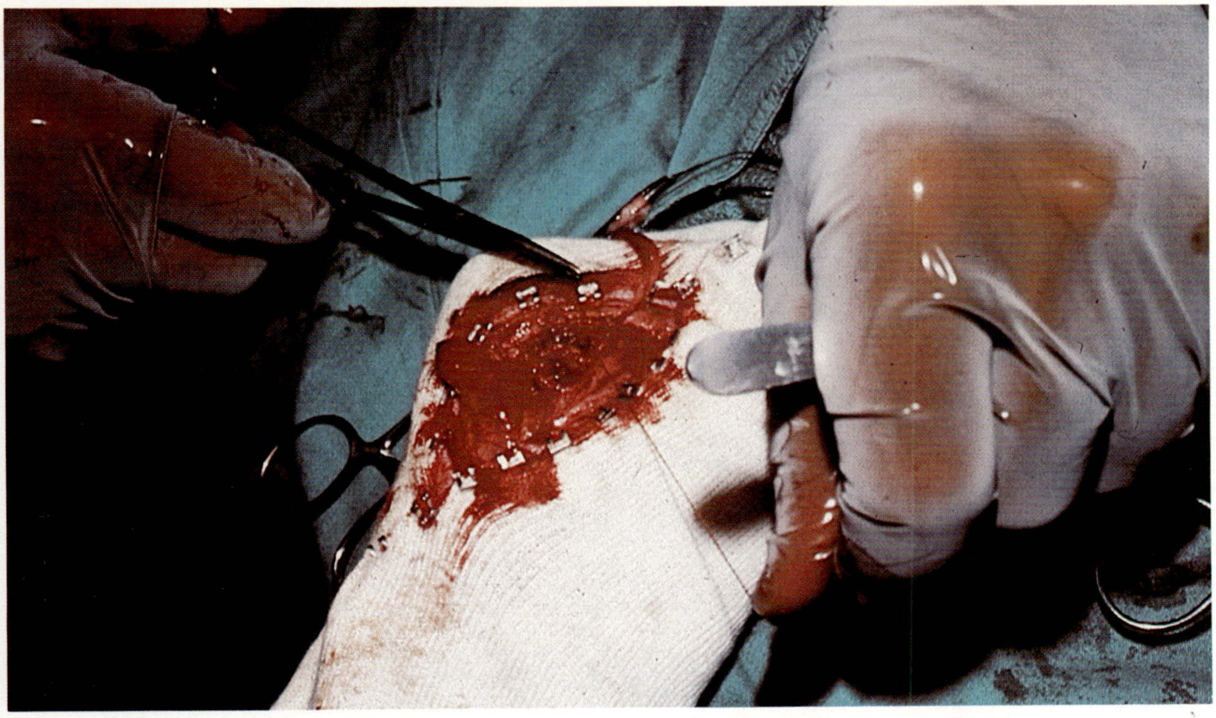

Figure 12
The head of the deep digital flexor is replaced using 2-0 chromic catgut.

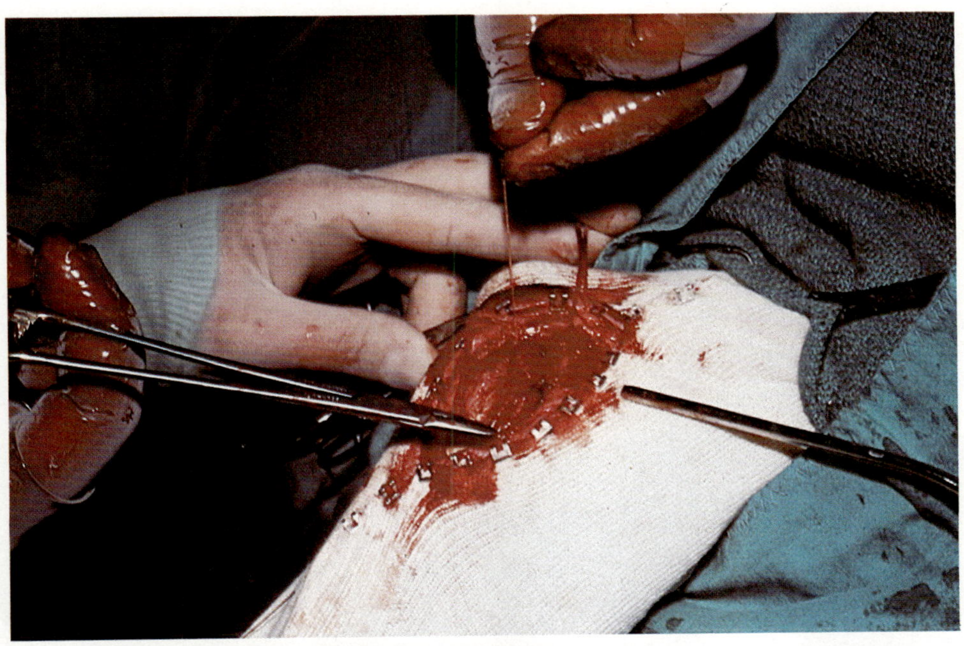

Figure 13
The head of the superficial digital flexor is replaced using 2-0 chromic catgut. The tape is removed from the ulnar nerve.

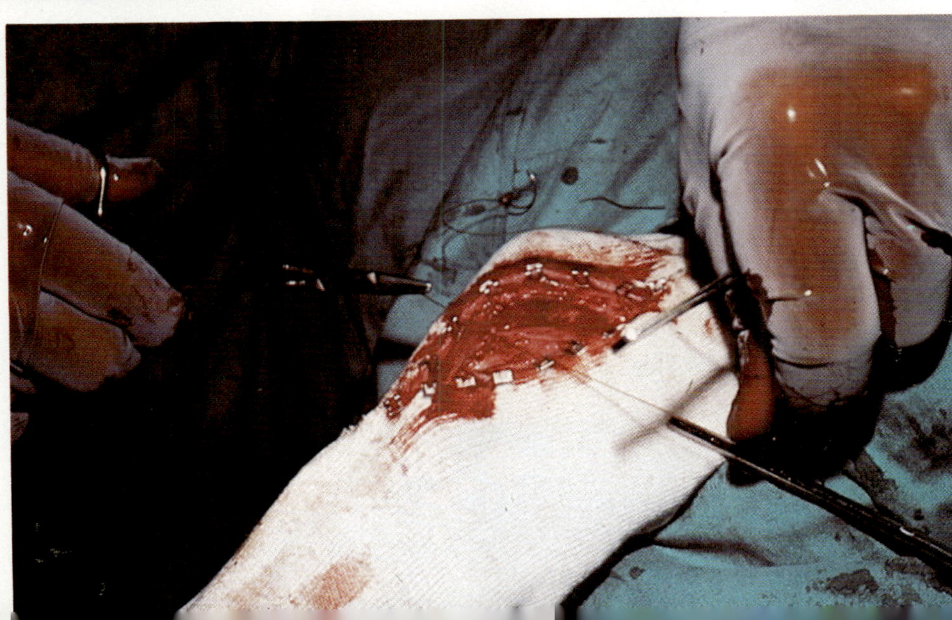

Figure 14
The fascia is closed.

subcuticular skin closure was done *(Figure 15).* The skin incision was closed with No. 30 Vetafil® (S. Jackson) *(Figure 16).*

No bandaging or splinting is required following this procedure. Possible postoperative sequellae are edema and formation of seromas.

REFERENCES

1. Aul, D.G.: Hinko, P.J.: A Review: Modified Approach for Surgical Treatment of Osteochondritis Dissecans in the Humeral Head. *Canine Practice 2:*28-30; 1975.
2. Birkeland R.: Osteochondritis Dissecans in the Humeral Head of the Dog. *Nord. Vet. Med. 19:*294-306; 1967.
3. Birkeland, R.: In *Proceedings of the 12th Nordic Veterinary Congress*, Reykjavik: 7-10 August, 1974. A/S Conf. Fr. Mortensen. Copenhagen, Denmark, 1974; pp 26-29.
4. Chaffe, V.W.; Knecht, C.D.: A Modified Posterior Approach to the Canine Scapulohumeral Joint. *JAAHA 12:*782-783; 1976.
5. Cordy, D.R.; Wind, A.P.: Transverse Fracture of the Proximal Humeral Articular Cartilage in Dogs (So-Called Osteochondritis Dissecans). *Pathologico Vet. 6:*424-436; 1969.
6. Dee, J.F.: A Simplified Approach to the Canine Shoulder for the Treatment of Osteochondritis Dissecans. *JAAHA 8:*111-114; 1972.
7. Griffiths, R.C.: Osteochondritis Dissecans of the Canine Shoulder. *JAVMA 156:*1733-1735; 1968.
8. Hohn, R.B.: Osteochondritis Dissecans of the Humeral Head. *JAVMA 163:*69-70; 1973.
9. Jones, D.G.C.; Vaughan, L.C.: The Surgical Treatment of Osteochondritis Dissecans of the Humeral Heads in Dogs. *J. Small Anim. Pract. 11:*803-812; 1970.
10. Leighton, R.L.: Osteochondritis Dissecans of the Shoulder Joint of the Dog. *Vet. Clinics of N. Am.1:*391-401; 1971.
11. Paatsama, S. *et al*: Changes in Osteochondritis of the Canine Humeral Head: *Scand. J. Clin. Lab. Invest. 27* (Suppl. 16): 29; 1971.
12. Paatsama, S.: Experimental Studies (in Dogs) of the Aetiology of Osteochondrosis. In *Proceedings of the 12th Nordic Veterinary Congress*, Reykjavik; 7-10 August, 1974. A/S Conf. Fr. Martensen. Copenhagen, Denmark, 1974; pp 24-25 (Abst. 6078).
13. Paatsama, S.*et al:*A Study of Osteochondritis Dissecans of the Canine Humeral Head Using Histological, OTC Bone Labeling, Microradiographic and Microangiographic Methods. *J. Small Anim. Pract. 12:*603-611; 1971 (Abst. 2019).
14. Smitch, L.W.; Stowater, J.L.: Osteochondritis Dissecans of the Shoulder Joint: A Review of 35 cases. *JAAHA 11:*658-662; 1975.
15. Vaughn, L.C.; Jones, D.G.C.: Osteochondritis Dissecans of the Head of the Humerus in Dogs. *J. Small Anim. Pract. 9:*983-994; 1968.
16. Wolfe, D.A.: Surgical Correction of Osteochondritis Dissecans of the Medial Humeral Condyle and Ununited Coronoid Process in a Dog. *VM/SAC 71:*1554-1557; 1976.
17. Wood, A.D.K.*et al:*Osteochondritis Dissecans of the Distal Humerus in a Dog. *Vet. Record 96:*489-490; 1975.
18. Grondalen, J.; Grondalen T.: Osteochondritis in the Knee Joints of Dogs. Comparative Aspects. In *Proceedings of the 12th Nordic Veterinary Congress*, Reykjavik; 7-10 August, 1974. U/S. Conf. Fr. Martensen. Copenhagen, Denmark, 1974; pp 30-31.
19. Herron, M.R.: Osteochondritis of the Femoral Head -- Diagnosis and Therapy. *Southwest. Vet. 23:*9-13; 1969.
20. Punzet, G. *et al:* Osteochondrosis Dissecans of the Stifle Joint in the Dog. *Kleintier-Praxis 20:*88-98; 1975.
21. Robins, G.M.: A Case of Osteochondritis Dissecans of the Stifle Joint in a Bitch. *J. Small Anim. Pract. 11:*813-817; 1970.

Figure 15—With the Autoclips removed and the subcutaneous closure made, subcuticular sutures are placed.

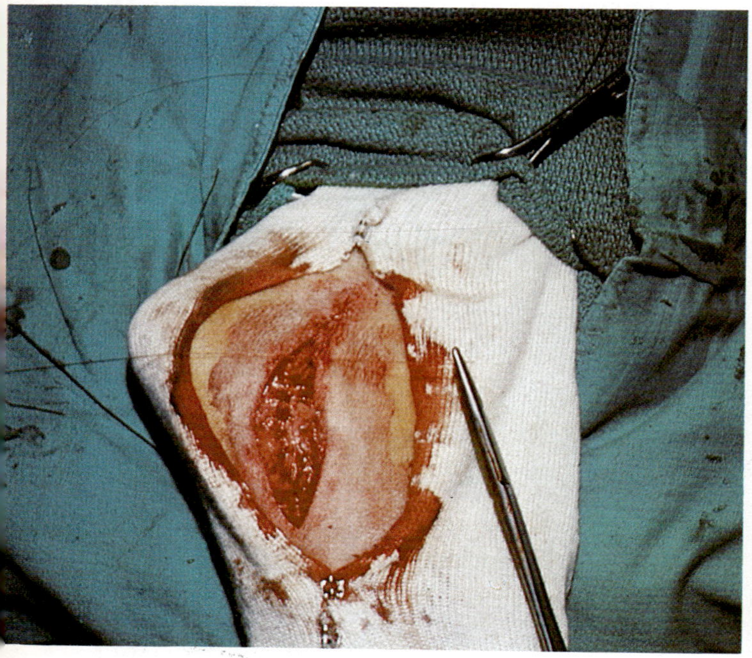

Figure 16—The skin is closed with No. 30 Vetafil® (S. Jackson).

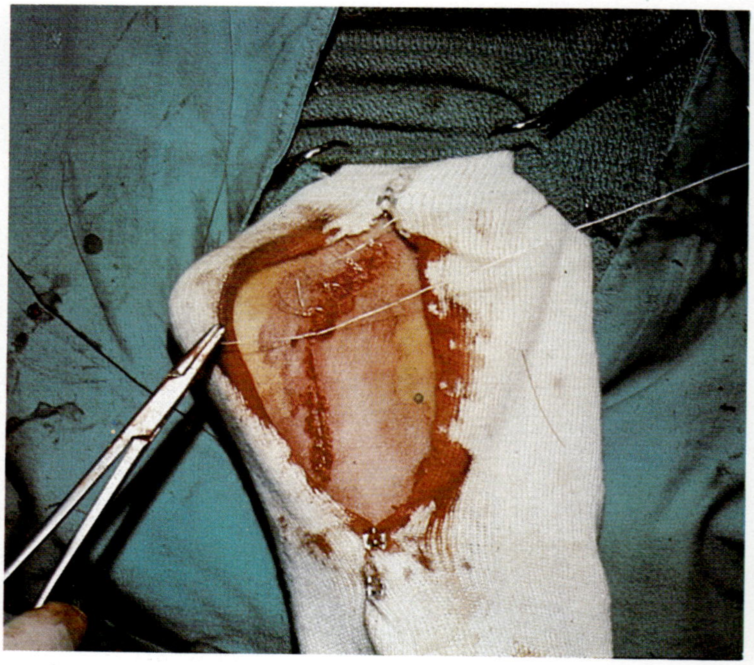

a technique for DECLAWING CATS

L. D. Rubin, VMD
D. C. Maplesden, DVM, PhD / Rhawnhurst Animal Hospital, 7905 Bustleton Avenue
Philadelphia, Pennsylvania 19152

ONYCHECTOMY is considered a relatively simple procedure.[1,3] However, the operation does not always go as smoothly as the surgeon would like. A few special techniques can help minimize bleeding and complications.

The patient is given a general anesthetic, usually ketamine. To prevent hemorrhage when removing the claws, the thumb of the left hand is pressed firmly against the metacarpal or metatarsal pad. Pressure is maintained on the ball of the thumb to control hemorrhage while the tip of the thumb is rolled forward to put pressure on the footpad of the individual third phalanx. Pressure is simultaneously applied on the dorsum of the digit with the index finger. This procedure completely exposes the claw and third phalanx and permits clean, neat removal of the claw.

A sterile, sharp nail clipper is carefully hooked over the third phalanx. The entire phalanx and appendages are removed by gentle traction on the clipper (*Figure 1*). All claws on the foot are removed. The cavities left after the claws are extracted are dusted with an antimicrobial powder (*Figure 2*). The foot is neatly and firmly wrapped with a Kling(R) bandage (Johnson & Johnson), which is placed above the carpus (*Figure 3*).

Four strips of 1-inch adhesive tape are applied. The first strip is applied starting dorsally above the carpus and continuing around the foot and on the ventral aspect to just above the carpus. The second strip is applied in a similar manner on the lateral and medial aspects of the foot. The remaining two pieces of adhesive tape are applied around the foot. The last strip should catch about ⅜ inch of the hair around the leg above the Kling bandage. This anchors the bandage to prevent it from slipping off the foot.

The bandages are removed in 24 hours. They are cut down the dorsal aspect using bandage scissors. When all four feet have been declawed, all four bandages should be split before any bandages are removed. If the bandages are removed from the hind feet before the bandages on the front feet are cut, the cat may attempt to claw with the hind feet and hemorrhaging may occur. Once all bandages are cut, they are easily slipped off, beginning with the front feet.

REFERENCES

1. Bojrab, M.J., ed.: *Current Technique in Small Animal Surgery.* Lea & Febiger, Philadelphia, Pa. 1975; pp 273-275.
2. Nagle, A.C.: A Technique for Feline Onychectomy. *VM/SAC* (ISSN 0042-4889) *71*(12):1685-1687; Dec. 1976.
3. Goodyear, M.D.: A Technique for Onychectomy in the Cat. *VM/SAC* (ISSN 0042-4889) *72*(4):569-572; Apr. 1977.

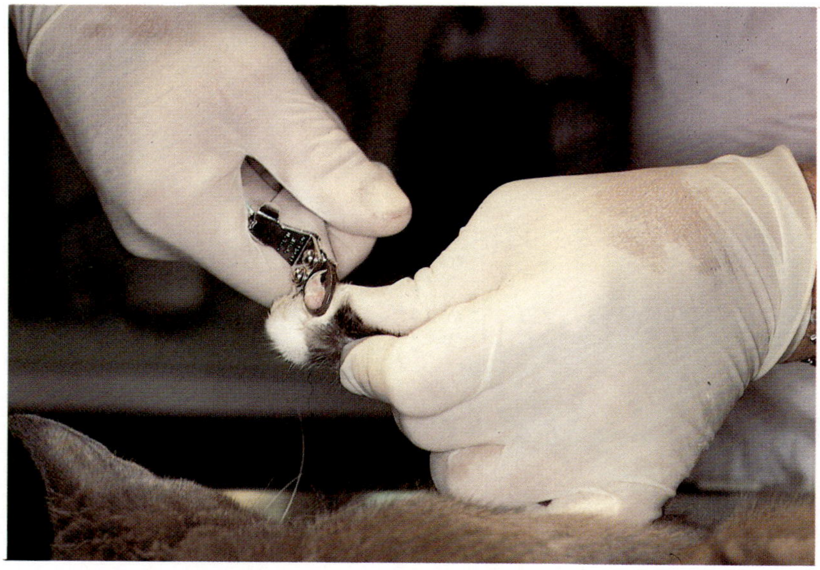

Figure 1
Hemorrhage is controlled by firmly pressing the thumb against the metacarpal pad while a sterile sharp nail clipper is hooked over the third phalanx.

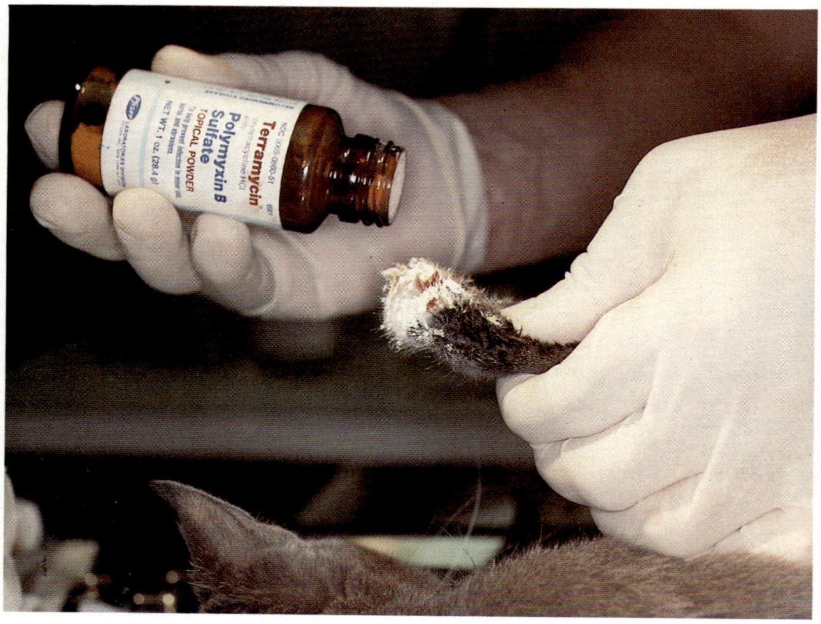

Figure 2
While hemorrhage is still controlled, the exposed cavities are dusted with an antimicrobial powder.

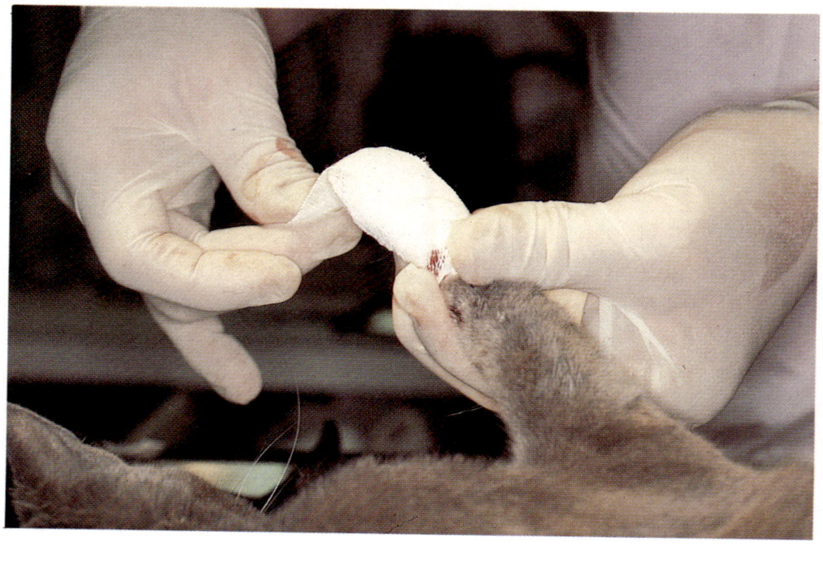

Figure 3
The foot is bandaged with a Kling bandage before adhesive tape is applied.

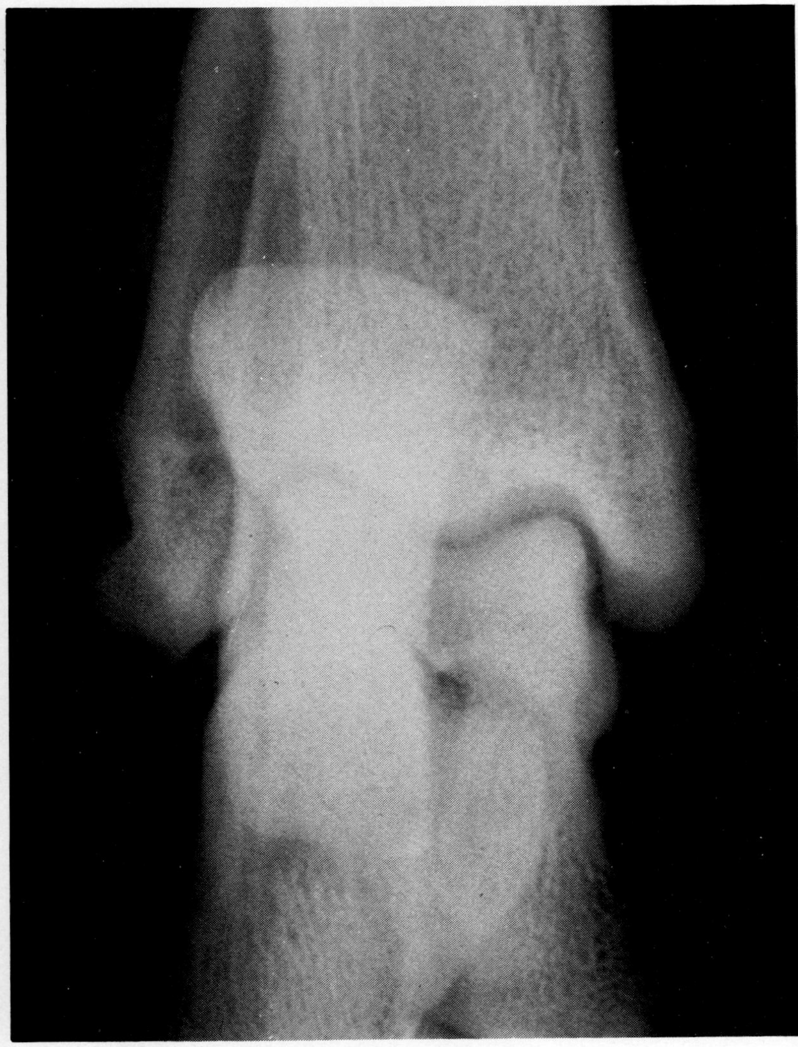

Figure 1
Anteroposterior radiographic view of a normal hock joint in a dog. Compare with Figure 2 *(next page)* showing a diseased hock joint.

Osteochondritis dissecans of the hock in a dog

Robert L. Leighton, VMD
School of Veterinary Medicine
University of California
Davis, California 95616

Osteochondritis dissecans in the shoulder, elbow, and stifle of the dog is well documented.[1,2] It occurs uncommonly in the hock, and as a cause of chronic lameness might be overlooked as a possibility in the differential diagnosis. Definitive diagnosis can be made by x-ray (*Figures 1 & 2*). Surgical relief is provided by an arthrotomy and curettage of the lesion, with removal of loose cartilage as foreign bodies. The approach is by a caudomedial incision which permits direct entry into the joint.[3]

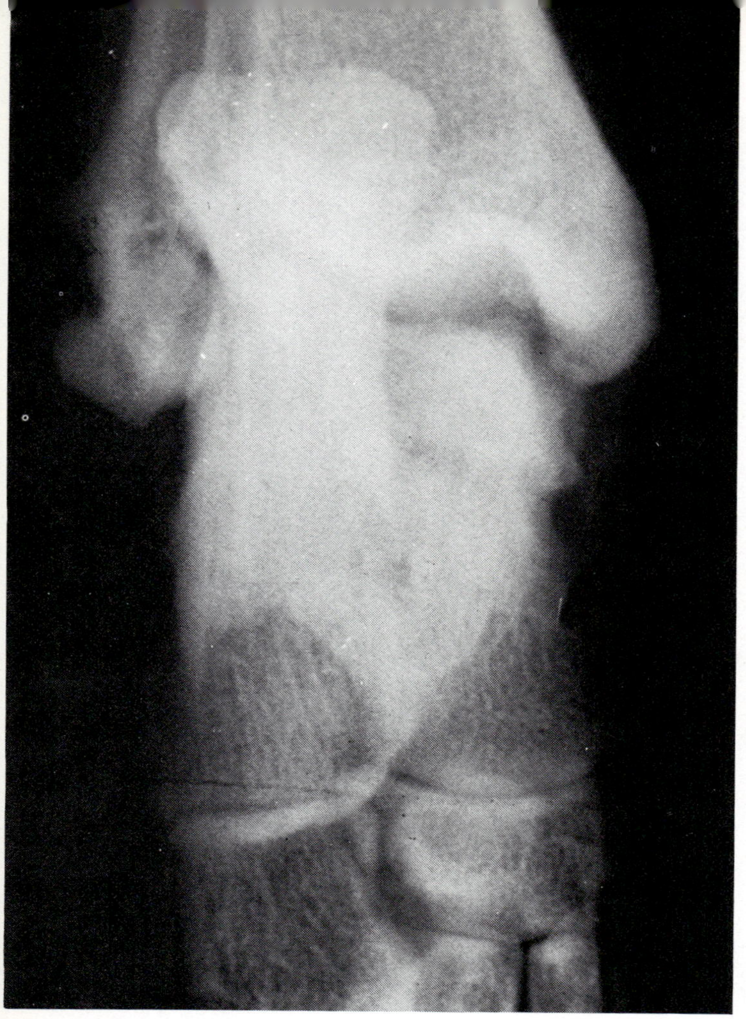

Figure 2
Anteroposterior radiograph of the hock showing the lesion situated caudomedially on the medial articular ridge of the tibiotarsal bone.

Case History

A 1-year-old black female Labrador Retriever was presented at the clinic of the Veterinary Medical Teaching Hospital because of a chronically developing lameness in the left hock that had been present since the dog was 10 weeks old. When the animal was 5 months of age, arthrocentesis was performed and radiographs were made without leading to a diagnosis. The lameness continued intermittently for several months until the dog became constantly lame. At that time the dog was referred to the Veterinary Medical Teaching Hospital. When the patient was examined, its left tarsus was found to be swollen and the joint filled with fluid. The report on fluid withdrawn from the joint showed the following:

Hazy, straw color

Good mucin clot test

Refractive index	1:3390
RBC	less than 2,000/ml
WBC	1,300/ml
No neutrophils	
Small mononuclear cells	13%
Large mononuclear cells	87%

Radiographs showed a defect in the medial trochlea of the left tibiotarsal bone. This was believed to be a

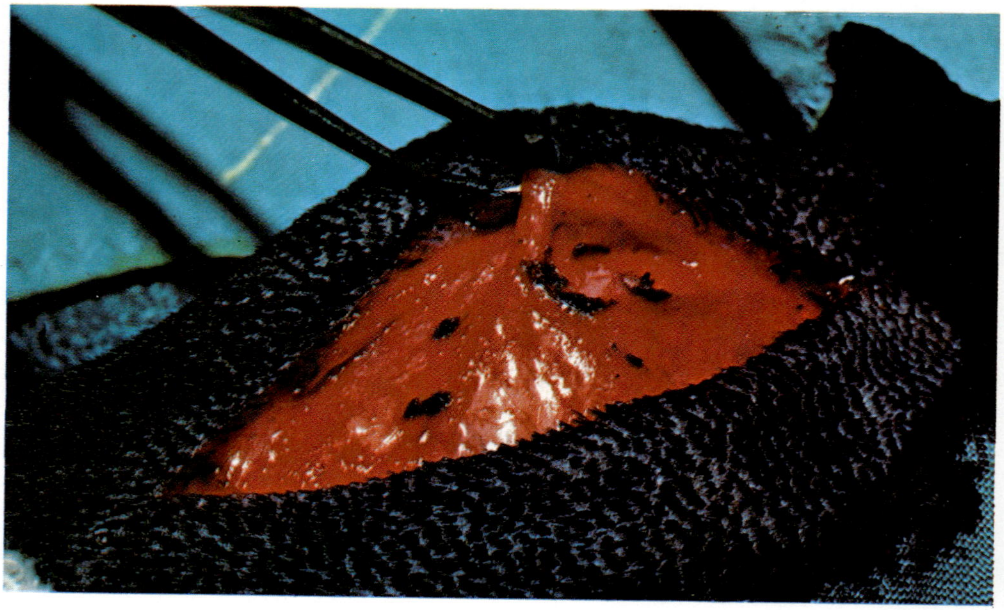

Figure 3
The incision in the skin and subcutaneous tissue is made over the caudomedial aspect of the hock and centered midway between the fibular tarsal bone and the medial malleolus.

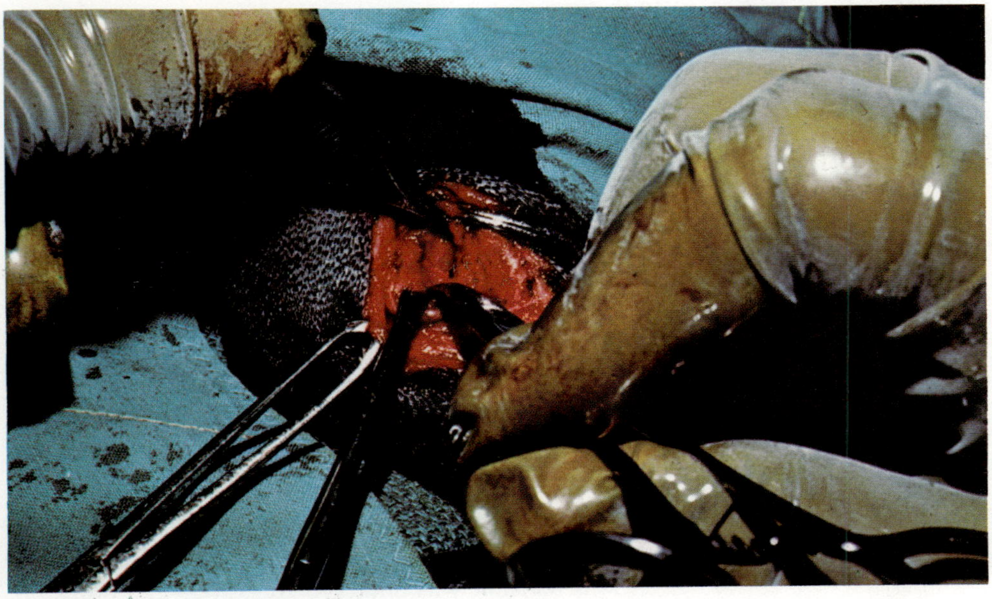

Figure 4
The incision has been carried into the hock joint by continued cutting with the scalpel.

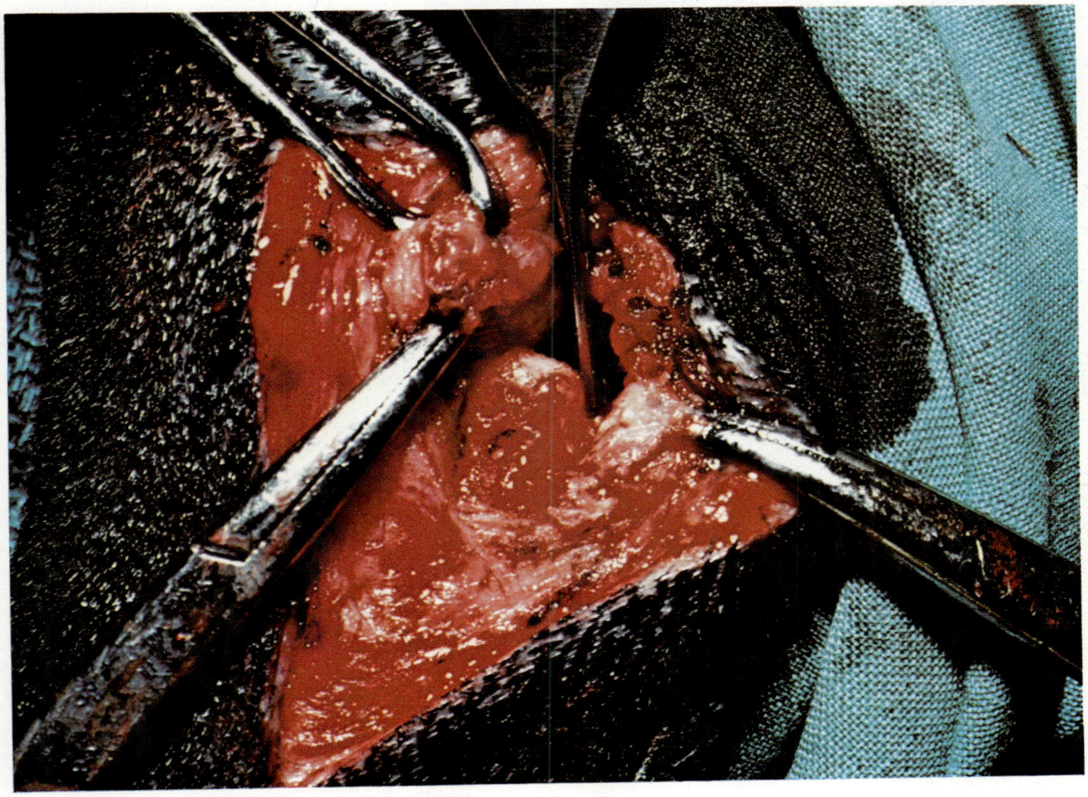

Figure 5
In this view the surrounding tissues have been cleared away, and the joint can be seen when lateral tension is applied to the foot.

Figure 6
The lesion of osteochondritis dissecans is curetted with a 2-mm curette.

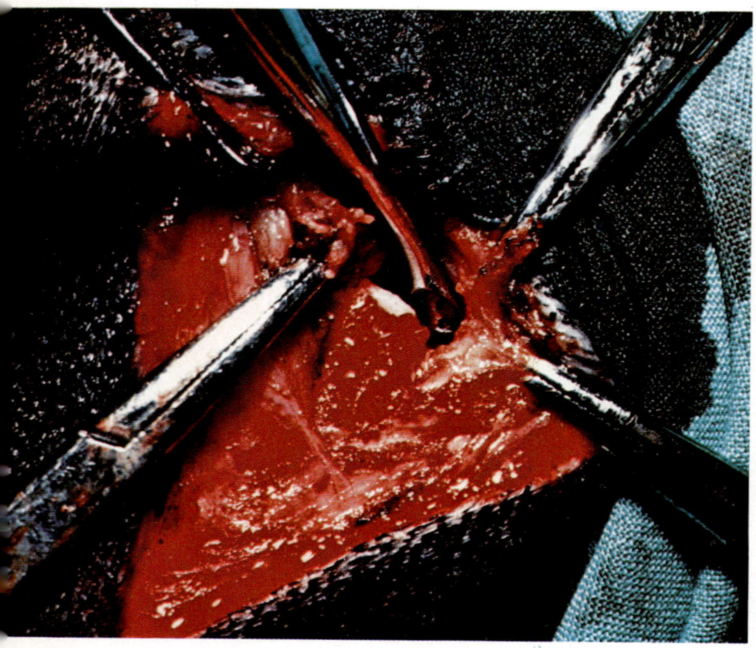

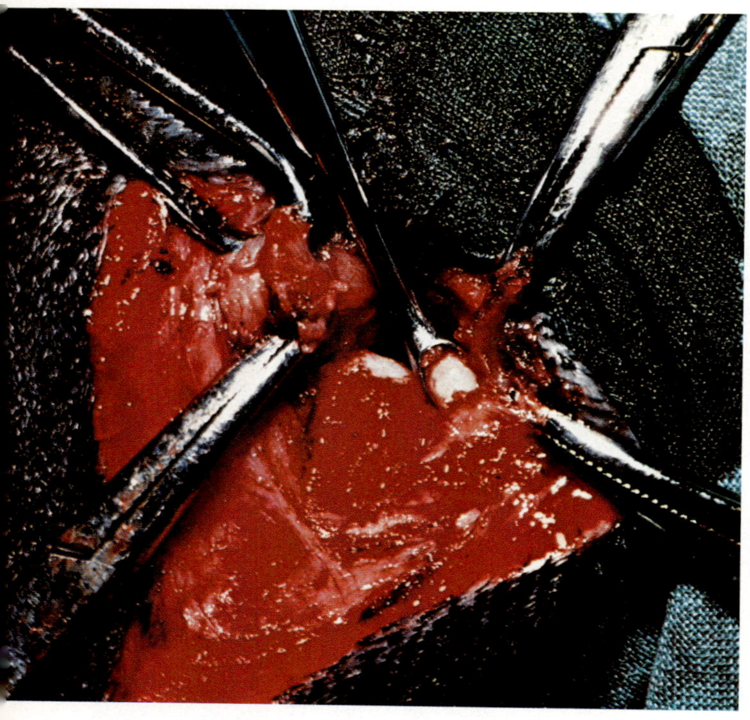

Figure 7
A loose body (seen in the curette) is removed.

defect in endochondral ossification, possibly due to early trauma.

The joint was entered surgically and the lesion curetted. A loose foreign body (joint mouse) was removed.

Surgical Technique

With the dog in left lateral recumbency under general anesthesia, the previously shaved and surgically prepared area of the left hock was blocked off with sterile towels. The foot was covered with a sterile stockinette and inserted through a fenestrated drape.

Midway between the fibular tarsal bone and the medial malleolus a longitudinal caudomedial incision, about 6 cm long, was made with the scalpel through the skin and subcutaneous tissue (*Figure 3*). The incision was continued with the scalpel until the joint was entered (*Figure 4*).

This incision was enlarged to expose the joint and the caudomedial aspect of the dorsal portion of the tibiotarsal articular surface (*Figure 5*). By application of lateral traction to the foot, the joint space could be opened to allow inspection and curettage of the lesion (*Figure 6*). A loose fragment (joint mouse) was removed (*Figure 7*) and the joint was flushed clean with saline solution (*Figure 8*).

Closure of the thickened joint capsule and fibrous connective tissue over the joint was achieved with 2-0 chromic catgut (*Figure 9*). Subcutaneous tissue was closed with 2-0 catgut, and the skin with Number 30 Vetafil® (S. Jackson).

The foot was bandaged in a modified Robert Jones splint for a few days. One week after surgery the dog was released. A good recovery ensued.

REFERENCES

1. Harrison, W.J.; Hohn, R.B.: Osteochondritis Dissecans. In *Current Techniques in Small Animal Surgery—I* (M.J. Bojrab, ed.). Lea & Febiger, Philadelphia, Pa., 1975; p 509.
2. Leighton, R.L.: Osteochondritis Dissecans of the Elbow in a Dog. *VM/SAC* 73(3):311-318; March 1978.
3. Piermattei, D.L.; Greeley, R.G.: Approach to the Distal End of the Tibia and the Hock Joint Through a Medial Incision. In *An Atlas of Surgical Approaches to the Bones and Joints of the Dog and Cat*. W.B. Saunders, Philadelphia, Pa., 1966; pp 118-119.

Figure 8

The joint is flushed with saline solution. The curetted lesion is seen at the lower left, directly dorsal to the tip of the hemostat.

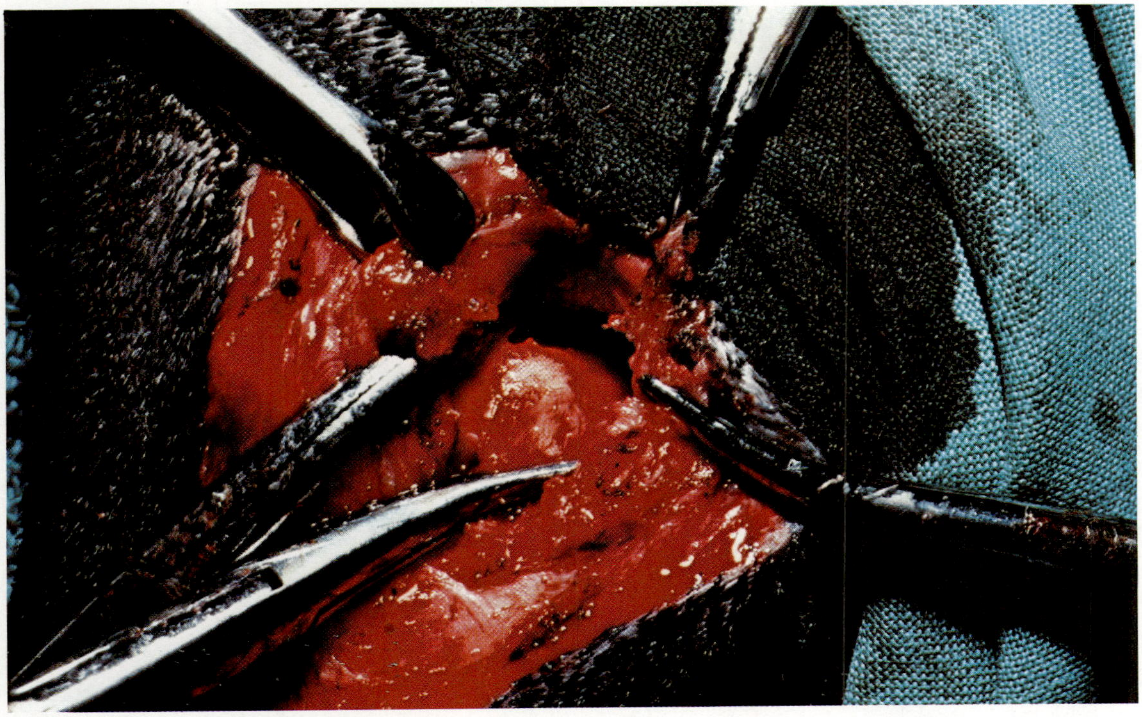

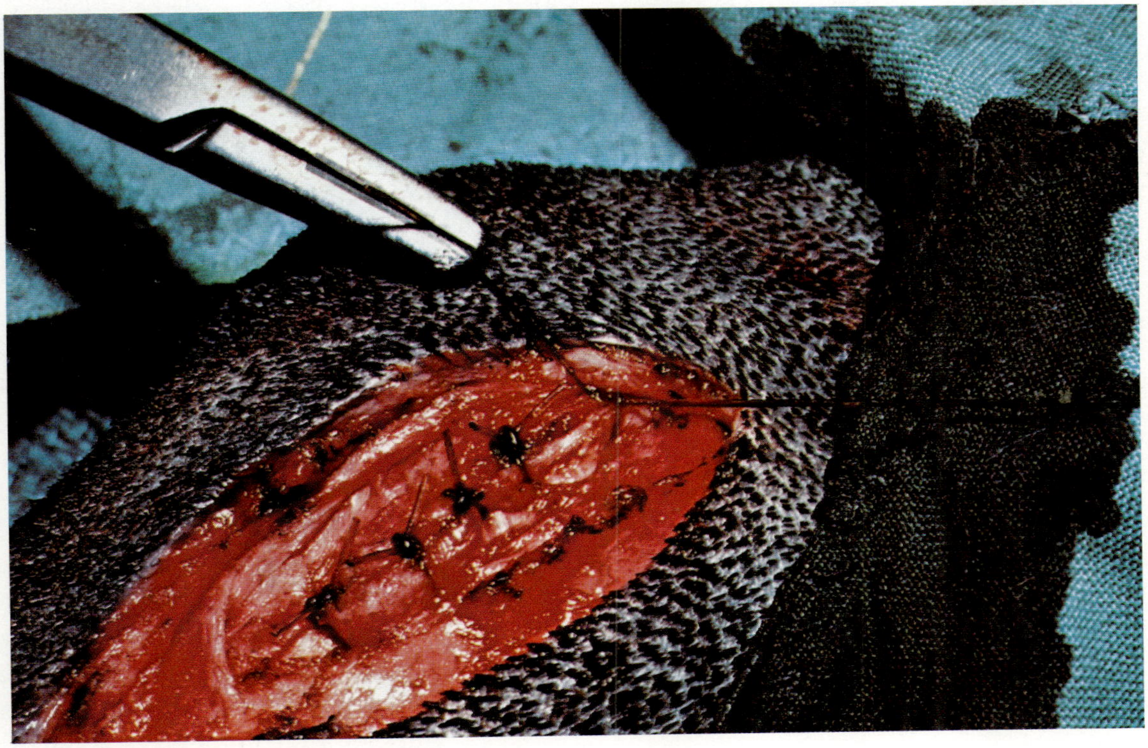

Figure 9

The joint capsule and thickened fascia are closed with 2-0 catgut. Other closure is routine.

OSTEOCHONDRITIS DISSECANS

of the shoulder joint: its surgical treatment

Roy T. Faulkner, DVM
Dept. of Small Animal Clinical Sciences
College of Veterinary Medicine
University of Minnesota
St. Paul, Minnesota 55108

OSTEOCHONDRITIS DISSECANS (OCD), a common orthopedic problem, can successfully be treated with gratifying results. Apprehension about performing joint surgery should not make the veterinary clinician reluctant to treat this disease. Osteochondritis dissecans is easily diagnosed radiographically. Although lesions of OCD can occur in the medial humeral condyle, lateral femoral condyle, medial condyle of the tibial tarsal bone, and end plates of the cervical vertebrae, the caudal aspect of the humeral head is most often affected.[1]

Incidence

Although some canine breeds are statistically more prone to OCD than others,[2,3] local incidence of the disease in a breed also depends on the breed's popularity in a given geographic area. Generally, the breeds affected are those that mature to weights greater than 60 lb. Other orthopedic diseases common to these breeds (hip dysplasia, panosteitis, ununited anconeal process, ununited coronoid process) should be ruled out. I have found that concurrent orthopedic diseases are not uncommon. One dog had unilateral OCD, bilateral subluxation of the coxofemoral joints, and panosteitis.

Most dogs presented because of foreleg lameness are less than 12 months old, the average being 8 to 10 months. The incidence of OCD in males has been reported to be two to five times greater than in females.[3,4] Bilateral lesions occur in 40 to 65% of reported cases.[2-4]

Clinical signs

Although OCD may be bilateral, the usual case presents with a unilateral foreleg lameness. Infrequently, animals in severe pain from bilateral lesions may be presented with the rear legs drawn forward, thus shifting more weight onto the hindquarters. Such cases might be mistakenly evaluated as problems of the hind legs.

A thorough, systematic examination starting at the distal leg is essential. The most consistent finding is the presence of pain when the shoulder joint is extended or flexed. A joint should be fully flexed and extended before it is pronounced free of pain. The shoulder joint should be isolated as much as possible during palpation and manipulation. Patients believed to have shoulder pain may be radiographically free of OCD but may have lesions of panosteitis. In cases of panosteitis, response to pressure on an overly sensitive distal humerus and proximal ulna during manipulation of the shoulder may be misinterpreted as evidence of shoulder pain. Many dogs with panosteitis react with well-defined signs of pain when digital pressure is applied to the bone.

Atrophy of the supraspinatus and infraspinatus muscles is often detected, especially when these muscles are compared to those of the contralateral leg. Joint effusion and crepitation are evident in longstanding cases in which the degree of osteoarthrosis has become significant.

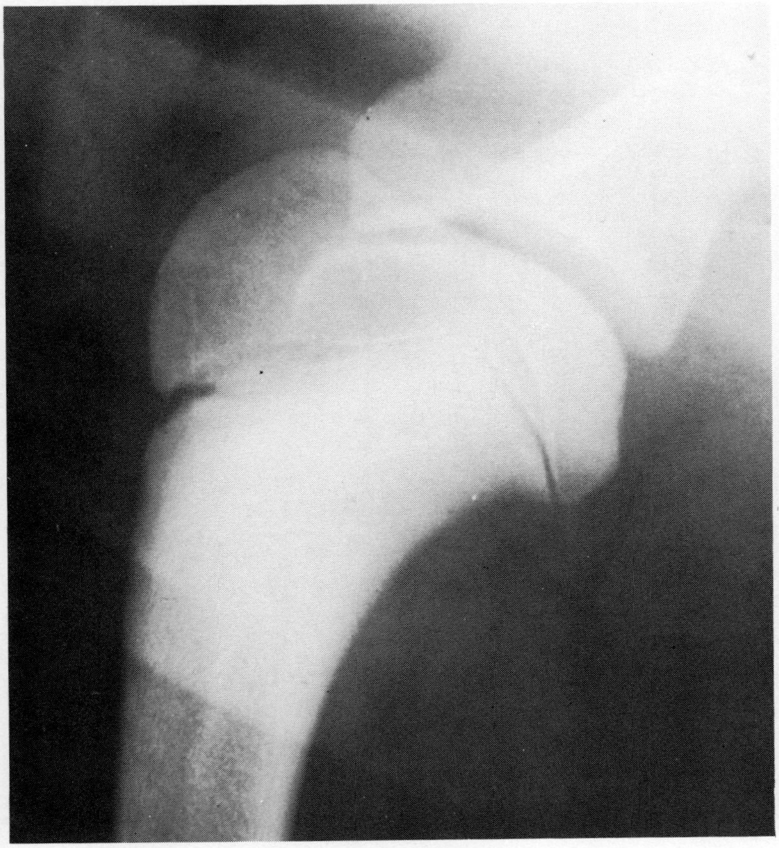

Figure 1—Typical dished-out appearance of the caudal humeral head in a case of OCD.

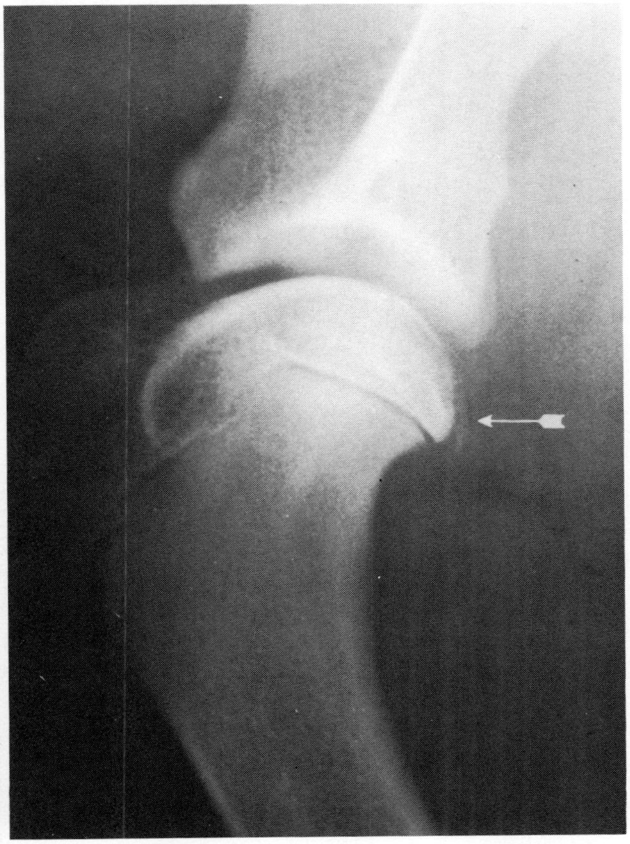

Figure 2—Radiographic appearance of an OCD lesion with an articular flap *(arrow)*.

Radiography

The essential elements for diagnosis of OCD are good-quality radiographs taken with the patient properly positioned. An ultrashort-acting anesthetic or narcotic agent must be used to obtain radiographs of diagnostic value. The affected leg is placed on the cassette for a mediolateral radiograph and the trunk of the animal's body is rotated to a 45 degree angle.[6] The leg should be fully extended forward. Slight lateral rotation of the distal leg will rotate the humeral head medially. Placing the head of the humerus over the trachea has been recommended as a means of achieving added radiographic contrast,[4] but good diagnostic radiographs can be made without this procedure.

The lesion seen radiographically is in the caudal part of the humeral head (*Figure 1*). It appears as a concave radiolucent area beneath the cartilaginous surface. An articular flap can sometimes be seen (*Figure 2*). If dislodged, the flap becomes a free joint mouse and can ossify (*Figure 3*). Radiographs should always be taken of the opposite shoulder.

Surgery

The decision to treat OCD surgically depends on the individual case and client. The severity of the clinical signs, size of the lesion, and presence of a cartilaginous flap or joint mouse should be considered. Lesions that are larger than 1.0 cm and have a cartilaginous flap, or have a joint mouse should be surgically treated. Dogs with smaller lesions but significant pain and discomfort also benefit from surgery.

The shoulder joint may be entered through one of three approaches:

1. Craniolateral: Cranial dissection of the acromial deltoideus muscle from the humerus, and reflection caudally.[6–8]
2. Lateral:
   a. Osteotomy of the acromion.[4,8,9]
   b. Tenotomy of the origin of the acromial deltoideus muscle.[8,10,11]
3. Caudolateral: Dissection between the spinous and acromial portions of the deltoideus muscle.[8,12]

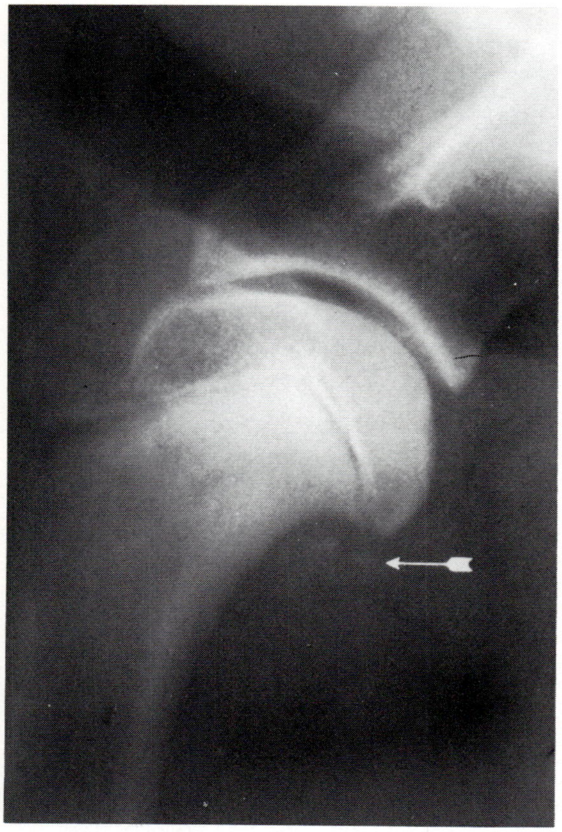

Figure 3—Radiograph showing slight irregularity of the caudal humeral head with the presence of a joint mouse *(arrow)*.

Figure 5—The superficial fascia has been reflected and the omotransversarius incised, exposing the acromion. (1) trapezius, (2) spinous deltoideus, (3) omotransversarius, (4) acromial deltoideus.

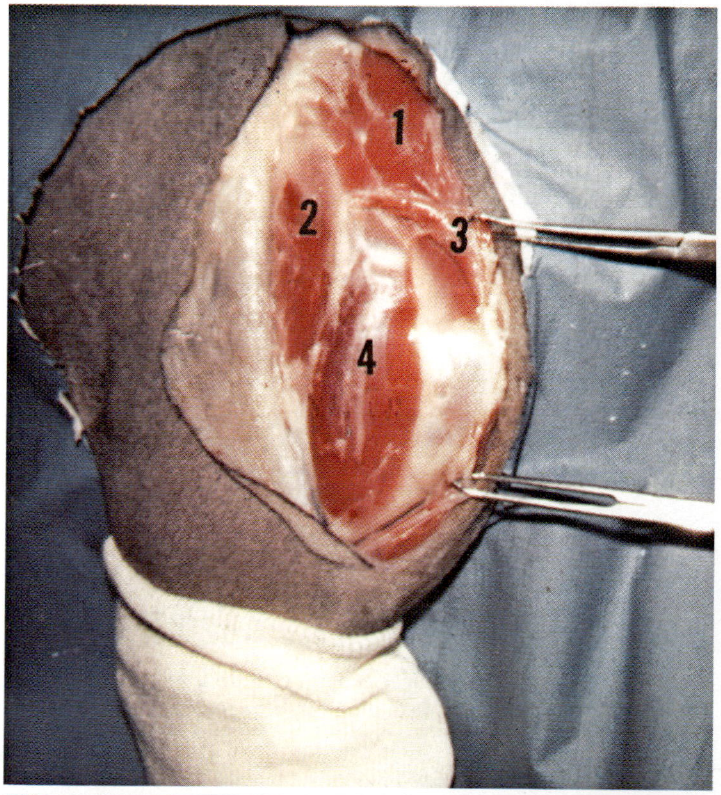

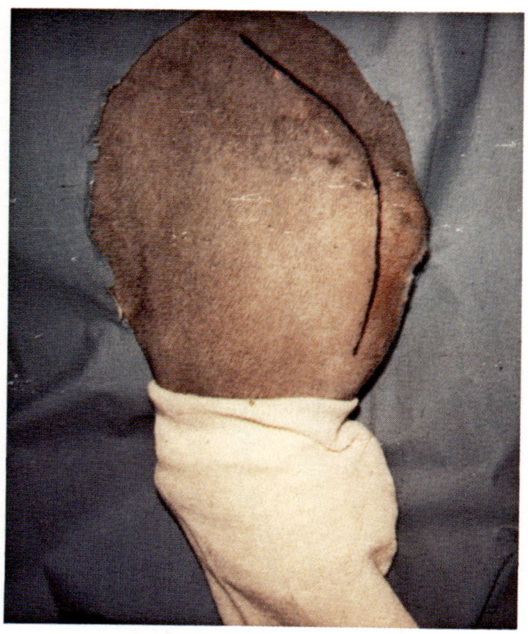

Figure 4—The initial skin incision shown on a cadaver.

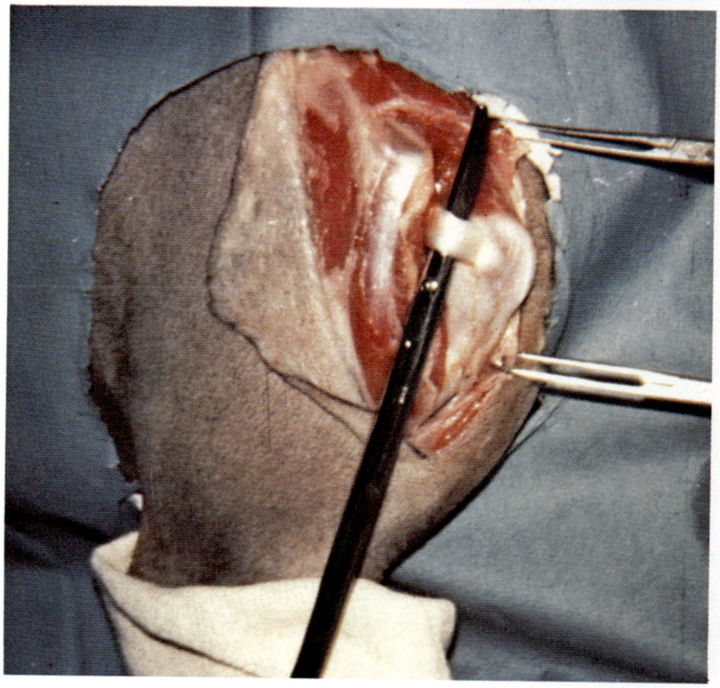

Figure 6—The deep fascia is incised and the infraspinatus tendon isolated.

Figure 7—The tendon of the infraspinatus is tagged and incised.

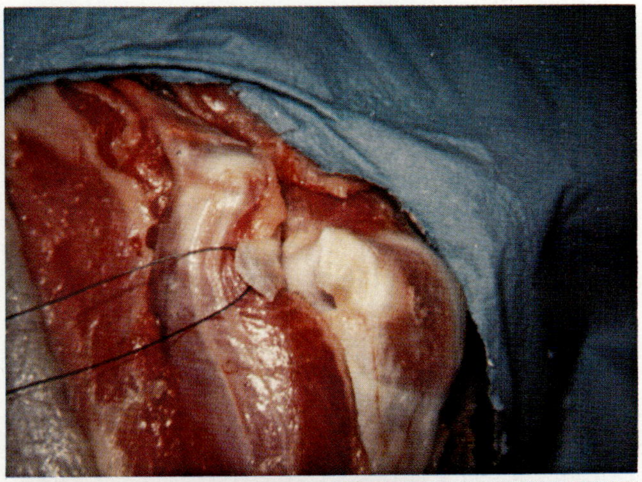

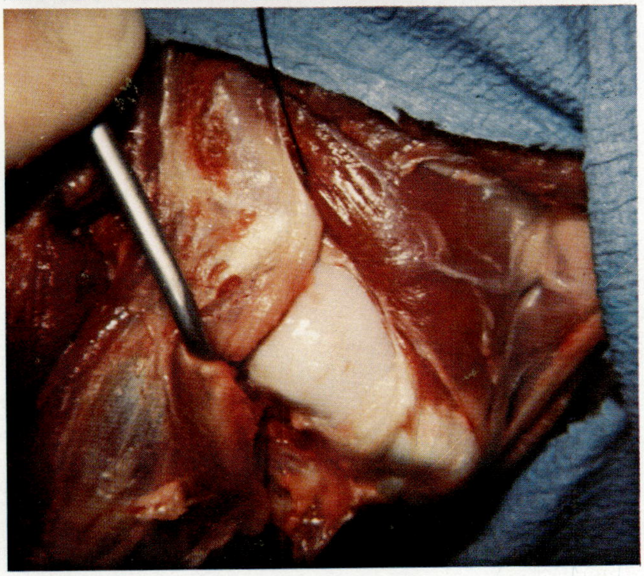

Figure 8—The joint capsule is incised between the glenoid rim and humeral head. The caudal head is exposed by internal rotation.

The approach used depends on the personal preference of the surgeon, size of the animal, size of the lesion, presence of joint mice, and the availability of a surgical assistant.

The skin incision is the same for each approach. A curved incision is started at the middle of the scapular spine and extended distally over the joint to the midpoint of the lateral humerus (*Figure 4*). The incision should be made so that it is not carried directly over the prominence of the acromion. After the skin and superficial fascia have been reflected, the muscles can easily be seen (*Figure 5*).

The craniolateral approach

The craniolateral approach is made by incising the deep fascia from the acromion and progressing distally over the cranial border of the acromial head of the deltoideus muscle. The omotransversarius may be incised along its attachment to the scapular spine and retracted cranially. The acromial deltoideus muscle is undermined and retracted caudally to allow observation of the tendon of insertion of the infraspinatus muscle (*Figure 6*). The tendon is tagged and a tenotomy is performed anterior to the suture (*Figure 7*). Caudal retraction of the acromial head of the deltoideus muscle is maintained. This permits exposure of the humeroscapular joint capsule, which is incised, exposing the head of the humerus (*Figure 8*).

The lateral approach

The lateral approach can be performed by osteotomy of the acromion or transection of the origin of the acromial deltoideus muscle. Only osteotomy of the acromion is described here. After the initial

Figure 9—The spinous deltoideus, omotransversarius, and trapezius are incised along the scapular spine. The deep fascia is incised distally to the cephalic vein.

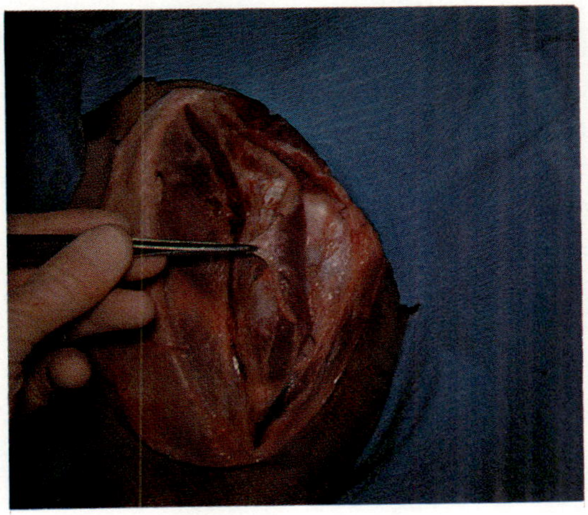

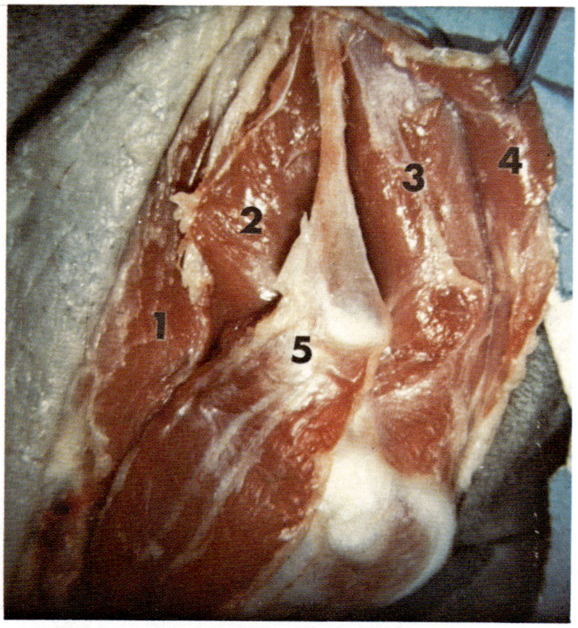

Figure 10—The acromion is exposed for osteotomy. (1) spinous deltoideus, (2) infraspinatus, (3) supraspinatus, (4) omotransversarius, (5) acromial deltoideus.

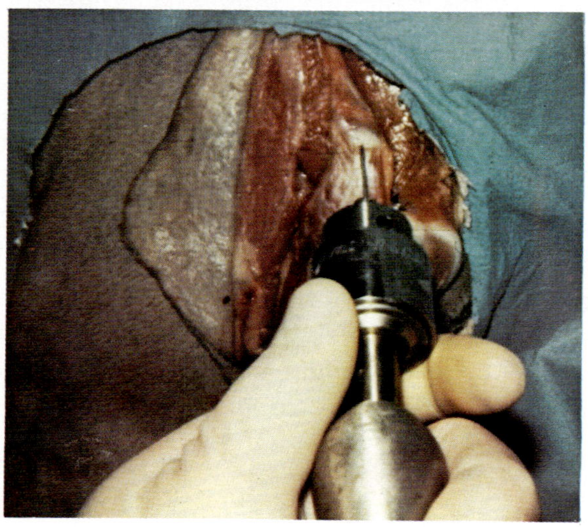

Figure 11—A 0.45 Kirschner wire is used to pre-drill the acromion before osteotomy.

Figure 12—Osteotomy of the acromion with an osteotome.

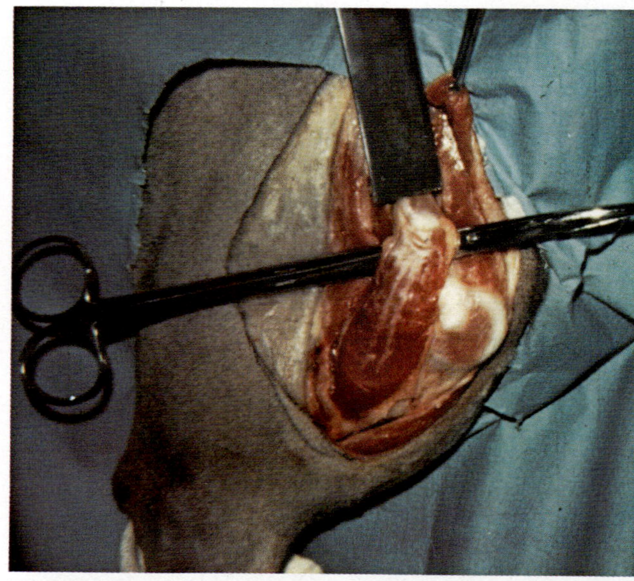

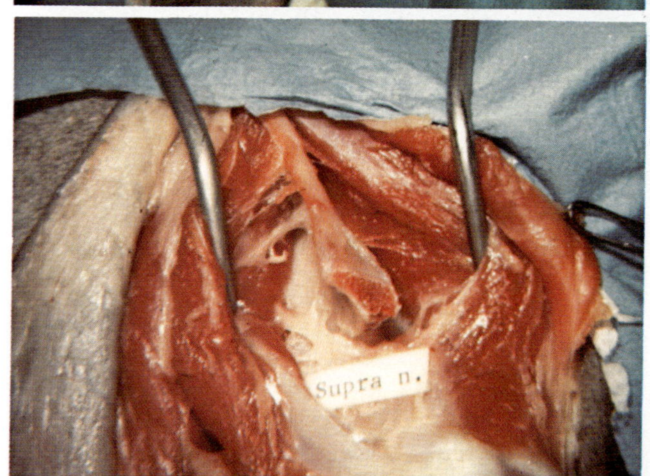

Figure 13—Location of the suprascapular nerve.

incisions in the skin and subcutaneous fascia, the attachments of the trapezius and omotransversarius muscles and the spinous head of the deltoideus muscle are incised along the scapular spine (*Figure 9*). The incision is continued distally through the deep fascia over the acromial head of the deltoideus muscle until the area of the cephalic vein is reached. The deep fascia is undermined and retracted from the acromial head of the deltoideus muscle. The omotransversarius and trapezius muscles are retracted cranially and the spinous head of the deltoideus muscle is retracted caudally, exposing the infraspinatus and supraspinatus muscles. The infraspinatus and supraspinatus muscles may be dissected free from the scapular spine for further exposure of the acromion (*Figure 10*).

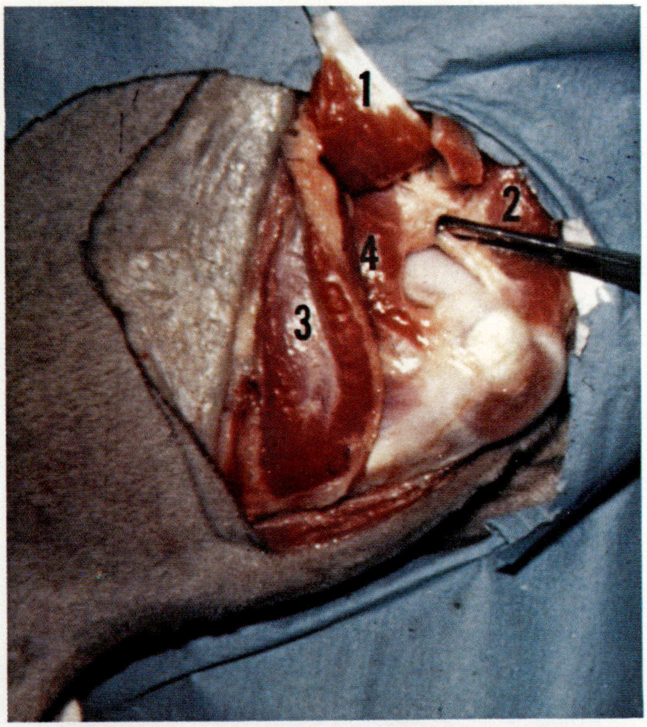

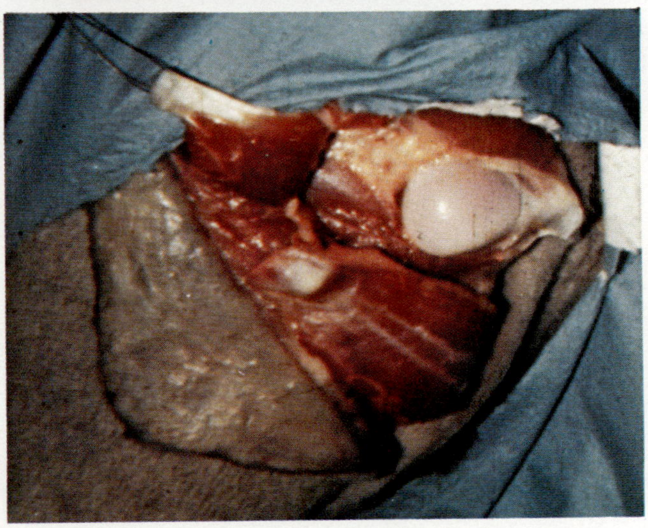

A small Kirschner wire can be used to pre-drill the acromion for later replacement and tension-band fixation (*Figure 11*). However, a larger pin should then be used for fixation. Once the acromion has been sufficiently exposed, it is osteotomized to include all of the acromial deltoideus muscle (*Figure 12*). The acromial head is reflected distally, thus exposing the tendons of the infraspinatus and teres minor muscles. The tendon of the infraspinatus muscle is incised as previously described, but no stay suture is required. The supraspinatus muscle may be dissected if needed for further exposure of the joint capsule. The location of the

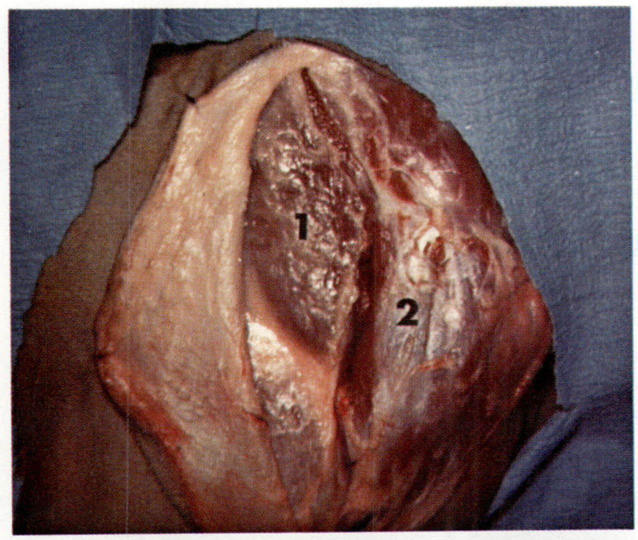

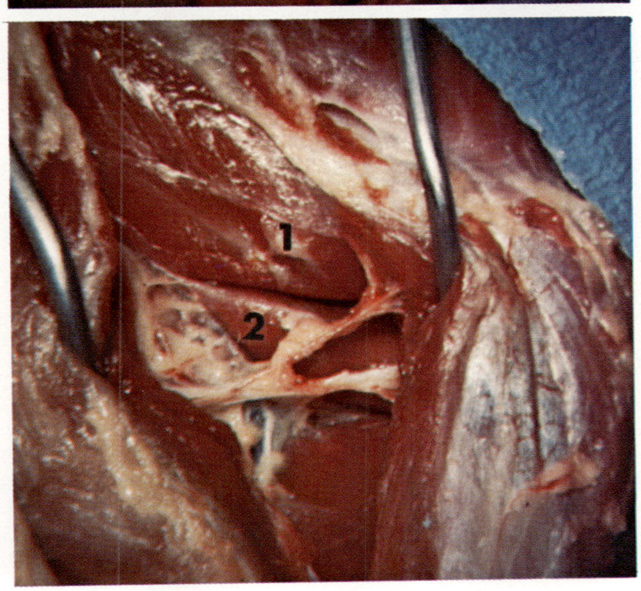

Figure 14—Joint capsule is incised. (1) infraspinatus, (2) supraspinatus, (3) acromial deltoideus, (4) teres minor.

Figure 15—Exposure of humeral head after osteotomy. The infraspinatus is retracted caudally with a stay suture.

Figure 16—A dissection plane is made between the two heads of the deltoideus muscle. (1) spinous deltoideus, (2) acromial deltoideus.

Figure 17—A muscular branch of the axillary nerve and the caudal circumflex vessels are shown. A dissection plane is created between the infraspinatus (1) and teres minor (2).

suprascapular nerve must be kept in mind during any dissection or manipulations in this area (*Figure 13*).

The joint capsule is incised midway between the rim of the glenoid and head of the humerus (*Figure 14*). Flexion and internal rotation of the humeroscapular joint allow exposure of the entire caudal aspect of the head of the humerus (*Figure 15*).

The caudolateral approach

The caudolateral approach is made by creating a dissection plane between the spinous and acromial parts of the deltoideus muscle (*Figure 16*). The spinous head is retracted caudally, and the acromial deltoideus muscle is retracted cranially. Dissection of the spinous deltoideus muscle from the scapular spine and the deep fascia over the acromial head of the deltoideus muscle helps provide more exposure. A muscular branch of the axillary nerve and accompanying caudal circumflex vessels is encountered in this approach and may have to be sacrificed (*Figure 17*). The infraspinatus and teres minor muscles can be seen and the latter may be tenotomized to provide further exposure of the posterior joint capsule (*Figures 18 & 19*). In some cases, the teres minor muscle may be dissected free and retracted without tenotomy.

After exposure of the lesion through the chosen approach, the cartilaginous flap, which is usually still attached along its medial edge, is incised with a No. 15 scalpel blade (*Figure 20*). The lesion is inspected for devitalized or loosely attached cartilage

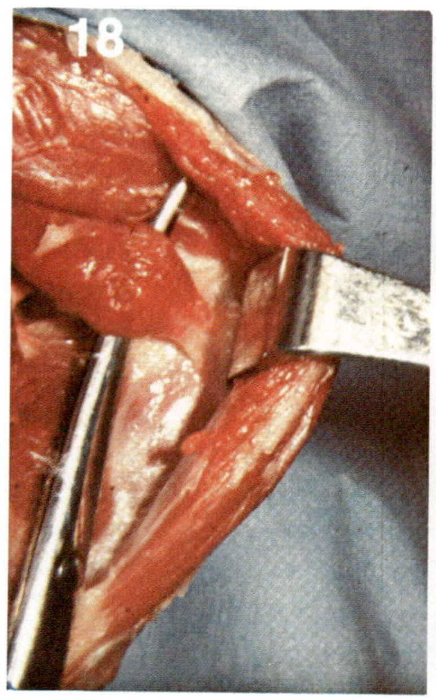

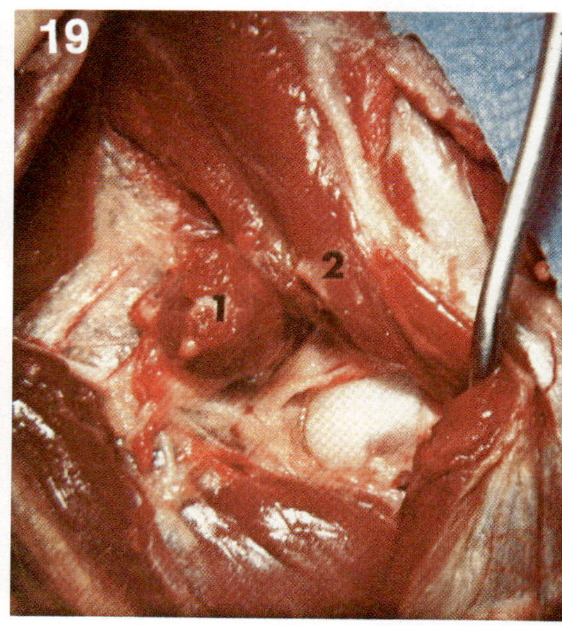

Figure 18—Isolation of the teres minor muscle before tenotomy.

Figure 19—The teres minor is tenotomized (1) and the joint capsule is incised. The infraspinatus is dorsal to the joint (2).

Figure 20—Cartilaginous flap on the humeral head.

Figure 21—Debridement of the periphery with a No. 15 scalpel blade.

Figure 22—The lesion is curetted to bleeding subchondral bone.

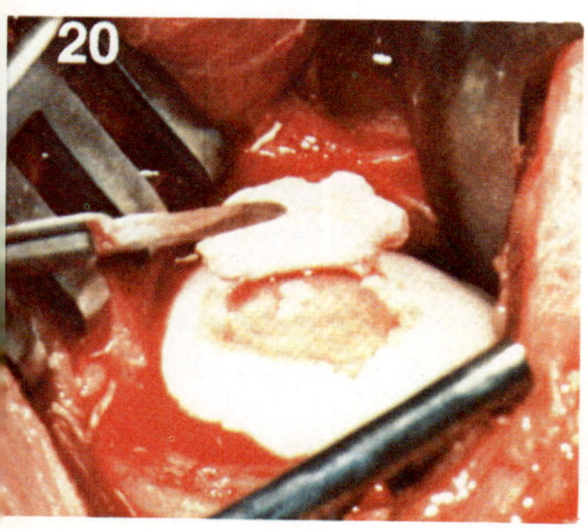

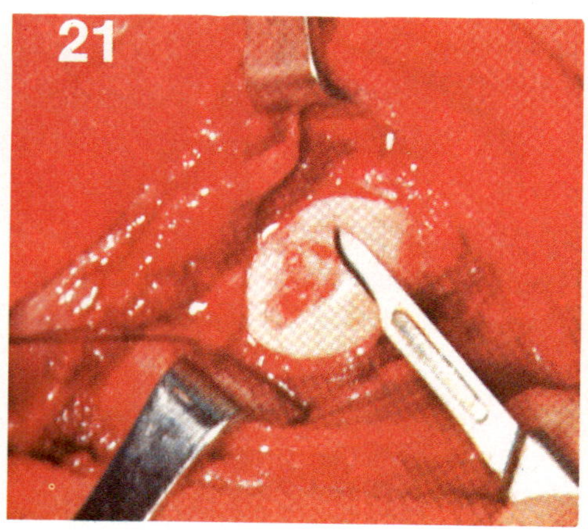

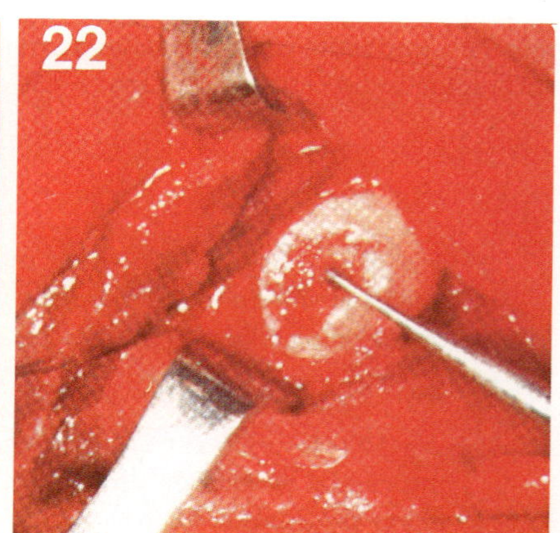

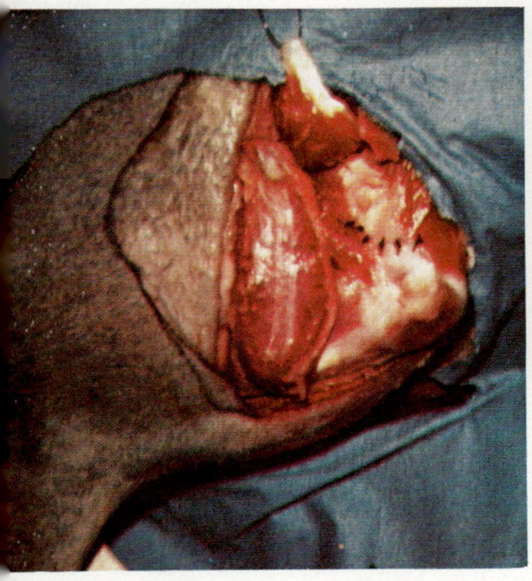

Figure 23—After liberal irrigation of the joint, the joint capsule is closed with simple interrupted absorbable sutures.

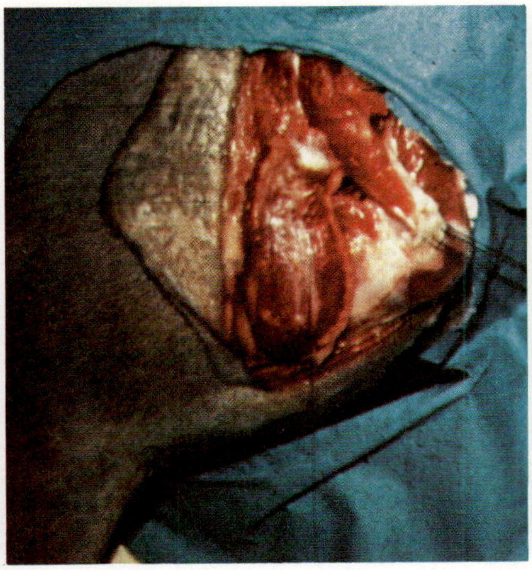

Figure 24—Two horizontal mattress sutures are placed to reappose the infraspinatus tendon.

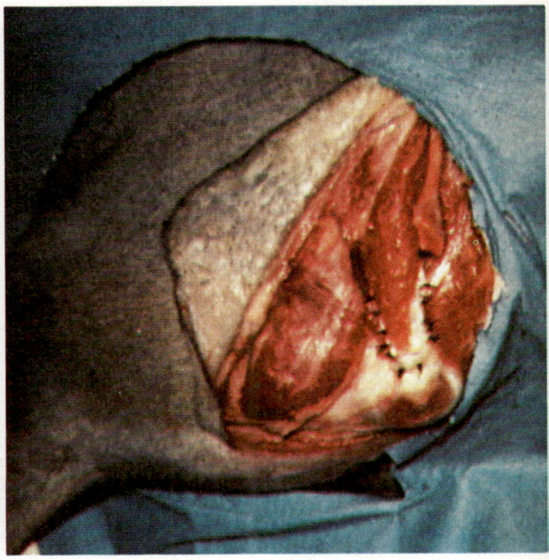

Figure 25—The tissue around the infraspinatus tendon is closed with simple interrupted absorbable sutures.

around the perimeter. The cartilage is trimmed around the periphery with a No. 15 scalpel blade so that only viable and firmly attached cartilage remains (*Figure 21*). The lesion is then curetted until fresh bleeding subchondral bone is reached (*Figure 22*). Intermittent flushing with sterile saline solution or lactated Ringer's solution, followed by aspiration, helps in viewing the area and removing curetted material. The caudomedial aspect of the joint is inspected for loose pieces of cartilage. The joint is liberally flushed with sterile irrigating solution and aspirated.

Absorbable suture (2-0) in a simple interrupted pattern is used to close the joint capsule (*Figure 23*). If an infraspinatus tenotomy was done, the tendon is repaired with two or three horizontal mattress sutures of 2-0 nylon (*Figure 24*). Tenotomy of the teres minor muscle can be repaired similarly. Tissue around the infraspinatus musculotendinous junction is closed with 3-0 absorbable suture (*Figure 25*). This helps close the bursa associated with the tendon.

The acromial osteotomy is repaired by placing a larger pin in the pre-drilled hole and reducing the acromion. The pin is advanced and seated into the spine of the scapula (*Figure 26*). If needed, a second pin of equal or smaller diameter may be placed for two-point fixation. A hole is made through the spine 2 to 3 cm proximal to the osteotomy site and 18- to 20-gauge orthopedic wire is passed through the hole (*Figure 27*). A figure-eight pattern is placed around the pin and positioned so that the wire can be tightened from two sides (*Figure 28*). The wire is alternately twisted until firm, solid reduction is achieved (*Figure 29*). The pin is bent proximally and cut. The hooked end of the pin is then rotated distally so that it overlies the orthopedic wire (*Figures 30 & 31*). The ends of the orthopedic wire are bent into the deeper tissues and should be thoroughly covered by muscle.

The trapezius and omotransversarius muscles are sutured to the spinous head of the deltoideus muscle using 2-0 absorbable material in a simple interrupted pattern (*Figure 32*). In each of the approaches, all muscle layers are closed routinely. Closure should be secure. All dead space should be obliterated to prevent formation of a seroma. The incisions in the subcutaneous tissue and skin are closed routinely.

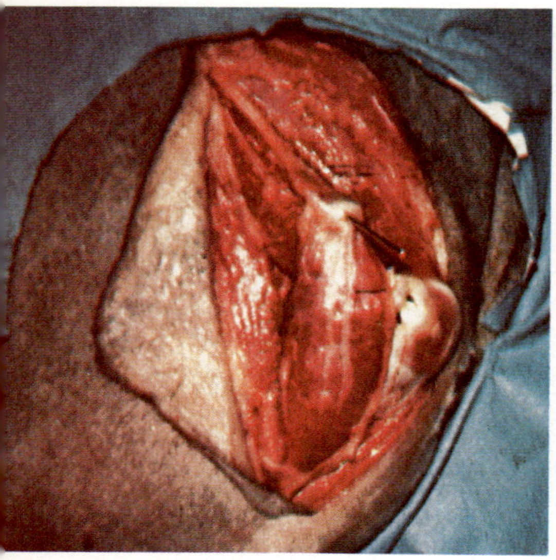

Figure 26—The osteotomy site is reduced and a larger Kirschner wire is passed through a pre-drilled hole in the acromion and seated in the spine.

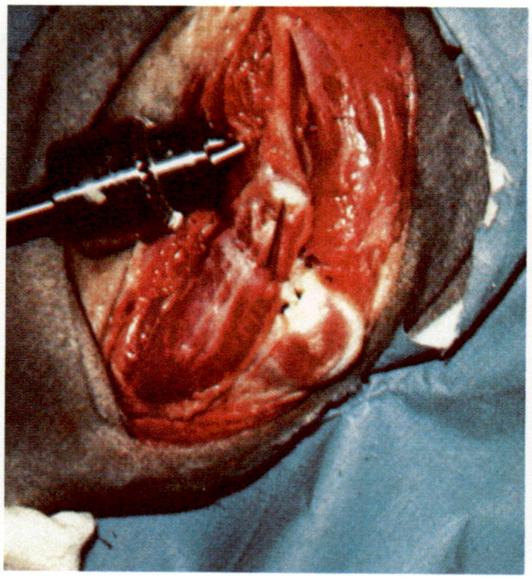

Figure 27—A hole is drilled in the scapular spine 2 to 3 cm proximal to the osteotomy site.

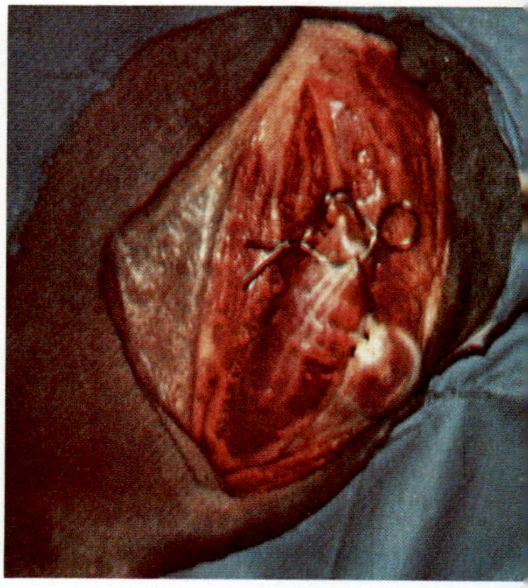

Figure 28—Orthopedic wire is passed through the hole and a figure-eight pattern is placed around the pin.

Postoperative care

Bandaging of the surgical area is optional. An elastic thoracobrachial bandage can be used to apply pressure and help prevent formation of a seroma. This may be maintained for 3 to 5 days. Seroma formation probably is influenced more by surgical technique than bandaging.

Initially the dog shows signs of pain and may carry the leg. However, gradual and marked improvement ensues during the next 3 to 5 days, after which the dog can be discharged. Activity should be restricted for 4 to 6 weeks after surgery. Exercise is gradually increased. At 8 to 12 weeks, full activity should be possible.

Discussion

Osteochondritis dissecans is a form of osteochondrosis that leads to separation of the articular hyaline cartilage from the underlying subchondral bone. The cause of the disease has not been determined. Over-nutrition, hormonal imbalances, genetic influences, accelerated growth, and avascular necrosis have been cited as possible factors.[2,9,13,14] However, trauma probably plays the most significant part in the development of OCD.[5,9,14,15]

The ultimate decision as to which surgical approach to use depends on the experience and personal preference of the surgeon. However, some practical aspects should be considered. The craniolateral approach involves minimal dissection, but a surgical assistant is usually required to maintain caudal retraction of the acromial part of deltoideus muscle. Also, access to the caudal aspect of the joint is limited for removal of joint mice.[8] An advantage of the approach is that it can easily be converted to a lateral approach if additional exposure and manipulation are required.

The caudolateral approach gives good exposure to the caudal part of the joint for removal of joint mice, but exposure of the lesion at the head of the humerus is more limited.[8] This could be a serious problem if a large lesion is present. Again, an assistant during surgery is helpful in maintaining exposure and during manipulative procedures. In some cases, tenotomy of the teres minor muscle may be avoided. The two other approaches require tenotomy of the infraspinatus muscle.

The lateral approach provides the best exposure of the joint, and an assistant is not required to provide retraction. Osteotomy of the acromion is preferred because the tension-band principle may be used to provide good rigid fixation. The use of this

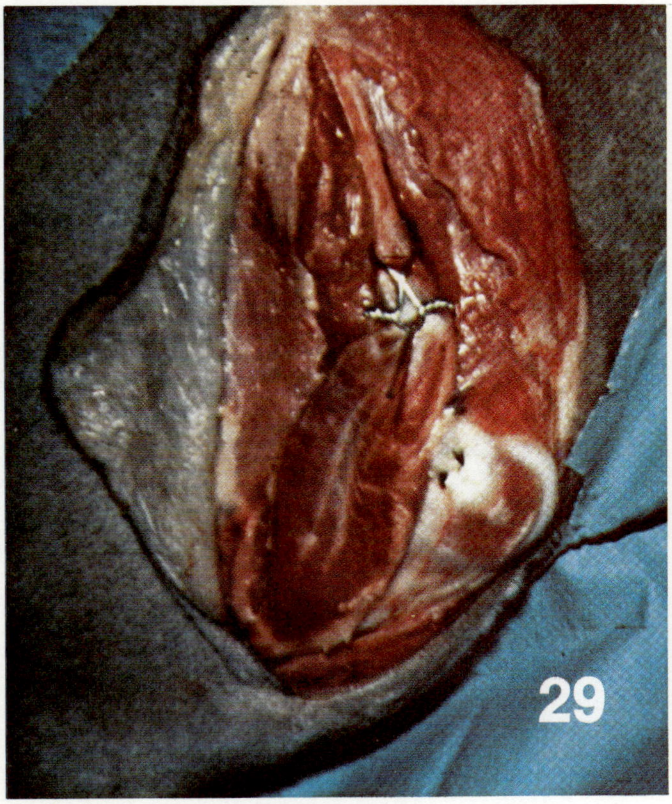

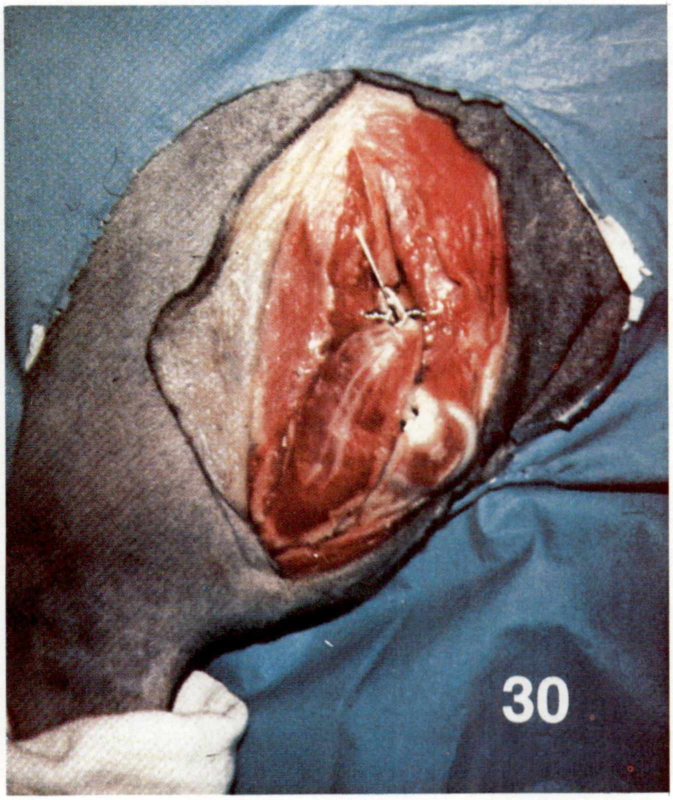

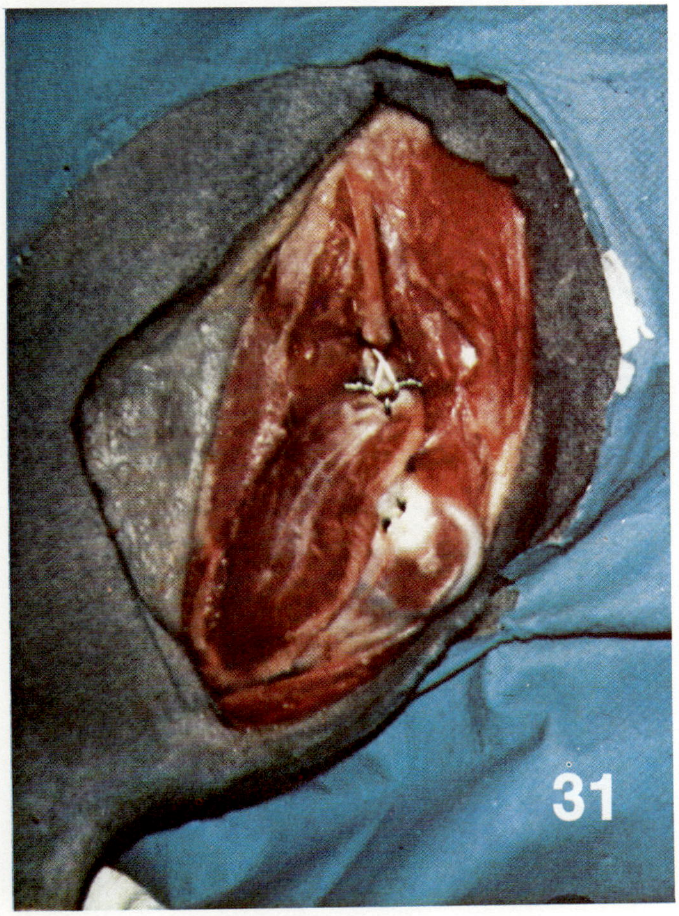

Figure 29
The orthopedic wire is alternately twisted to provide solid fixation.

Figure 30
The pin is bent proximally before it is cut.

Figure 31
The pin is cut and the hooked end twisted so that it overlies the wire.

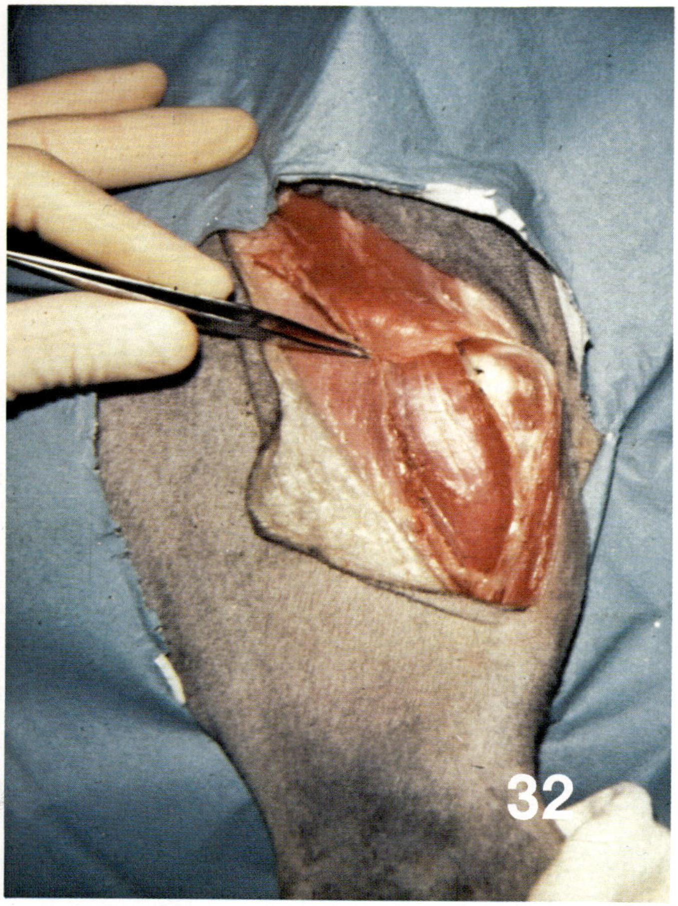

Figure 32
The trapezius and omotransversarius muscles are sutured to the spinous deltoideus muscle so that the wire and pin are thoroughly covered with soft tissue.

approach to provide good exposure for debridement of devitalized cartilage, curettage of the lesion, and removal of joint mice may be advantageous for an inexperienced surgeon. After becoming familiar with the technique and the anatomy, the surgeon may progress to one of the other approaches. An obvious disadvantage is the need for creating a fracture, which requires some additional instruments. Placement of the tension band lengthens the time required for closure.

I have not seen nor been aware of any difference in recovery from the various approaches. The rate of recovery of normal leg function probably depends more on the severity of the lesion. Radiographs should be taken postoperatively to evaluate placement of the pin and reduction of the osteotomy site. Recently, the drilling of holes through the defect toward the metaphysis has been proposed as a way to stimulate neovascularization of the area and accelerate healing with fibrocartilage.[13]

REFERENCES

1. Olsson, S.E.: Osteochondrosis in the Dog. In *Current Veterinary Therapy*-VI (R.W. Kirk, ed.). W.B. Saunders, Philadelphia, Pa., 1977; pp 880-886.
2. Griffiths, R.C.: Osteochondritis Dissecans of the Canine Shoulder. *JAVMA 153*:1733-1735; 1968.
3. Smith, C.W.; Stowater, J.L.: Osteochondritis Dissecans of the Canine Shoulder Joint: A Review of 35 Cases. *JAAHA 11*:658-662; 1975.
4. Whittick, W.G.: *Canine Orthopedics*. Lea & Febiger, Philadelphia, Pa., 1974; pp 154-157.
5. Craig, P.H.; Riser, W.H.: Osteochondritis Dissecans in the Proximal Humerus of the Dog. *J. Am. Vet. Radiog. Soc. 6*:40-49; 1965.
6. Harrison, J.W.; Hohn, R.B.: Osteochondritis Dissecans. In *Current Techniques in Small Animal Surgery*-I (M.J. Bojrab, ed.). Lea & Febiger, Philadelphia, Pa., 1974; pp 504-509.
7. Hohn, R.B.: Osteochondritis Dissecans of the Humeral Head. *JAVMA 163*:69-70; 1973.
8. Piermattei, D.L.; Greely, R.G.: *An Atlas of Surgical Approaches to the Bone of the Dog*, 2nd ed. W.B. Saunders, Philadelphia, Pa., 1979; pp 62-71.
9. Leighton, R.L.: Osteochondritis Dissecans of the Shoulder Joint of the Dog. *Vet. Clin. N. Am. 1*:391-401; 1971.
10. Herron, M.R.: Osteochondritis Dissecans and Epiphysitis in a Young Pointer. *VM/SAC 65*:991-993; 1970.
11. Rehmel, R.A.: Approach to the Shoulder. In *Small Animal Surgery: An Atlas of Operative Techniques* (W.E. Wingfield and C.A. Rawlings, eds.). W.B. Saunders, Philadelphia, Pa., 1979; pp 176-181.
12. Birkeland, R.: Osteochondritis Dissecans in the Humeral Head of the Dog. *Nord. Vet. Med. 19*:294-306; 1967.
13. Berzon, J.L.: Osteochondritis Dissecans in the Dog: Diagnosis and Therapy. *JAVMA 175*:796-799; 1979.
14. Knecht, C.D. *et al*: Osteochondrosis of the Shoulder and Stifle in 3 of 5 Border Collie Littermates. *JAVMA 170*:58-60; 1977.
15. Cordy, D.R.; Wind, A.P.: Transverse Fracture of the Proximal Humeral Articular Cartilage in Dogs. *Path. Vet. 6*:424-436; 1969.

Use of an allogeneic bone graft to enlarge the pelvic outlet in a cat

Ivor Evans, DVM
Evans-Keatts Veterinary Hospital
5603 West Canal Drive
Kennewick, Washington 99336

ONE COMPLICATION of unreduced pelvic fractures is a narrowing of the pelvic outlet which impairs the passage of feces. The result is chronic constipation. Many animals with this problem are euthanatized. In this report I describe an apparently practical alternative to sacrificing affected animals.

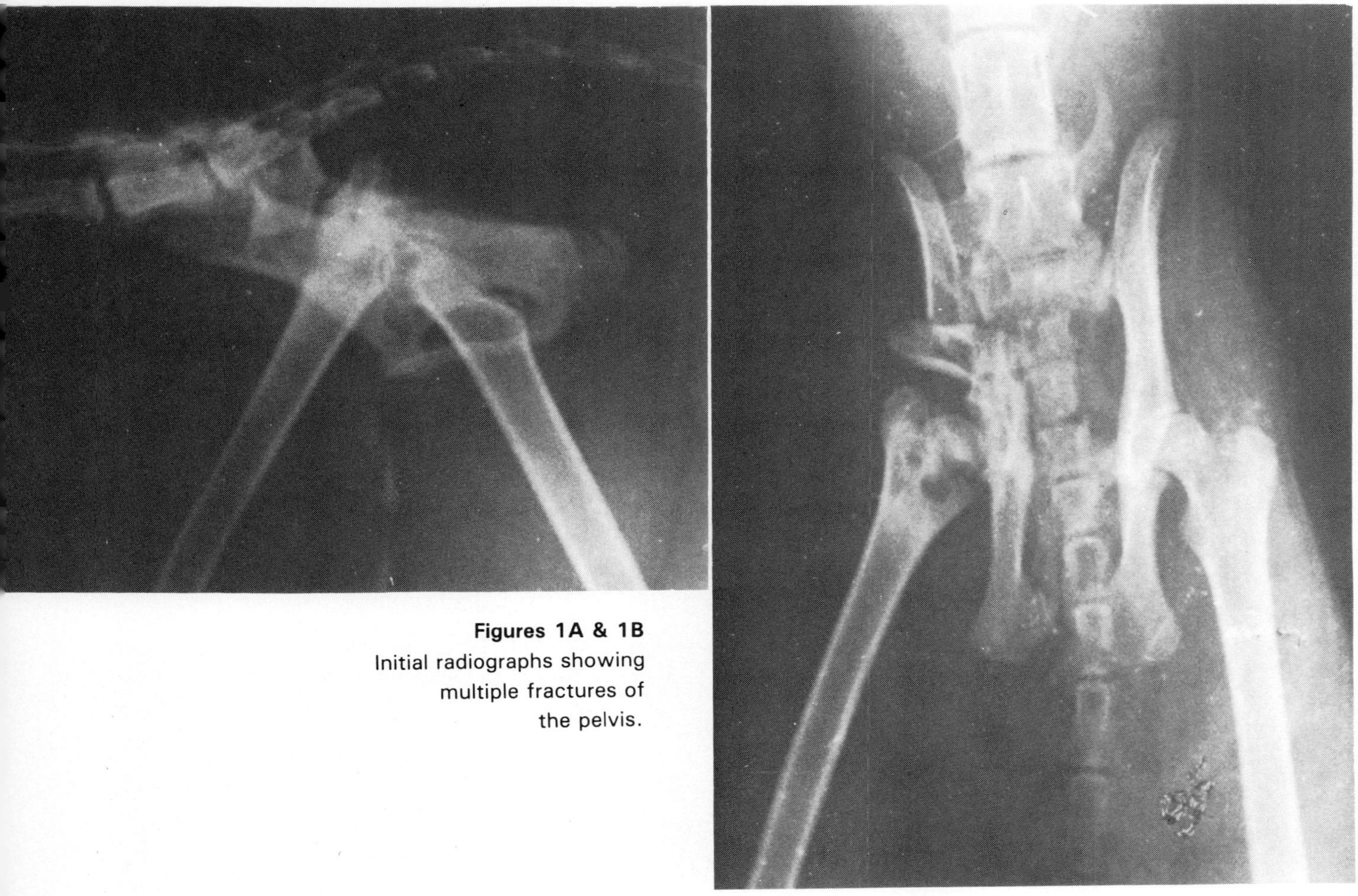

Figures 1A & 1B
Initial radiographs showing multiple fractures of the pelvis.

Case history

In June of 1978, a 1-year-old male cat was presented to the hospital after it had been hit by a car four days previously. Radiographs showed multiple fractures (*Figures 1A & 1B*). The owner decided against surgical repair and the cat was discharged after three days.

On July 29, 1978, the cat was returned to the hospital because it had been constipated for three days. Attempts to break up the fecal mass with commercially prepared enemas were unsuccessful. The next day the cat was anesthetized and the mass was massaged. Finally, on July 31 the mass was manually broken down and eliminated. Palpation of the bowel indicated no abnormality, so the cat was discharged.

On August 10 the cat was again presented, this time because of severe straining when attempting to defecate. A fecal mass could be palpated at the pelvic inlet. The owner requested that the cat be euthanatized if we could not permanently relieve the problem.

The decision was made to attempt surgical correction. The next morning the cat was anesthetized with a 2% solution of thiamylal sodium and intubated. Surgical anesthesia was maintained with methoxyflurane (Metofane™—Pitman-Moore). The entire ventral pelvic area was clipped and prepared for aseptic surgery.

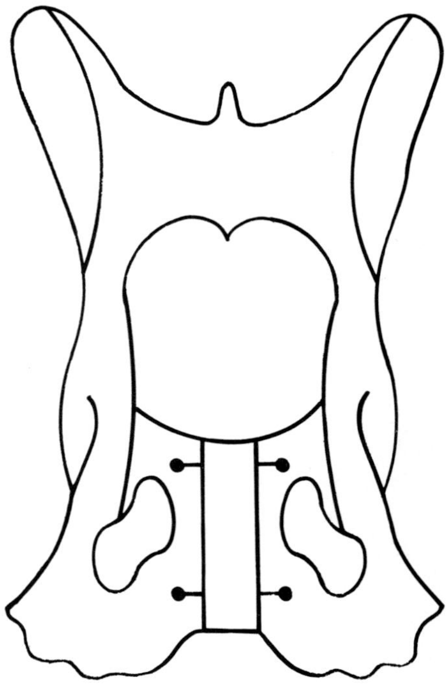

Figure 3

Schematic showing placement of the graft.

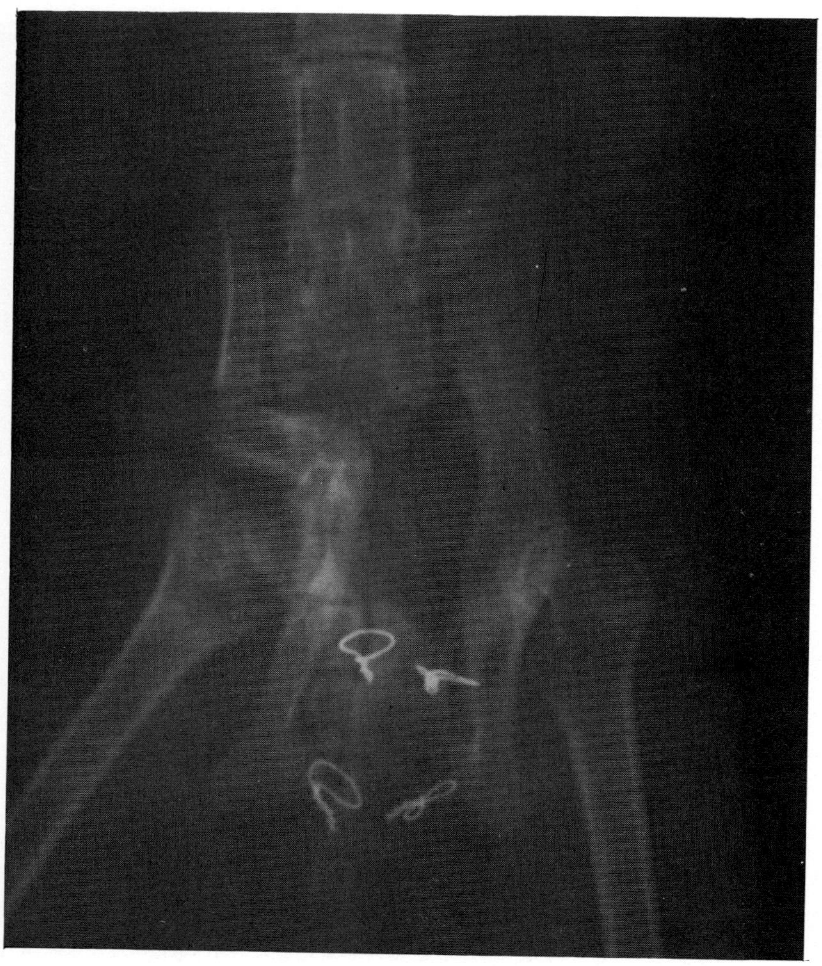

Figure 2

Postoperative radiograph showing the graft in place and secured with orthopedic wire.

I had seen only a brief reference to surgical enlargement of the pelvic outlet[1] but, after the radiographs were reviewed we decided to attempt that procedure, using a graft 1 cm wide × 4 cm long from the wing of the ileum. Because of the large size of the graft required, we felt a donor cat was needed. A piece of bone of proper size was taken from the wing of the ileum of the donor cat and immersed in saline solution until used.

A midline incision was made directly over the pelvic symphysis. Then, by means of a small chisel, the symphysis was separated along its entire length. Four holes were drilled through the pubis, two on each side of the separated symphysis and 5 mm from it. Matching holes were drilled through the graft, on each side. The symphysis was spread with forceps, the graft inserted in the separation and secured by orthopedic wire passed through the holes (*Figures 2 & 3*). Closure of the subcutaneous tissue and skin was routine.

The next day the patient was ambulatory, with only slight stiffness of gait. When the stitches were removed from the skin incision eight days postoperatively, the cat was walking normally. Constipation had not recurred.

Nine months after the operation the cat walks and runs normally. It eats a normal diet and has shown no signs of difficult defecation.

REFERENCES

1. Bojrab, J.M.: *Current Techniques in Small Animal Surgery—I.* Lea & Febiger, Philadelphia, Pa., 1975; p 422.

Small Animal Surgery

GENITO-URINARY

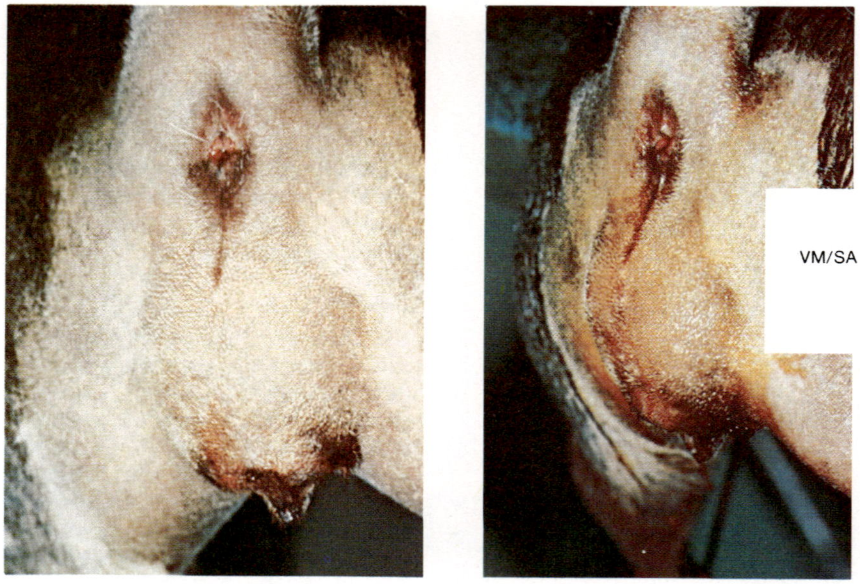

Figures 1a and 1b—Enlargement of the perineum in a 2½-year-old female dog of mixed breed.

Transmissible Venereal Tumor in a Dog

George A. White, DVM
Captain, USAF, VC
Udorn RTAFB, Thailand

TRANSMISSIBLE venereal tumor (known also as venereal granuloma, histiocytoma, or transmissible sarcoma) occurs most commonly on the external genitalia of sexually mature dogs. In the male, they are usually seen on the penis or prepuce. They can, however, invade the scrotum and perineum. In the female, they occur on any part of the vagina. Although not common in the United States, these neoplasms are seen frequently in Southeast Asia.

This type of tumor is unique in that it can be transmitted, usually by coitus. Experimentally, transplantation of neoplastic cells to a susceptible host will produce growth. The lesions vary in size, ranging from one to several centimeters in diameter. The lesion is singular or multiple, with a gray-to-red color and a lobular texture. The lesions often ulcerate, causing hemorrhage.

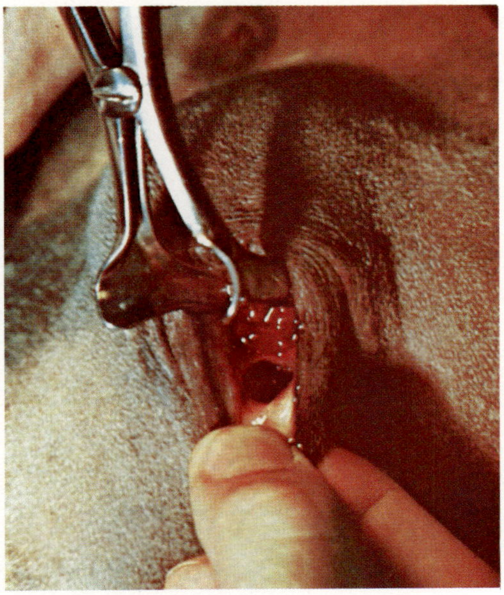

Figure 2—Appearance of the tumor within the vagina. The ventral opening is the clitoral fossa. Note the hemorrhagic surface.

Although spontaneous regression may occur, surgical removal is the treatment of choice. Radiation therapy has been used with some success.

Case History

On May 14, 1975, a 2½-year-old female of mixed breed was presented with a complaint of an intermittent bloody vaginal discharge that had been present since August of 1974. A sizable bulge was visible in the perineal area (*Figures 1A & 1B*). When the vagina was examined a mass could be seen lying just anterior to the clitoral fossa (*Figure 2*).

By surgical resection (*Figures 3-8*) the tumor was found to be divided into two parts. The larger portion partially circumscribed the vaginal canal and was attached to the dorsal lateral walls. The smaller segment arose from the floor of the vagina at the level of the urethral orifice.

Figure 3—Growth occurred along the lateral and dorsal walls of the vagina and from the vaginal floor.

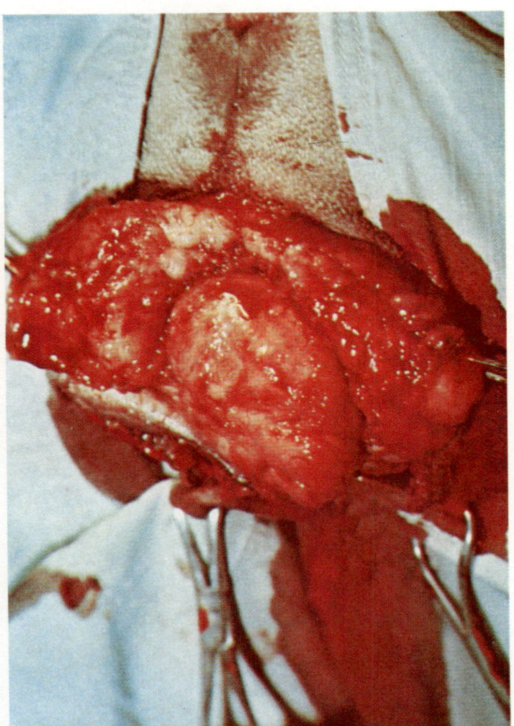

Figure 4—Catheterization of the urethral orifice. Note the area of normal vaginal mucosa.

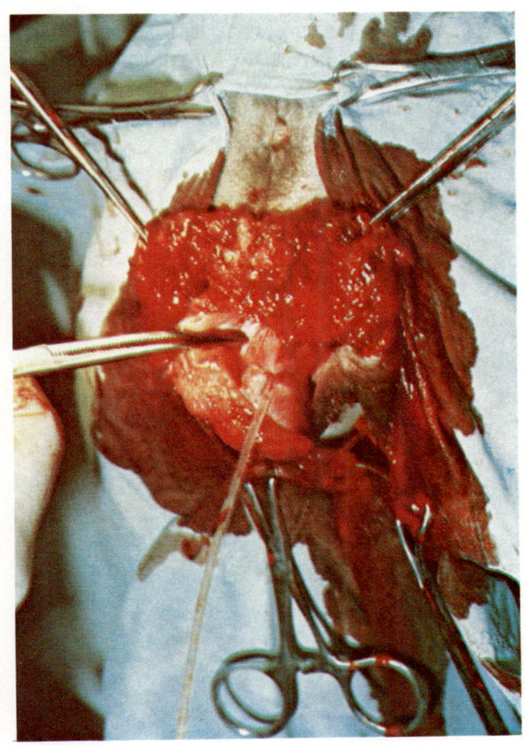

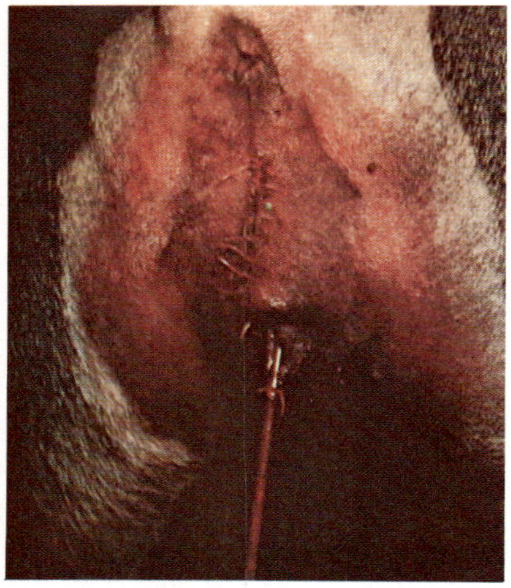

Figure 7—Closure of the episiotomy incision.

Figure 8—Appearance of the surgical site 10 days after surgery.

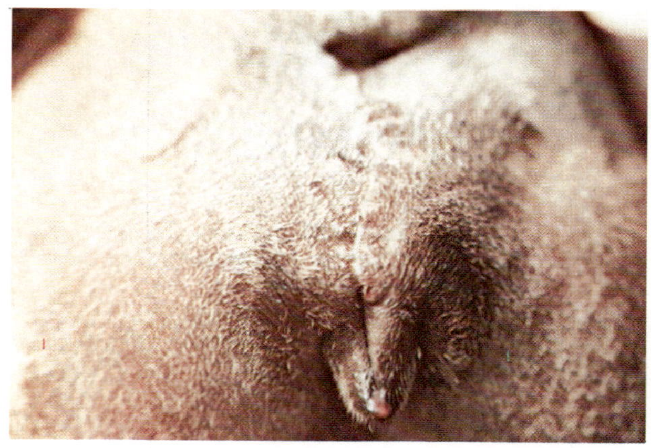

When the dog was examined rwo months after surgery, no recurrence of the tumor was seen.

REFERENCES

1. Gilmore, C.E.: Tumors of the Urogenital System; in *Current Veterinary Therapy III*, R. W. Kirk ed. W. B. Saunders Co., Philadelphia, Pa. 1968; pp 663, 666.
2. Smith, H.A.; Jones T.C.: *Veterinary Pathology*. Lea and Febiger, Philadelphia, Pa., 1966; pp 220.

Figure 5—Appearance of the affected site after resection of the tumor.

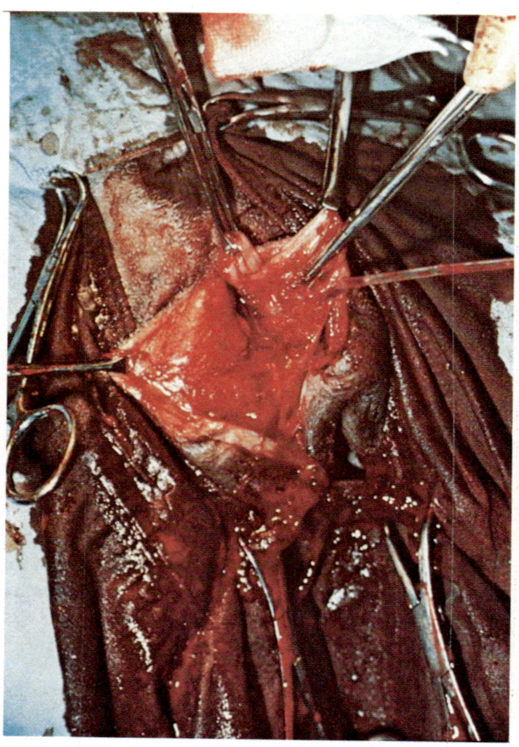

Figure 6—Repair of the vaginal mucosa.

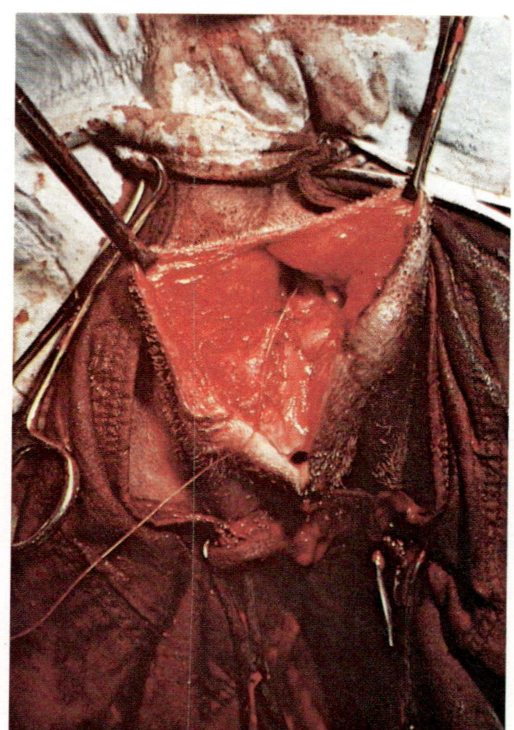

an alternate approach for

Castration of the Dog

Charles D. Knecht, BS, VMD, MS
Small Animal Clinic
School of Veterinary Medicine
Purdue University
West Lafayette, Indiana 47907

An alternate surgical approach is presented for castration in the dog where a perineal incision is also indicated. The caudolateral approach permits castration without repositioning of the patient and allows use of the same surgical instruments for both procedures. There is no increase of hemorrhage or difficulty of operation.

PRESCROTAL incision for castration has been successfully and quickly performed in the dog for many years.[1] Results are universally good if proper procedures are followed. The primary disadvantage is the cosmetic appearance of the empty scrotum postoperatively. Castration with scrotectomy to eliminate this disadvantage has been described.[2]

Castraction may be performed in young animals to prevent male behavior and later for removal of testicular neoplasm or inflammation of the testicle or prostate.[1] Castration is also performed to retard the growth of perianal adenomas and to prevent recurrence of surgically treated perianal adenoma and perineal hernia. In the latter two instances the effects are intended to lessen the androgen response of the neoplasm and prostate, respectively.

When castration is performed in conjunction with perineal surgery, differing positions and approaches are frequently used. When surgery has been performed on the perineal region in the dog in upright, flank-suspended position, the patient must be repositioned in dorsal recumbency and rescrubbed for castration. A new instrument set should be used for the castration and the surgeon should reglove. Repositioning is time-consuming, more dangerous for the patient and more expensive in that it requires more anesthetic and an added surgical pack.

An alternative approach for castration is described which does not require repositioning for repair of perineal hernia.

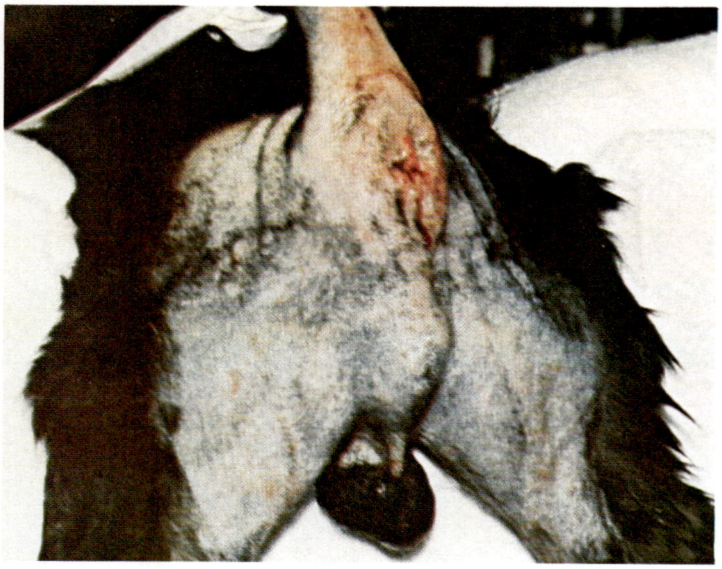

Figure 1—The animal is placed on a padded perineal hernia board and the tail is taped forward.

Figure 2—The site for the scrotal and perineal incisions is four-corner draped. Accessory draping is used over the anus.

Figure 3—The scrotum and scrotal tunic are incised on the caudolateral aspect.

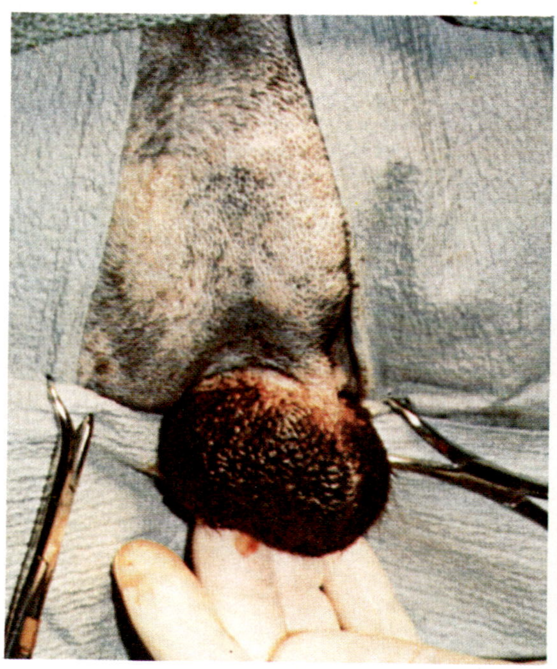

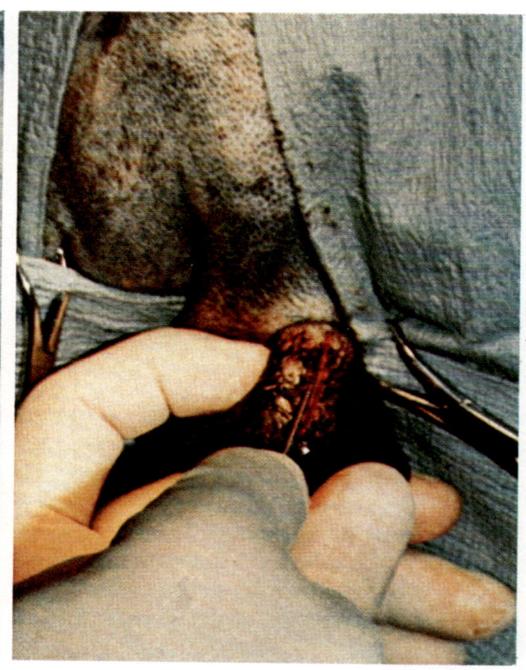

Technique

The animal is clipped and scrubbed for aseptic surgery. A purse-string suture may be placed in the anus if indicated. The animal is placed on a padded perineal hernia board or over the padded edge of a tilted surgery table. The tail is fixed in dorsoflexion with adnesive tape (*Figure 1*).

The surgical field is rescrubbed and rinsed with an antiseptic. Four corner drapes are applied, exposing the operative site and the scrotum. Secondary draping is used to cover the anus during castration (*Figure 2*).

An incision is made in the caudolateral scrotum ventral to the perineal skin. The lateral incision is made to avoid the cremaster muscle. The this scrotal fascia is incised to expose the vaginal tunic (*Figure 3*). The testicle, enclosed in the vaginal tunic, is forced through the incision by pressure applied on the cranial aspect (*Figure 4*).

The gubernaculum testis is incised, the testicle retracted caudally and the parietal and visceral layers of the vagina tunic incised with sharp and blunt dissection (*Figure 5*). The testicular vessels and ductus deferens are triple-clamped and double-ligated with 00 catgut (*Figures 6 & 7*). The testicle is excised.

Figure 4—The testicle is exposed by pressure applied cranially.

Figure 5—The proper and visceral vaginal tunics are incised.

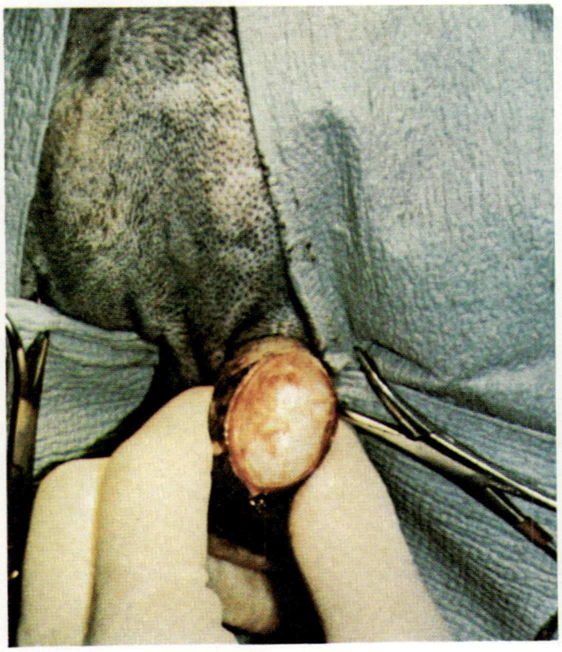

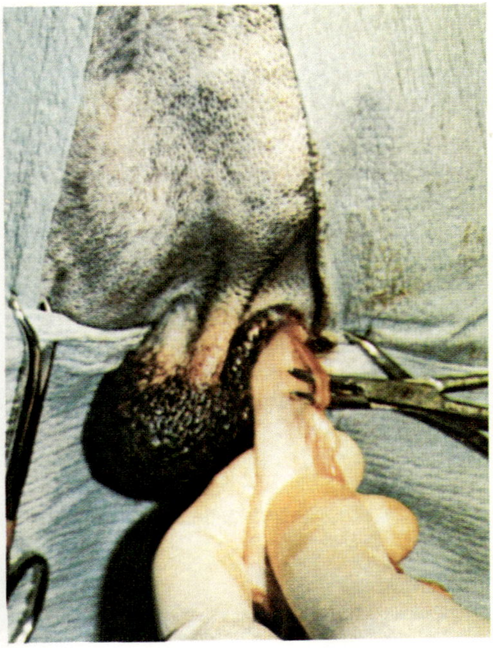

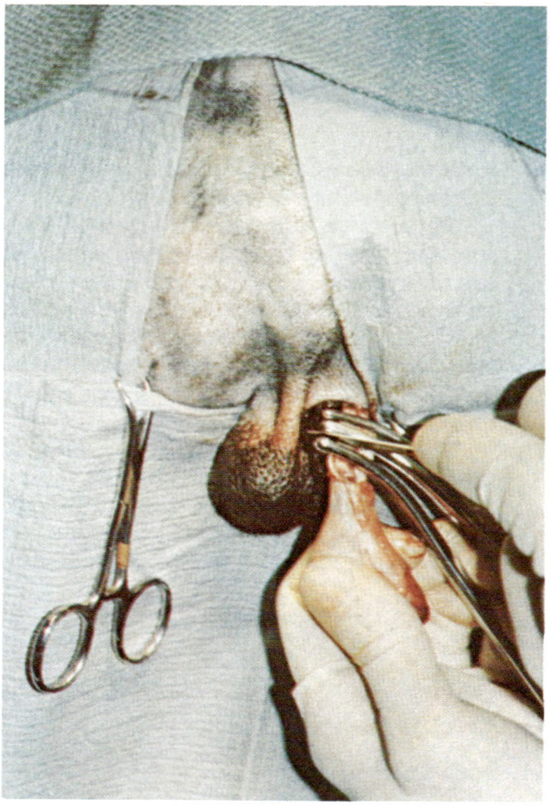

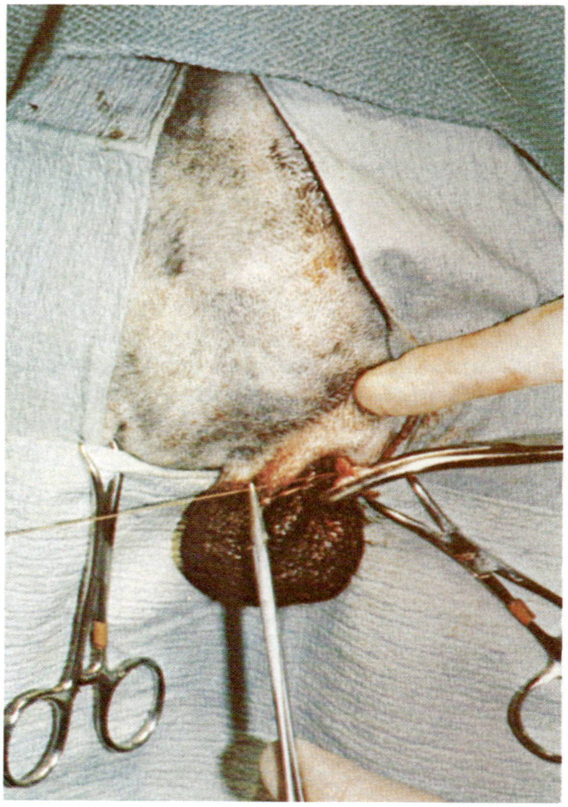

The opposite testicle is exposed by pressure applied from the cranial aspect and incision of the thin midline raphe (*Figure 8*). This testicle is excised as the vessels and ductus are ligated (*Figure 9*).

Each set of ligations is checked for hemorrhage and replaced in the scrotum. The scrotal incision is apposed with sutures of nonabsorbable material in a simple interrupted or mattress pattern (*Figure 10*).

Accessory draping is removed to expose the site for perineal incision (*Figure 11*).

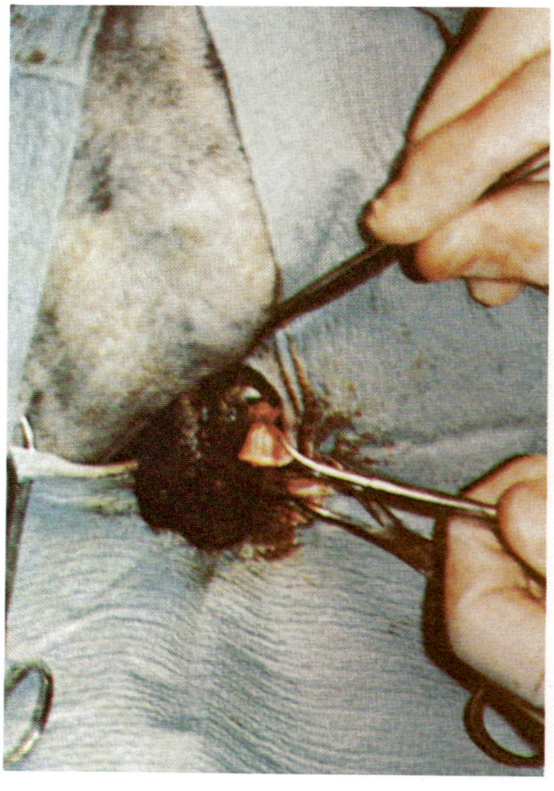

REFERENCES

1. Johnston, D.E.; Archibald, J.: The Testes. In *Canine Surgery*, 1st Archibald Ed., Am. Vet. Publications, Santa Barbara, Calif., 1974; pp 720-729.
2. Harvey, C.E.: Scrotal Ablation and Castration in the Dog. *JAAHA* 9:170-171; 1973.
3. Pettit, G.D.: Perineal Hernia in the Dog. *Cornell Vet.* 52:261-179; 1962.

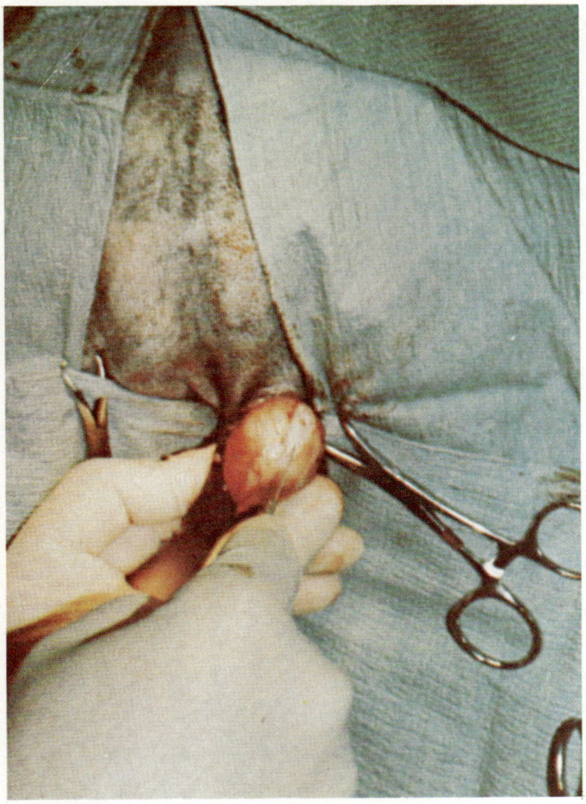

Figures 6, 7, 8 *(left to right)*

Figure 6—Three forceps are applied and the spermatic cord is incised between the distal two forceps.

Figure 7—The testicular vessels and ductus are doubly ligated with catgut.

Figure 8—The opposite testical is exposed by digital pressure and incision of the thin medial raphe.

Figures 9, 10, 11 *(left to right below)*

Figure 9—The second testicle is excised and the stump double ligated.

Figure 10—The skin incision is apposed with interrupted nonabsorbable sutures.

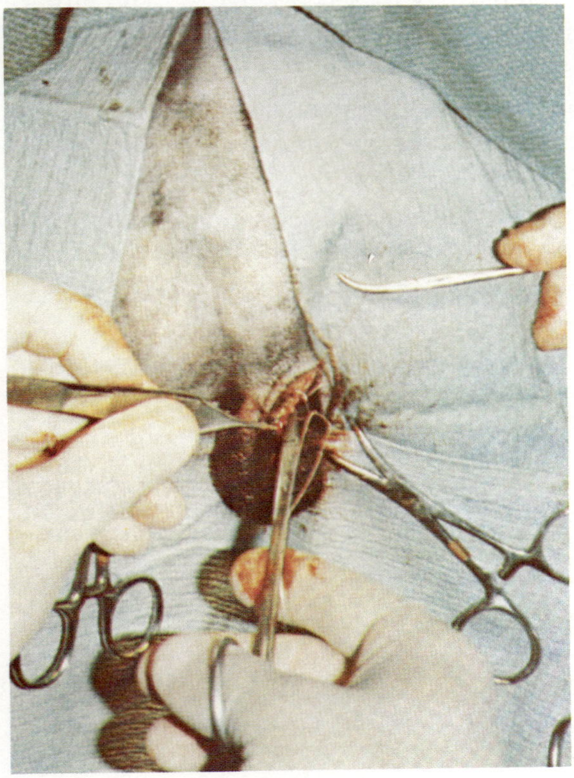

Figure 11—Castration is completed and perineal surgery can be started.

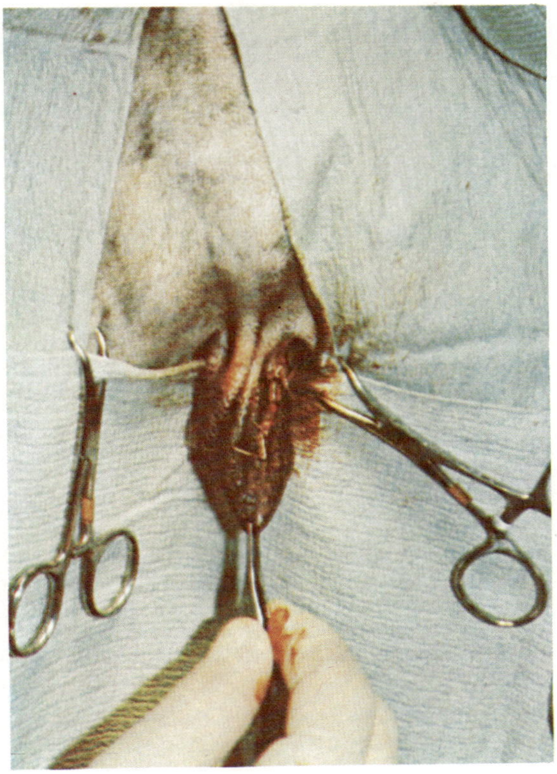

a technique for

VASECTOMY in DOGS

Leon D. Rubin, VMD
Douglas C. Maplesden, DVM, PhD
Rhawnhurst Animal Hospital
7905 Bustleton Avenue
Philadelphia, Pennsylvania 19152

The technique for vasectomy described here varies from the standard method. The vascular network along the ductus deferens (deferent artery and vein) is dissected and a length of ductus measuring 5 to 6 cm is removed without prior crushing with forceps or subsequent ligation or cauterization. The operation produces rapid healing with minimal postsurgical inflammation and no unfavorable sequelae.

VASECTOMY is indicated when a sterile dog with normal libido is desired or when the owner, for cosmetic, anthropomorphic, or other reasons, requests a vasectomy rather than castration.

The operation has been succinctly and clearly described.[1,2] Another author[3] has described a modification of the standard procedure whereby the ductus deferens is divided by electrosurgery, and the cut ends are cauterized.

General anesthesia is induced, starting with intravenous administration of surital sodium followed by intubation[4] and balanced inhalation anesthesia.

The ventral midline area cranial to the scrotum is prepared for aseptic surgery. An incision 2 to 3 cm long is made on the midline cranial to the scrotum and parallel to the spermatic cords. One spermatic cord is exposed by blunt dissection and brought through the incision (*Figure 1*). The cord is rotated and the ductus deferens is identified by its ivory-colored, cord-like structure.

The tunica vaginalis parietalis is incised and the ductus deferens is exposed (*Figure 2*). The minute vascular network running along the ductus (deferent artery and vein) is removed from the ductus by blunt dissection for 6 to 7 cm along the ductus, care being taken that the delicate artery and vein are not ruptured.

The usual procedure for dividing the ductus is to apply crushing forceps to the ductus, ligate, and cut. Another method is to divide the ductus by electrosurgery.[3]

In the procedure described here, a section of the ductus 5 to 6 cm long is removed without the use of crushing forceps or the application of ligatures (*Figures 3 & 4*). Because the deferent vein and artery have been stripped from the ductus, little if any bleeding occurs, and because of the length of the ductus removed, there is no chance that the cut ends will anastomose. Since ligatures are not used, no foreign substance that can cause irritation is buried. In addition, the delay in healing typically encountered after electrocautery[5] is avoided.

The small incision in the tunica is not sutured. The cord is repositioned by slight caudal tension on the testicle and the operation is repeated on the other cord. The single skin incision is closed with interrupted sutures using 32-gauge monofilament stainless steel sutures. Virtually no tissue reaction occurs, and healing is rapid. The sutures are removed in seven days.

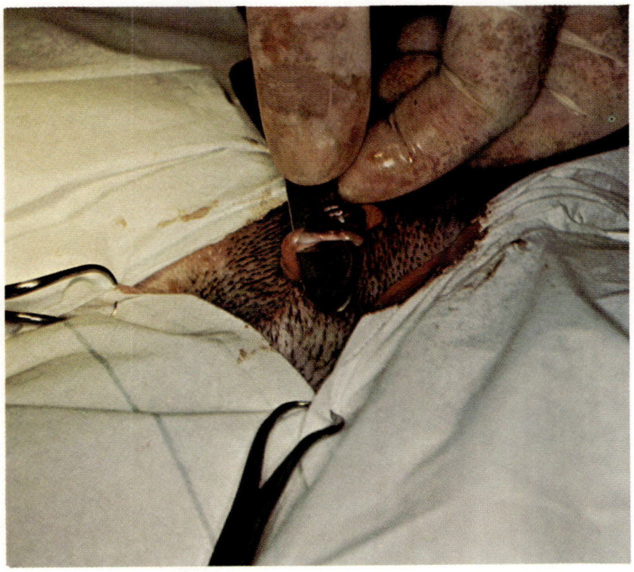

Figure 1
The spermatic cord after exposure by blunt dissection. Note the ivory-colored ductuc deferens.

The client should be told that ejaculates from bilaterally vasectomized dogs may comtain spermatozoa for as long as 21 days after vasectomy,[6] and thus the dog is potentially fertile for that period of time.

REFERENCES

1. Archibald, J., ed.: *Canine Surgery*, 3nd Archibald ed. American Veterinary Publications, Inc., Santa Barbara, Calif., 1974; p 725.
2. Wilson, G.P.: *Vet. Clinics of N. Am.* 5(3):545-546; 1975;
3. Clinton, R.K. *et al:* Canine Vasectomy: A Modern Solution to an Age-Old Problem (A Photographic Essay). *VM/SAC 67*:1097-1099; 1972.
4. Rubin, L.D.; Maplesden, D.C.: A Simplified Technique for Endotracheal Intubation in Gogs. *JAVMA* (in press).
5. Knecht, C.D. *et al: Fundamental Techniques in Veterinary Surgery. W. B. Saunders, Philadelphia, Pa., 1975; p 3.*
6. *Pineda, M.H. et al*: Disappearance of Spermatozoa from the Ejaculates of Vasectomized Dogs. *JAVMA 168*:502-503; 1976.

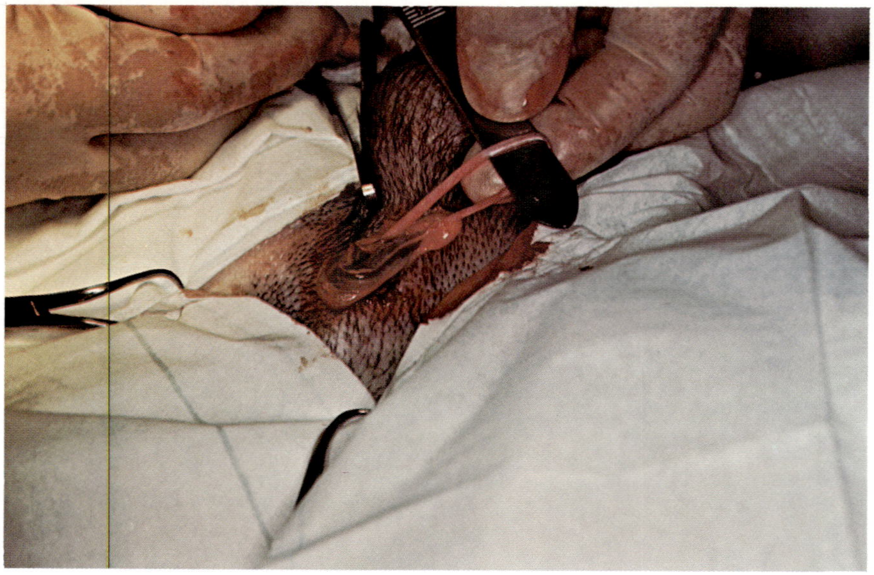

Figure 2
The ductus deferens is separated and incised.

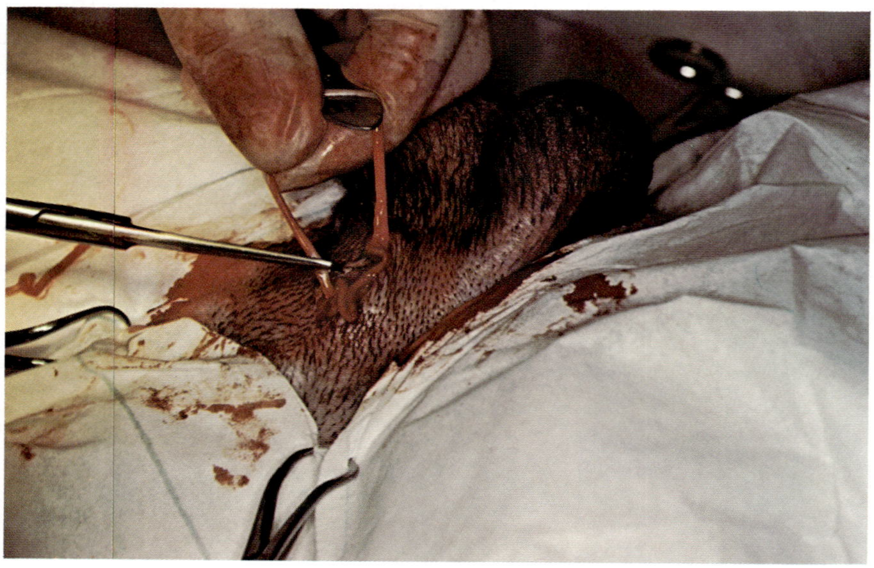

Figure 3
The ductus deferens is incised.

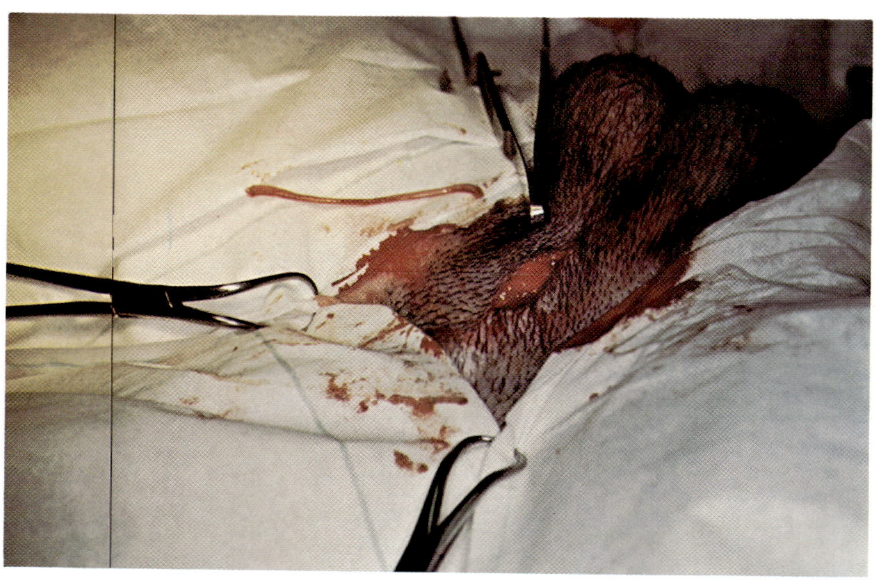

Figure 4
A section of the ductus deferens 6 cm long is laid out on the drape. The incision is ready for closure with interrupted sutures of stainless steel wire.

Transmissible venereal tumor: surgery and chemotherapy

(a case report)

Lawrence T. McAfee, DVM
John T. McAfee, DVM
McAfee Animal Hospital
R.R. 13, Box 265
Valparaiso, Indiana 46383

TRANSMISSIBLE veneral turmors commonly affect the mucosa of the genital organs of young, sexually mature animals.[1] The tumors are usually spread by coitus.[2] In this paper we report treatment of a transmissible venereal tumor with a combination of surgery and chemotherapy.

Case Report

A 1½-year-old intact male West Highland White Terrier was examined because pus and blood had been draining from its prepuce for several weeks. Appetite and activity were reportedly normal. The dog had been used for stud service three times; most recently, only three weeks earlier. Micturition was normal and no incontinence had been noticed. The urine was clear and odorless.

Physical Examination

The dog weighed 17.16 lb (7.8 kg) and appeared active and alert. When the bladder and the kidneys were palpated no abnormalities were found, although mild cystodynia was evident. A foul-smelling serosanguincous pus exuded from the prepuce (*Figure 1*). When the penis was extended from the prepuce, numerous bright-red, lobulated, hyperemic, ulcerated masses were seen along the penile shaft (*Figure 2*). These masses hid the glans penis (*Figure 3*). The prepuce had no gross lesions, nor did the scrotum or perineum.

Clinical Evaluation

A cystogram showed no abnormalities. Results of uninalysis and hemanalysis were within normal limits. The dog was deemed a good surgical risk, and immediate extirpation and histopathology of the tumor were undertaken.

Surgical Procedure

The dog was anesthetized with thiamylal sodium (Bio-tal® —Bio-Ceutic). An endotracheal tube was passed and anesthesia was maintained with halothane. Due to the friability and high vascularity of the masses, electrocautery with coagulation setting was chosen to remove the tumor. We also felt that the use of electrocautery would minimize the chance of normal tissue beeing reinoculated with tumorous tissue.

A medium-point electrode was attached to a Miller electroscalpel. Hot coagulation was achieved by placing hemostats at the base of the tumouour mass, flush with the normal penile tissue (*Figure 4*), and slowly electrocoagulating and removing the extremely friable masses (*Figure 5 & 6*). This technique resulted in total gross extirpation of the masses with no resultant active hemorrhage from the penis (*Figure 7*). At this time the normal anatomy of the glans penis could be seen (*Figure 8*).

The penis and prepuce were thoroughly flushed with sterile saline solution, and irrigation with gentomicin sulfate (Gentocin® —Schering) was begun. The prepuce was flushed with 20 cc of the antibiotic, which was massaged thoroughly into the sheath. Panolog® (Squibb) was dispensed for application to the penis twice daily for seven days.

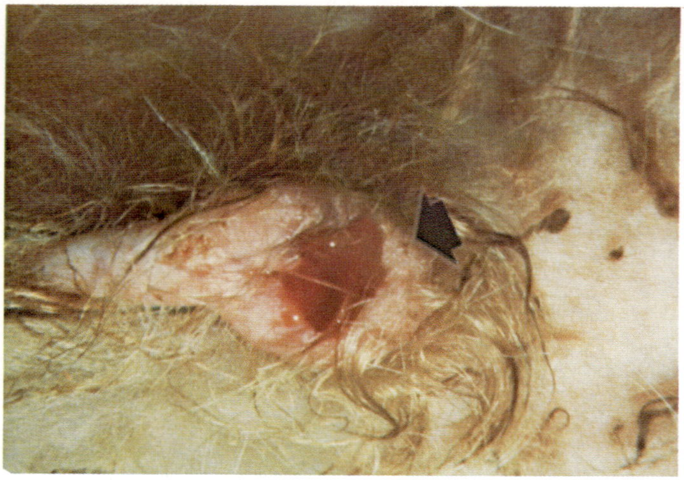

Figure 1

Sanies exuding from the penile sheath. Notice the matted hair and inflamed prepuce (*arrow*).

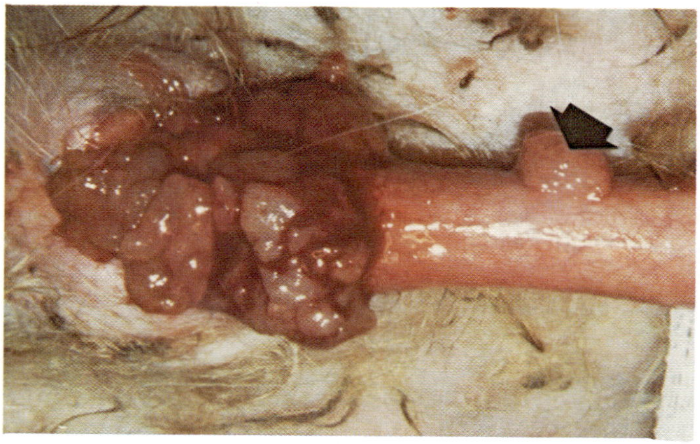

Figure 2

A moderately ulcerated, hyperemic, firmly lobular mass adhering to the surface of the shaft (*arrow*).

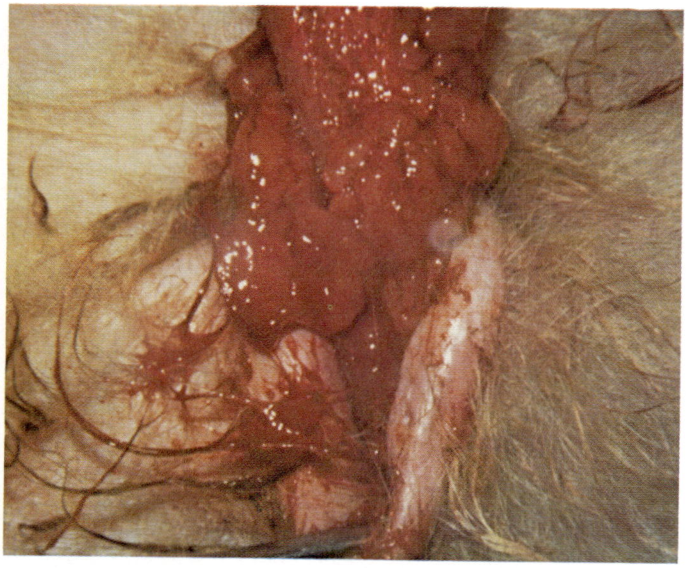

Figure 3

The glans penis, with extremely vascular tissues covering its surface. Notice the bright red of the neoplastic masses.

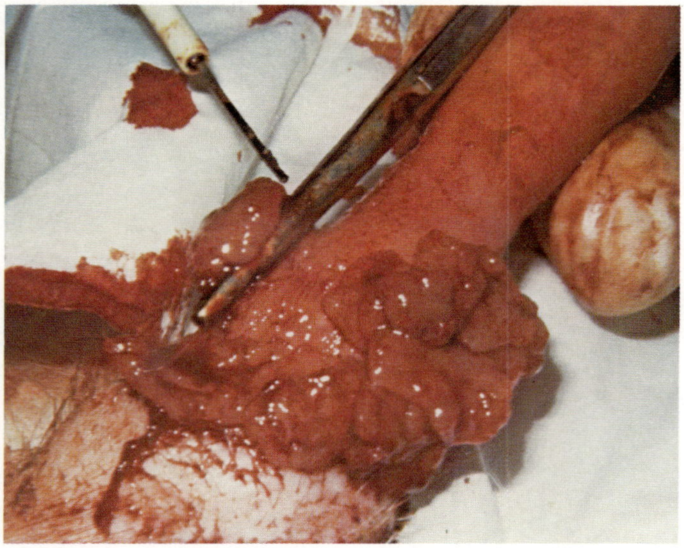

Figure 4
The penis has been extruded from the sheath. Hemostats are being used to separate the tumor from the penile base in preparation for electrocautery.

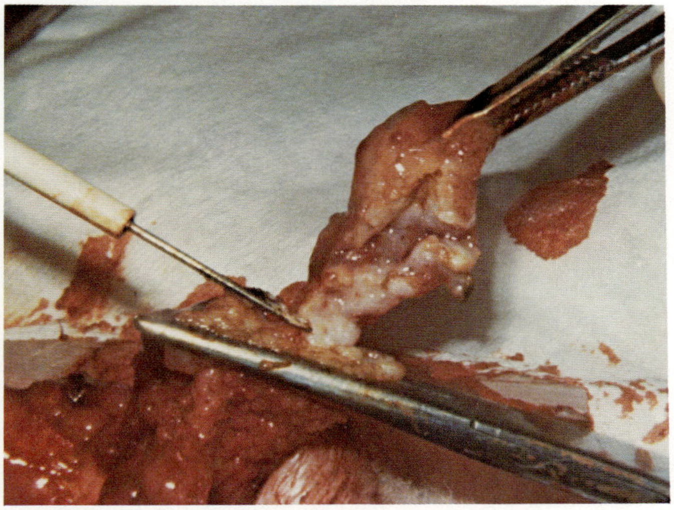

Figure 5
The electroscalpel is used to remove one of the masses. The yellow and blanched appearance is caused by the thermocautery.

Figure 6
One of the extirpated masses. Formalin, used as a fixing medium, distorts the venereal tumor cell and causes it to lose characteristics vital to its identification. Thus impression smears and needle aspiration are recommended as quick and accurate methods of establishing a clinical diagnosis. Histopathologically, the mass was characterized by cords exhibiting a moderately high mitotic index. Plasma cells were also found within the mass.

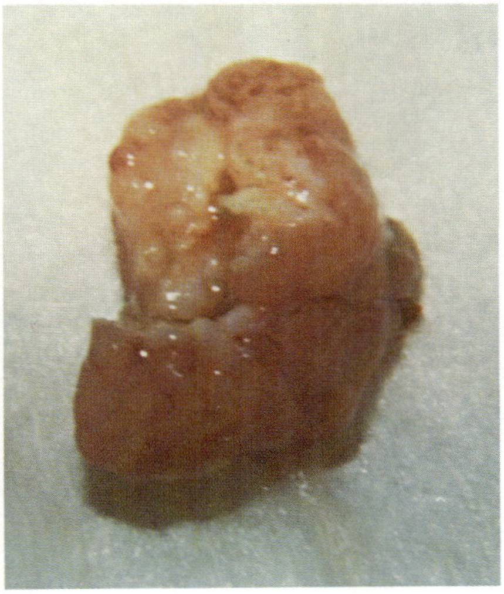

A tissue section was submitted to a laboratory and confirmed histopathologically as a transmissible veneral tumor.

Surgical excision provides immediate relief, but does not prevent the possibility of metastatic foci elsewhere.[3] Also, transmissible veneral tumors often recur.[4] Therefore, a regimen of chemotherapy was initiated on the third postoperative day.

To ensure that toxic signs would be minimal and to attack the veneral tumor cells at several stages of mitosis[3], three drugs were used. Vincristine sulfact (Oncovin® —Lilly) was given intravenously once weekly at a dosage of 0.5 mg/m². Oral medication consisted of Methotrexate (Lederle) at a dosage of 2.5 mg/m² and cyclophosphamide (CYtoxan® —Mead-Johnson) at a dosage of 50 mg/m² given alternately every other day.

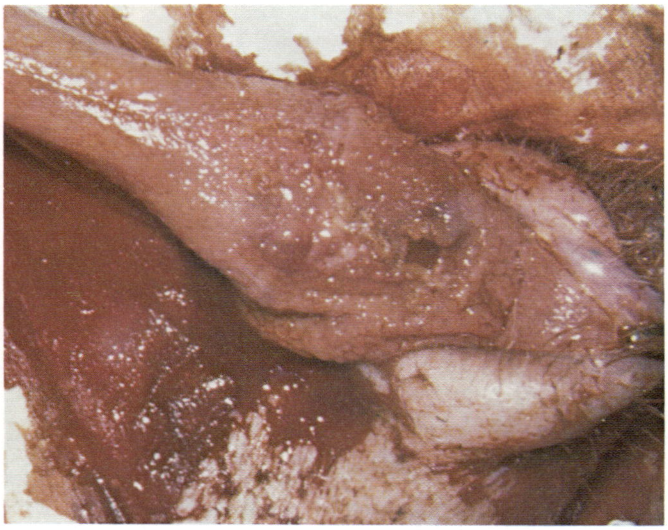

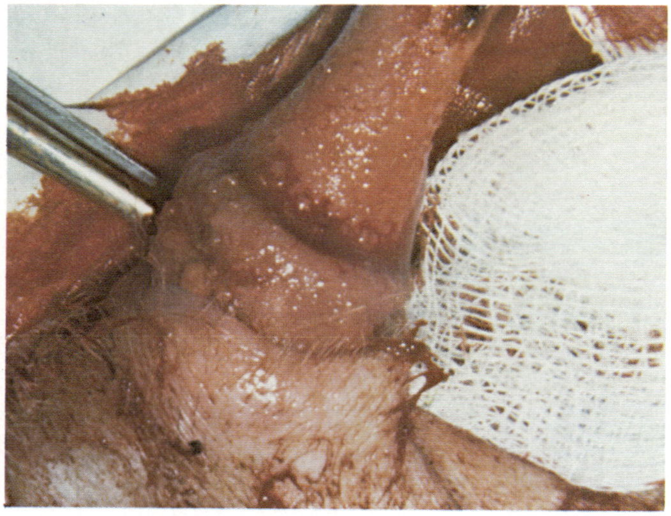

Figures 7 & 8—The penis after removal of the masses. There is no active hemorrhage.

The most common adverse reactions to these drugs are alopecia, leukopenia, constipation, nausea, and vomiting. These side effects can be treated if deemed necessary.

The chemotherapy was continued for eight weeks. Each week, before the Oncovin was administered, hemanalysis was performed to determine if leukopenia was present. The white blood cell level never fell below 8000/cm³. If leukopenia, accompanied by a decrease of white blood cells to less than 2000/cm³ had developed, administration of Onocovin would have been discontinued.

Three weeks after surgery, regression of the tumor appeared to be complete (*Figures 9-11*). When chemotherapy was discontinued a tissue impression from the penis, stained with Wright's stain, was sent to our consulting laboratory. Shown on the stain were erythrocytes and squamous epithelial cells in various stages of keratinization. Neoplastic cells were not seen.

Two months postoperatively, the patient was an active stud with normal penile anatomy and function.

A 3-year-old West Highland Terrier bitch living in the same household had previously been bred to the patient. Impression smears from the female's vulva and vagina were negative for transmissible venereal tumor.

Discusion

Transmissible veneral tumors are commonly found on the exterior genitalia of both sexes.[4] Little evidence to date supports a virus as the cause; transmission is thought to be due to cellular implants.[5] Apparently the biologic behavior of this tumor varies strikingly. Sometimes the tumor remains localized and spontaneous regression occurs; other times metastasis occurs—usually to regional lymph nodes and the eye, resulting in the animal's death. For this reason all cases should be considered malignant. We recommend surgery to treat the localized tumor and chemotherapy to treat the metastatic tumor.

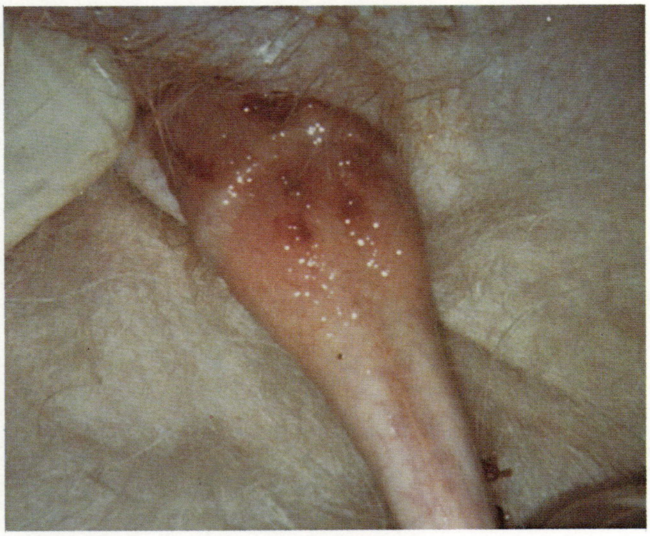

Figure 9
The penis one week postoperatively.

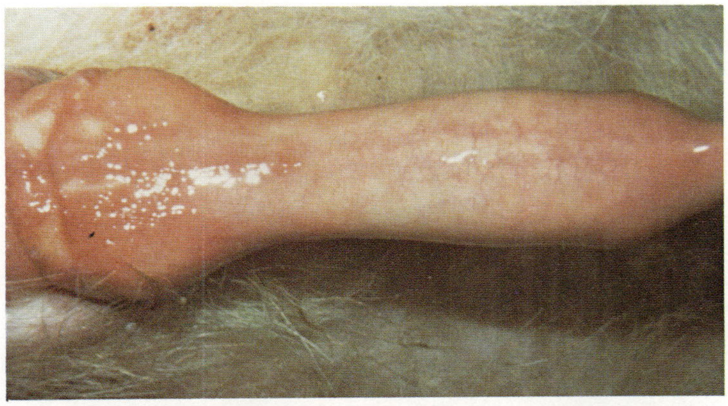

Figure 10
The penis two weeks postoperatively.

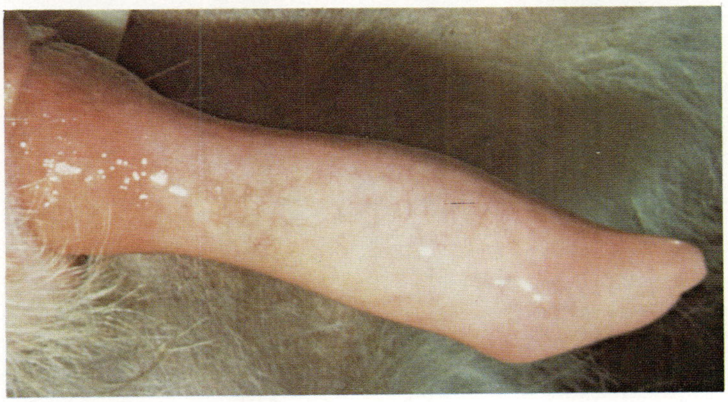

Figure 11
The penis three weeks postoperatively. The gross appearance is now normal.

ACKNOWLEDGMENT
Compliments are extended to the Animal Disease Diagnostic Laboratory of Purdue University for rapid and accurate diagnosis of submitted specimens; and to Nancy Jo McAfee and Isolde McAfee for manuscript preparation.

REFERENCES

1. Ettinger, S.J.: *Textbook of Veterinary Internal Medicine.* W.B. Saunders Co., Philadelphia, Pa., 1975; pp 1072-1073.
2. Roberts, S.J.: *Veterinary Obstetrics and Genital Diseases*, 2nd ed. Stephen J. Roberts, Ithaca, N.Y., 1971; p 594.
3. Kirk, R.W.: *Current Veterinary Therapy V.* W.B. Sauncers Co., Philadelphia, Pa., 1974; pp 933-934.
4. Bojrab, M.J.: *Current Techniques in Small Animal Surgery.* Lea & Febiger, Philadelphia, Pa., 1975; p 254.
5. Siegmund, O.H., ed.: *The Merck Veterinary Manual*, 4th ed. Merck & Co., Inc., Rahway, N.J., 1973; pp 849-850.

a sterile surgical procedure for FELINE CASTRATION

(a photographic essay)

Lester Mandelker, DVM
Community Veterinary Hospital
1631 West Bay Drive
Largo, Florida 33540

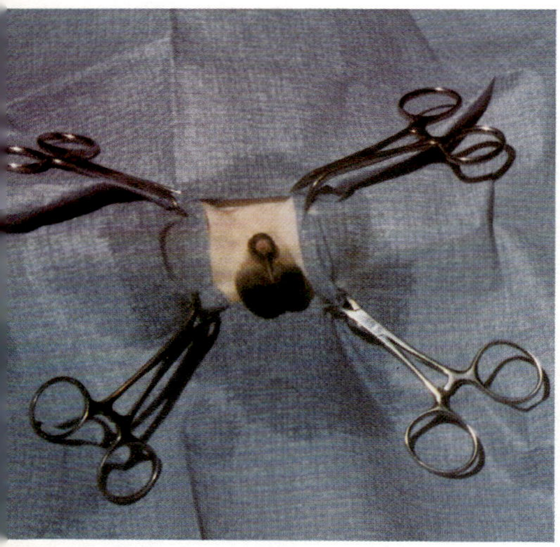

Figure 1—The surgical site is prepped and draped for surgery.

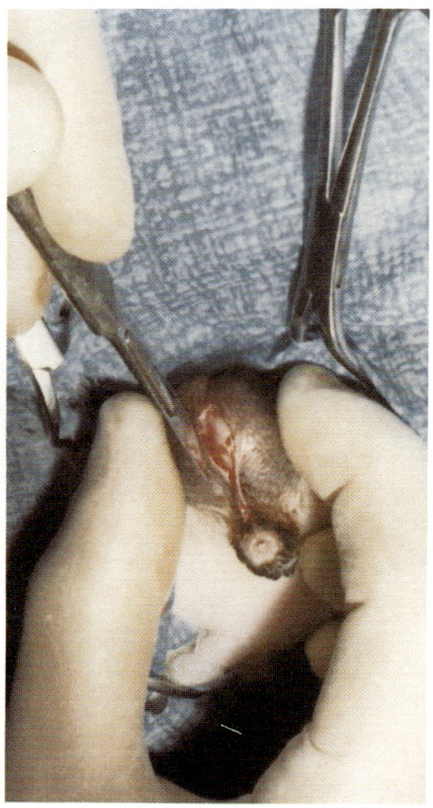

Figure 2—A midline incision is made in the scrotum.

CASTRATION of the cat is one of a few surgical procedures routinely performed in veterinary medicine without sterile technique. The procedure illustrated here makes use of sterile technique but requires only a few minutes more than do other procedures for feline castration.

The mature cat is given a combination intravenous injection of 0.5 cc each of ketamine (Vetalar® —Parke-Davis; Ketaset® —Bristol), piperacetazine (Psymod® — Pitman-Moore), and atropine. Intubation is optional. On a short-haired cat, the surgical site is clipped; on a long-haired cat, the site is plucked. The site is scrubbed with povidone-iodine solution (Betadine® — Purdue Frederick) and sprayed with alcohol. With the animal in dorsal recumbency, the surgical area is draped (*Figure 1*).

Next, a midline incision is made in the scrotum (*Figure 2*). One testicle is brought through the incision with sufficient tension being applied to expose the entire spermatic cord. Then the vas deferens is carefully separated from the spermatic cord (*Figure 3*), and the vas is used in a double square knot to tie off the spermatic vessels (*Figure 4*).

After both testicles have been removed in this way, the scrotum is sutured as shown in Figure 5. Only two or three sutures are needed (*Figure 6*).

This method is simple, provides good asepsis, causes no hemorrhage, and minimizes trauma to the genital tissue. Among the more than 100 cats I have castrated this way, there have never been any complications. For some reason the cats never bother the stitches. Healing is evident in a few days. The stitches are removed in seven to 10 days.

The extra time (two to three minutes) required for this procedure is more than compensated by its clean, cosmetically pleasing appearance. Although the fee for the surgery has to be a little higher, clients seem not to mind the extra cost, if they are aware of it. ■

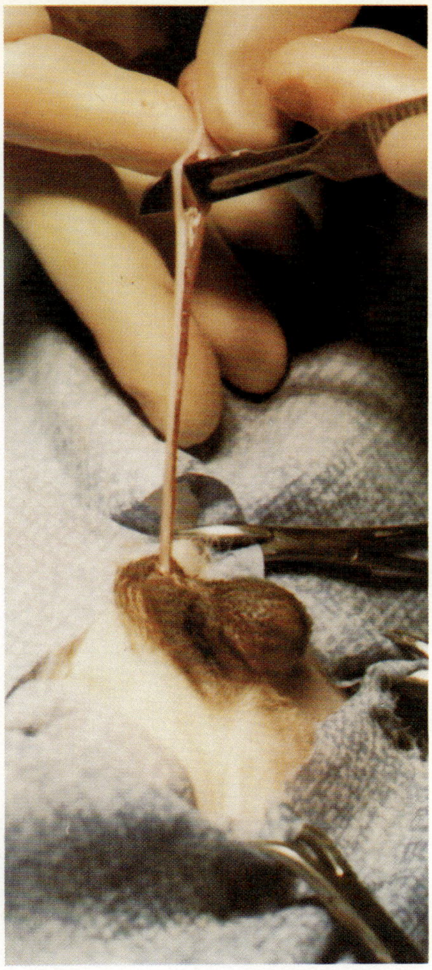

Figure 3—The vas deferens is separated from the spermatic cord.

Figure 4—After the vas has been separated from the spermatic cord, it is used in a double square knot to tie off the spermatic vessels.

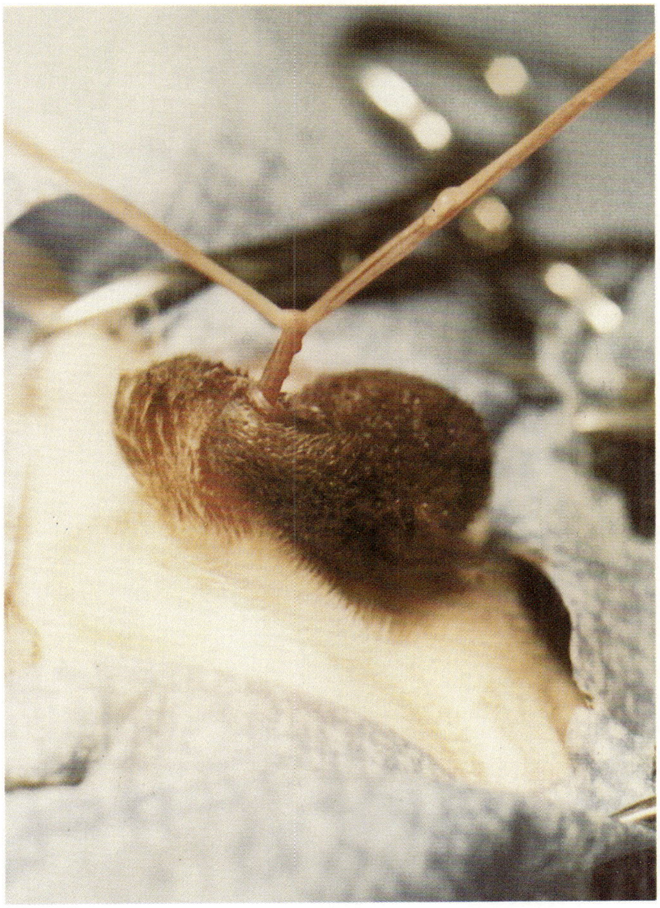

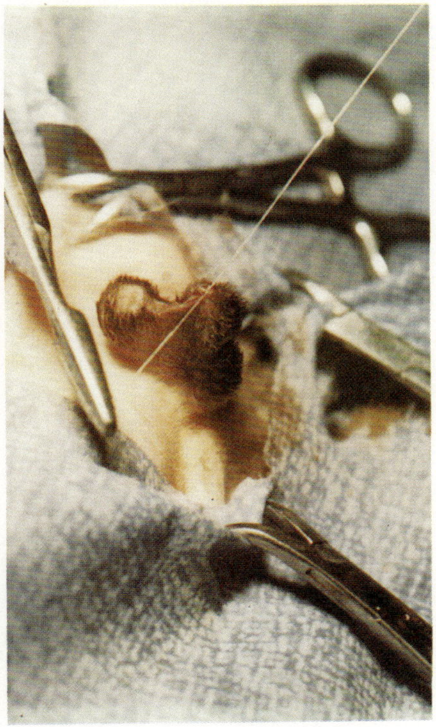

Figure 5—The incision is closed.

Figure 6—The completed surgery.

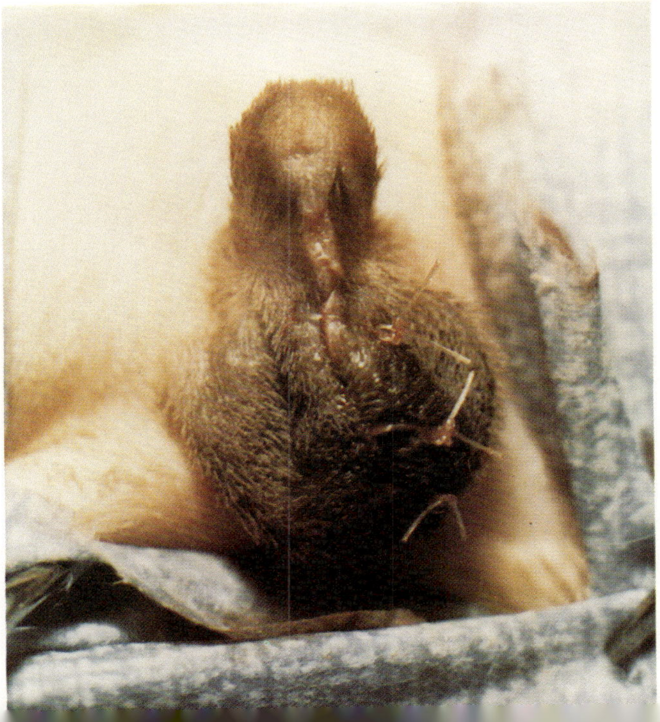

Small Animal Surgery

OPTIC

use of a corneoscleral homograft to treat

PROLIFERATIVE EPISCLERITIS in the dog

R. L. Peiffer, Jr., DVM
Comparative Ophthalmology
College of Veterinary Medicine
University of Minnesota
St. Paul, Minnesota 55108

K. N. Gelatt, VMD
R. M. Gwin, DVM
Comparative Ophthalmology
College of Veterinary Medicine
University of Florida
Gainesville, Florida 32610

Supported in part by NIH Fellowships 1F22 EYO197701 (Peiffer) and 1F22 EYO310001 (Gwin).

PROLIFERATIVE DISEASES of the canine uvea, cornea, conjunctiva, and/or sclera frequently require excisional biopsy as an aid to determining appropriate therapy and a diagnosis. Lamellar or full-thickness excision of the fibrous coats of the eye may be necessary, depending on the extent of the pathologic process. In a full-thickness excision, a fresh full-thickness homograft from a donor animal can provide satisfactory cosmetic and functional results.

Case Report

A 2-year-old male Boston Bull Terrier exhibited a limbal mass that had been noticed about four weeks before the animal was presented for examination. The referring veterinarian had attempted excision and had treated the lesion postoperatively with topical antibiotics and corticosteriods (Vetropolycin HC®—Pitman-Moore™). Recurrence was noticed two weeks later and the animal was referred to the Ophthalmology Section of the University of Minnesota Veterinary Hospital.

When presented, the dog appeared healthy. Pathologic findings were limited to the right eye, where a limbal mass 2 cm in diameter was seen temporally. The cornea, sclera, and bulbar conjunctiva were infiltrated by pink, fleshy, proliferative tissue. Extension into the cornea was characterized by a leading edge of corneal edema (*Figure 1*).

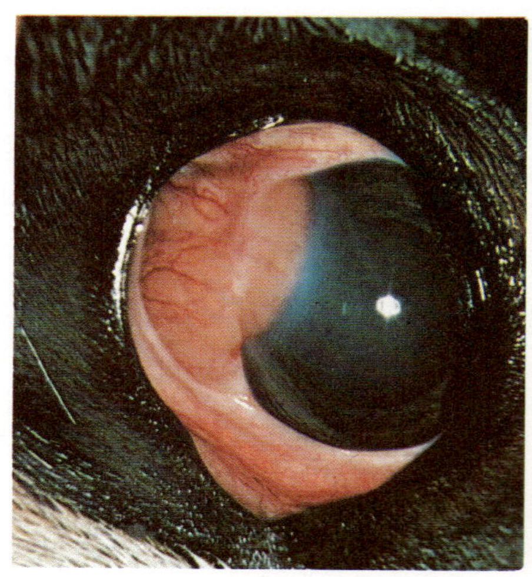

Figure 1—Limbal tumor in the right eye of a 2-year-old Boston Terrier with involvement of the temporal cornea, sclera, and bulbar conjunctiva.

Fine-needle aspiration biopsy of the mass and impression smears showed numerous lymphoblasts. Based on these findings, a tentative diagnosis of lymphosarcoma was made. Gonioscopy with the Tronsco goniolens demonstrated a narrowed and hypermic temporal angle due to infiltration and depression of the overlying cornea and sclera; however, the inner limbus and the anterior chamber appeared free of involvement. Thoracic radiographs were normal. Complete blood count,

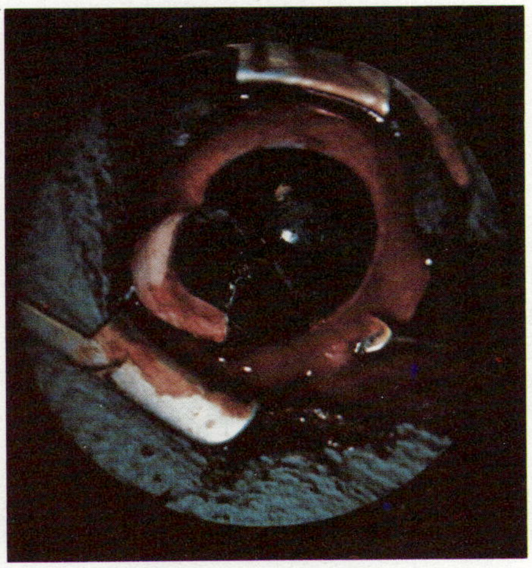

Figure 2—Full-thickness excision of the involved tissues was performed. Note the shaped and trimmed homograft.

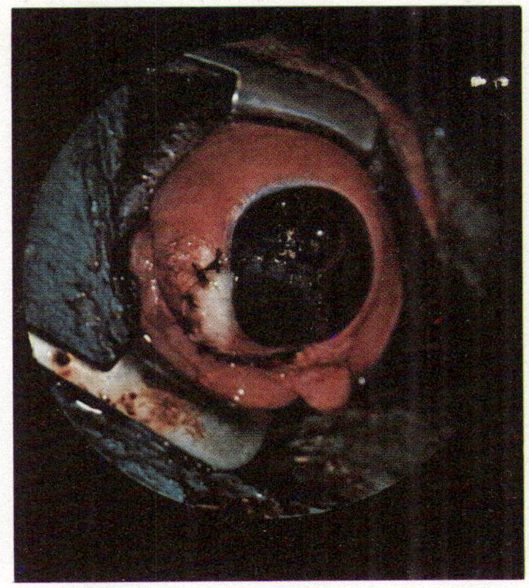

Figure 3—A fresh homogenous corneoscleral graft was sutured in place and the anterior chamber was reformed with an air bubble. Adjacent conjunctiva was undermined and sutured to the limbus with simple interrupted 6-0 chromic collagen.

blood urea nitrogen, alkaline phosphatase, and urinalysis were within normal limits.

Treatment

Because of the potentially malignant nature of the tumor, lamellar excision was decided upon. With the dog under general anesthesia, the margins of the tumor were outlined, including the full thickness of involved bulbar conjunctiva to a depth of one-third the corneal and scleral thickness. After lamellar resection, gross involvement of deeper cornea and sclera was present. Impression smears again demonstrated numerous lymphoblasts, and lymphosarcoma was still suspected.

The decision was made to perform a full-thickness corneoscleral excision. The cornea and sclera were incised, a deep cylodialysis was performed, and the involved tissue was excised by gentle separation from the underlying uvea (*Figure 2*). A fresh graft of cornea and sclera was prepared from the enucleated eye of a canine blood donor. The graft was trimmed to match the excised tissue and sutured in place with simple interrupted sutures of 6-0 chromic collagen. Bulbar conjunctiva was undermined and pulled over the graft to the limbus where it was affixed with the same suture pattern and material (*Figure 3*). The anterior chamber was reformed with an air bubble.

Postoperative treatment consisted of 250 mg of oral ampicillin t.i.d. as a prophylaxis against infection, and 2 mg of dexamethasone given intramuscularly b.i.d. to temper surgically induced iridocyclitis and possible rejection of the graft. Topical 1% atropine and 10% phenylephrine were administered q.i.d. to prevent ciliary spasm and synechiae associated with the intraocular inflammation. A topical antibiotic/corticosteroid suspension (Maxitrol® —Alcon) was also administered q.i.d. to enhance the effects of the systemic drugs. Hospitalization and treatment continued for seven days.

Six days after surgery the graft was edematous. Two of the sutures had untied, but integrity of the anterior chamber was maintained. The host cornea was edematous centrally. An irregular central ulcer involving the epithelium was attributed to surgical trauma and exposure (*Figure 4*). The anterior chamber was well-formed. Lens, vitreous, and fundus appeared normal.

Topical administration of Maxitrol was continued despite the ulceration, because the ulcer was superficial and appeared uninfected.

Oral antibiotics were discontinued 10 days after surgery. Oral dexamethasone (15 mg b.i.d.) and topical Maxitrol were continued for three weeks. At this time the ulcer had epithelialized. The graft

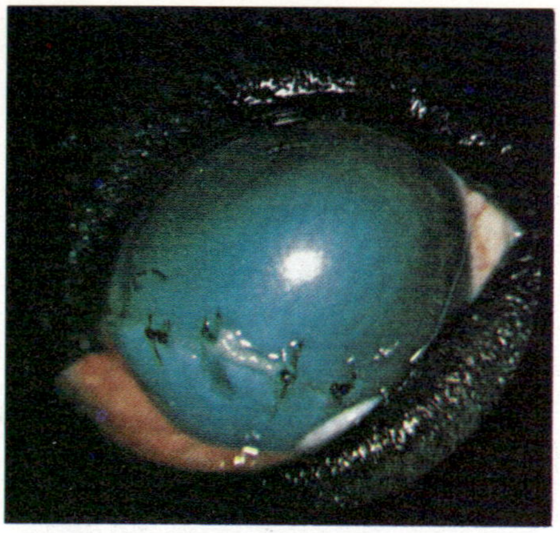

Figure 4—The eye six days after surgery. One suture was gone and another untied. The donor tissue was diffusely edematous; moderated edema of the central host cornea and an epithelial ulcer were present.

Figure 5—Eight months after surgery. The grafted tissue was vascularized and the transplanted cornea translucent. The eye was otherwise normal.

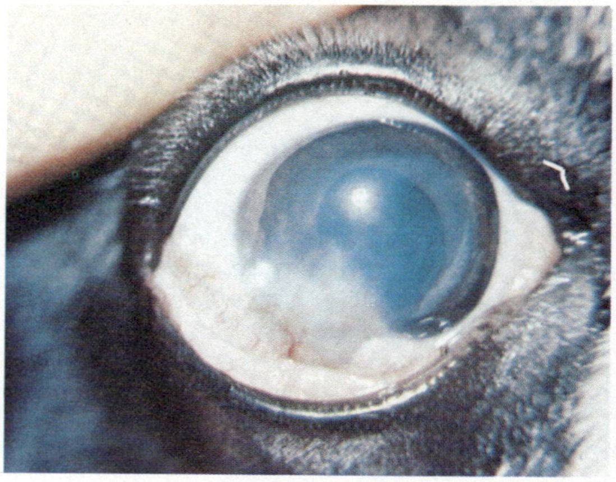

appeared intact but was edematous and partially vascularized. Fluorescein retention was negative. Oral steroids were discontinued but topical therapy was continued for three more weeks.

Eight months after surgery the grafted cornea was translucent, edematous, and scarred. On its surface was an extensive vascular network. The grafted sclera could not be directly examined; overlying conjunctiva demonstrated hypervascularity (*Figure 5*). Complete ophthalmic examination including tonometry and indirect ophthalmoscopy demonstrated no abnormalities. Good functional vision was present.

Histopathology

The clinical diagnosis of malignancy was not confirmed by histopathologic examination of the surgically excised tissue. The specimen consisted of numerous fibroblasts with an infiltration of lymphocytes and histiocytes (*Figure 6*).

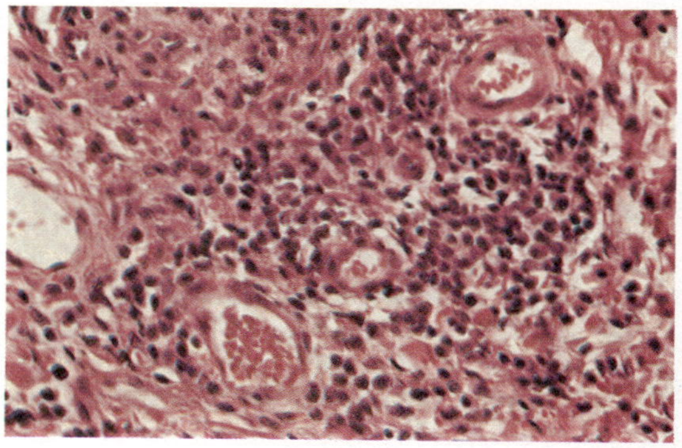

Figure 6—The excised tissue was characterized by many fibroblasts, collagen fibers and ground substance, and a nongranulomatous inflammatory response consisting of lymphocytes and plasma cells. The tissue was well vascularized and the inflammatory cells were organized in a perivascular pattern.

Discussion

A proliferative mass at the limbus in a young dog presents a challenging diagnostic problem. Neoplastic processes need to be differentiated from inflammatory disease, and extent of involvement must be determined before a prognosis and course of management can be established.

Nodular fasciitis is a benign lesion that has been reported to occur in man[1-7] The etiopathogenesis is uncertain. Pathologic findings consist of fibroblasts (often exhibiting miotic figures), histiocytes, lymphocytes, and unorganized collagen. The proliferative tissue is well vascularized and, while thought to originate from Tenon's capsule, may invade adjacent tissues.[1,3-5,7] The pathologic process appears to be a collagen disease that elicits an inflammatory response. In the dog, the term *proliferative episcleritis* is perhaps more applicable than *nodular fasciitis* because 1) involvement cannot be definitely related to Tenon's capsule, and 2) the condition is characterized by broad proliferation and infiltration rather than nodular outgrowth.[6]

Proliferative episcleritis can be difficult to differentiate clinically from malignant tumors. Histopathologic interpretation can also be challenging because the condition can be mistaken for sarcome orlymphoid neoplasm. We have seen partial regression of similar lesions in a few cases after treatment with corticosteriods, but generally the lesions are unresponsive to medical therapy.

Surgery was performed in this case because malignancy was suspected, based on clinical observations and biopsy information. Examination of a frozen section during surgery, after partial lamellar excision, might have made the radical full-thickness removal unnecessary.

The use of full-thickness homogenous corneoscleral grafts in the dog has been described.[8] Eight-0 Nylon suture would have been less reactive and the knots more stable than the 6-0 chromic collagen used in this case. While the majority of ocular tumors warrant consideration of enucleation, use of the technique discussed in this paper can provide rewarding results.

REFERENCES

1. Font, R.D.; Zimmerman, L.E.: Nodular Fasciitis of the Eye and Adnexa. *Arch. Ophthal. 75:*475-481; 1960.
2. Hufter, R.V.P. *et al:* Fasciitis: A Report of 70 Cases with Follow-up Proving Benignity of the Lesion. *Cancer 15:*992-995; 1962.
3. Price, E.B. *et al:* Nodular Fasciitis: A Clinicopathologic Analysis of 65 Cases. *Am. J. Clin. Path. 35:122-136; 1961.*
4. *Tolls, R.E. et al:* Benign Nodular Fasciitis Originating in Tenon's Capsule. *Arch. Ophthal. 75:*482-483; 1966.
5. Bellhorn, R.W.; Henkind, P.: Ocular Nodular Fasciitis in a Dog. *JAVMA 150:*212-213; 1967.
6. Gwin, R.M. *et al:* Unpublished data.
7. Lavignette, A.M.; Carlton, W.W.: A Case of Ocular Nodular Fasciitis in a Dog. *JAAHA 10:*503-506; 1974.
8. Gelatt, K.N. *et al:* Excision of an Adenocarcinoma of the Iris and Ciliary Body in a Dog. *JAAHA 6:*59-70; 1970.

Enucleation of the eye by subconjunctival ablation

ENUCLEATION by subconjunctival ablation has been previously described.[1] This procedure has an advantage over exenteration in that it preserves the conjunctiva, extrocular muscles, and other intraorbital structures. There is usually less hemorrhage, thus less postsurgical accumulation of serum. Also, less retraction of skin into the orbital cavity gives a more acceptable cosmetic appearance. Using this technique, the optic nerve and accompanying vessels have only occasionally been difficult to expose for ligation.

Eugene L. Kuhns, DVM, MS
Wyoming Animal Hospital, Inc.
2754 Burlingame SW
Wyoming, Michigan 49509

Case Report

A 4-month-old, female German Shepherd-cross was admitted for examination of the right eye, which had been severely traumatized six weeks earlier. The cornea was opaque (*Figure 1*) and the globe was in a state of advanced buphthalmos. Clinical evidence strongly suggested permanently destroyed vision. The patient showed signs of discomfort by occasionally pawing and rubbing the affected eye. The decision to enucleate the eye was based on such factors as humane and cosmetic considerations, expense to the owner, and permanence of treatment.

After induction of general anesthesia with thiamylal sodium (Surital®—Parke-Davis) anesthesia was maintained with methoxyfulrane (Metofane™—Pitman Moore) given in a closed system. The cul-de-sac was irrigated with a 10% Betadine® solution (Purdue Frederick) followed by rinsing with a physiological saline solution. A 1% chloramphenicol ophthalmic ointment (Chloromycetin® —Parke-Davis) was applied topically and

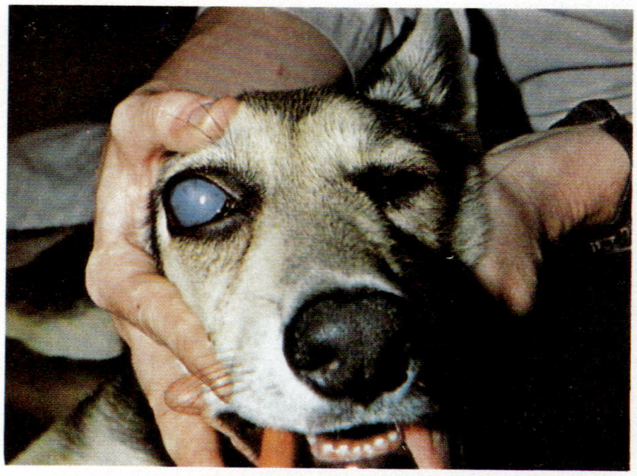

Figure 1—A 4-month-old German Shepherd-cross exhibiting a severely traumatized right eye with advanced buphthalmos.

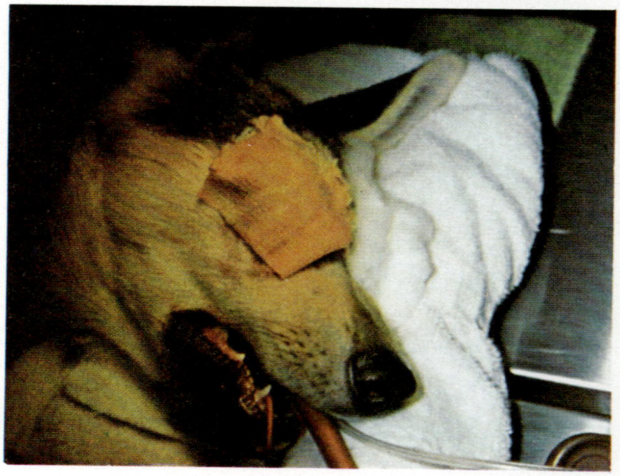

Figure 2—After the eye was prepared for enucleation, a gauze sponge impregnated with a 10% Betadine® Solution (Purdue Frederick) was applied over it while the surgeon scrubbed and gowned.

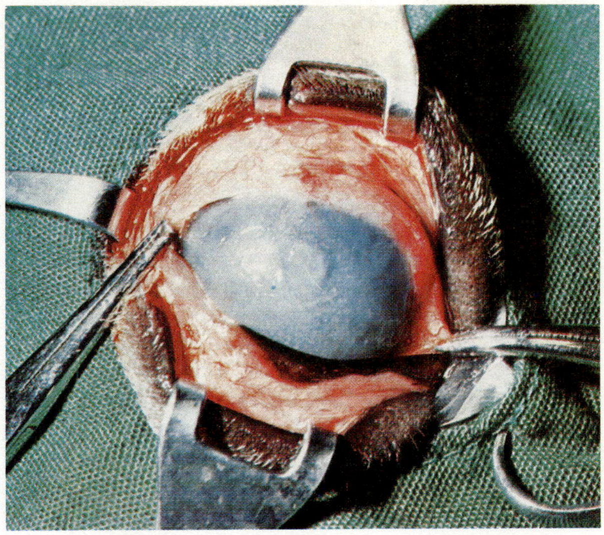

Figure 4—A Park-Guyton eye speculum (Lawton Instrument Co.) was applied and the globe stabilized with two rat-toothed mosquito forceps.

Figure 3—A lateral canthotomy was performed to facilitate exposure of the surgical site.

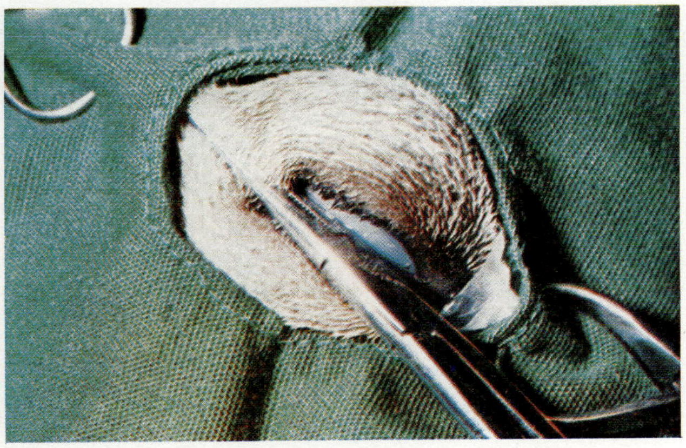

Figure 7—Blunt scissors were introduced under the first attachment of the extraocular muscle.

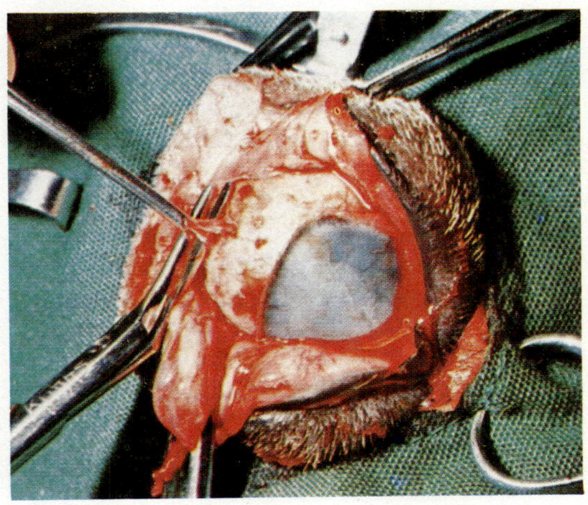

the eyelids and adjacent tissues were scrubbed. During the scrub-and-gowning phase, a gauze sponge impregnated with 10% Betadine solution was applied over the surgical area (*Figure 2*). The eye was irrigated again with physiological saline solution and draped for aseptic surgery.

Figures 3 through 25 illustrate the surgical procedure.

Postoperatively, ampicillin was given at a dosage of 10 mg/lb body weight, t.i.d. for seven days. The sutures were removed 14 days after surgery.

Recovery was uneventful.

ACKNOWLDEGMENT

Gratitude is expressed to Mary D. Bloye, Certified Animal Technician, for her assistance with the photography.

REFERENCE

1. Magrane, W.G.: *Canine Ophthalmology*, 2nd ed. Lea & Febiger, Philadelphia, Pa., 1971.

PHOTOGRAPHIC TECHNIQUE

Camera: Nikkormat FTN; *lens:* Micro-Auto-Nikkor 55 mm f.3.5 plus one M2 extension ring; *film:* Kodachrome ASA 25; *light:* Kako High Beam II electronic flash; *exposure:* f.16 at 1/60 sec.

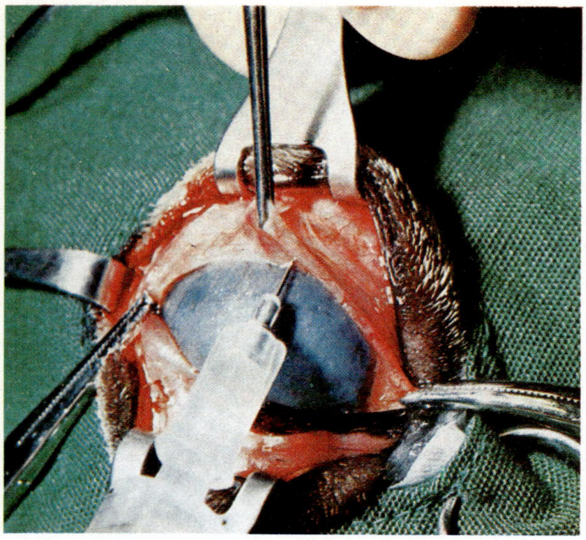

Figure 5—To aid in the initial phase of dissection and to reduce hemorrhage, the limbal area was infiltrated with 1:10,000 epinephrine. The use of epinephrine at this stage is not always necessary.

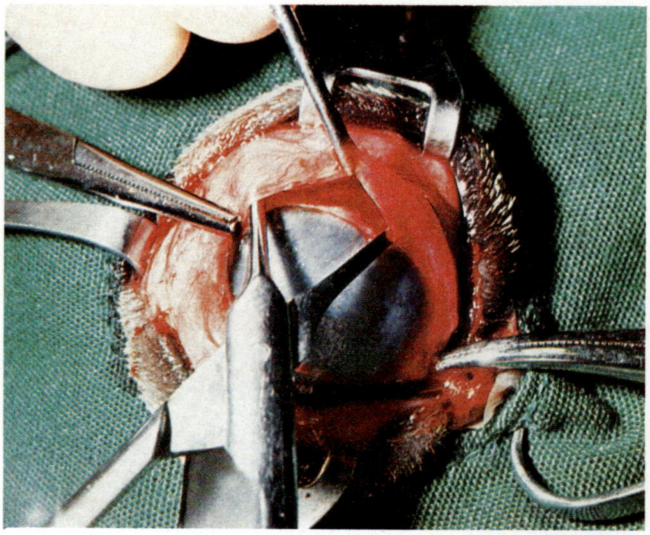

Figure 6—An incision was made just behind the limbus, through the conjunctiva and Tenon's capsule, down to the sclera. The dissection was extended around the circumference of the limbus, with the undermined tissues being reflected caudally until the first attachments of the extra-ocular muscles were exposed.

Figure 8—Further dissection was accomplished by opening the scissor blades to stretch the muscle attachment.

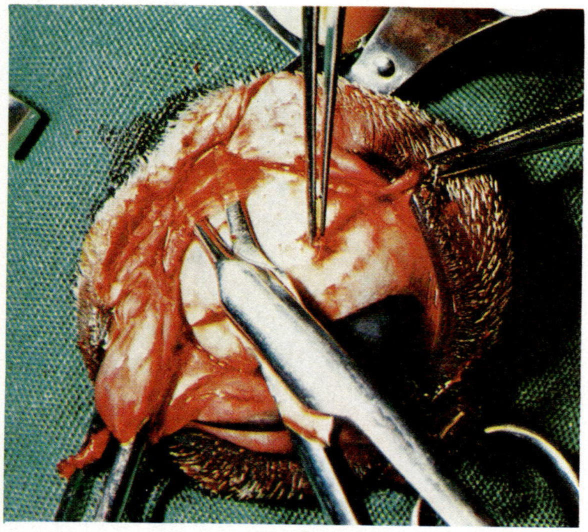

Figure 9—The muscle attachment was grasped with a small thumb forceps and elevated.

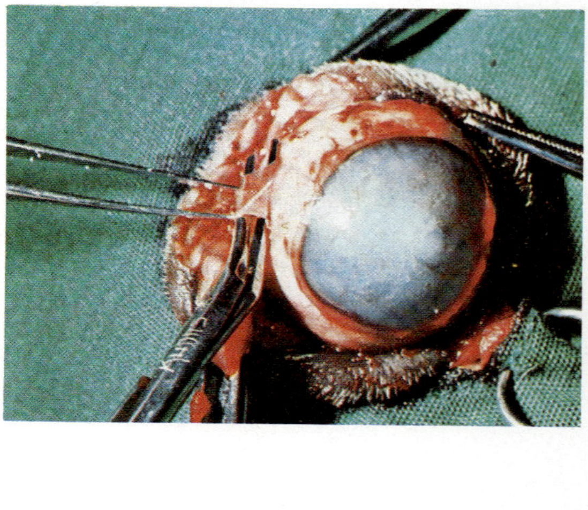

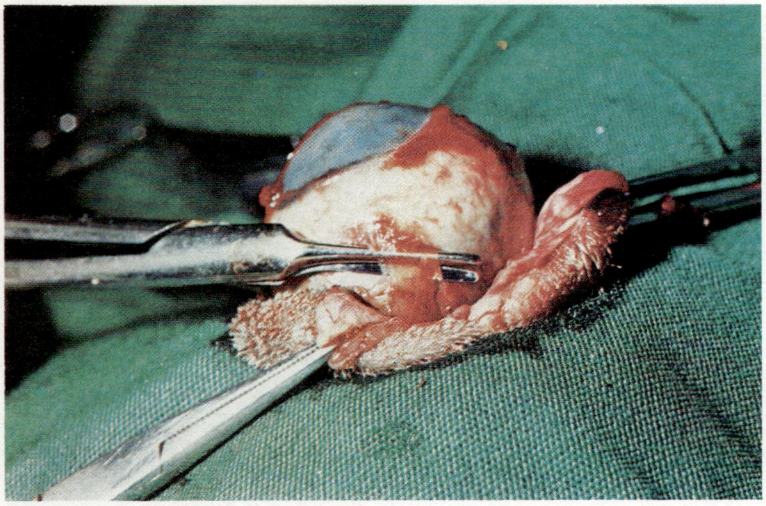

Figure 10—Scissors were reintroduced and the muscle attachment dissected.

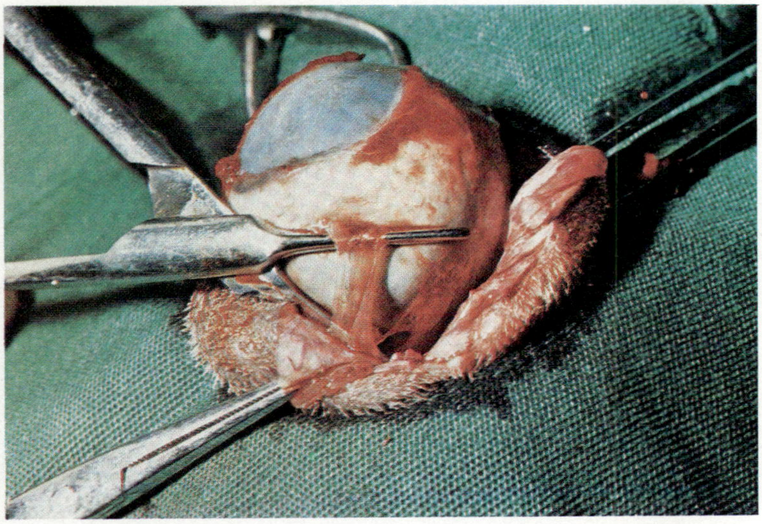

Figure 11—As each muscle was severed, the globe protruded further from the orbit, exposing other muscle attachments.

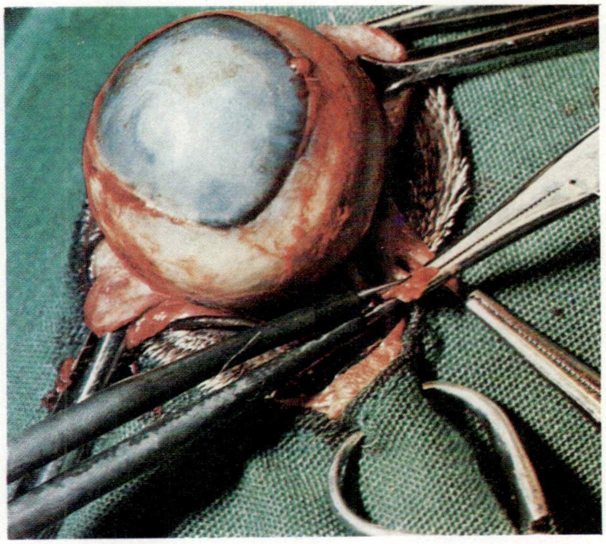

Figure 12—When needed, electrocautery forceps (Cameron-Miller) were used to control hemorrhage.

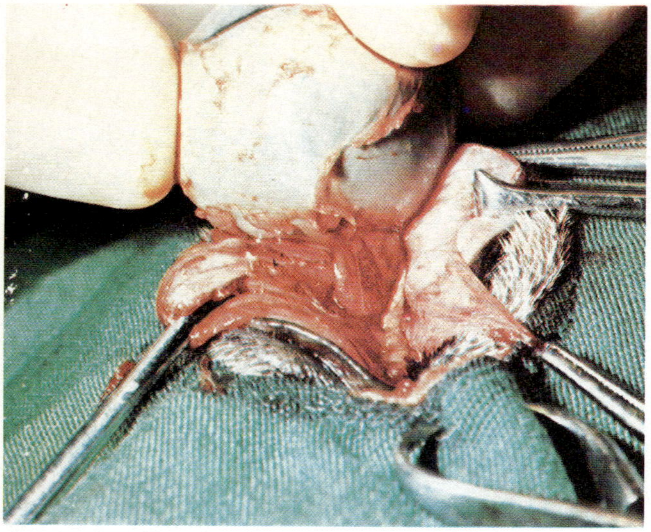

Figure 13—The globe is shown attached only by the retractor bulbi muscle and the optic nerve.

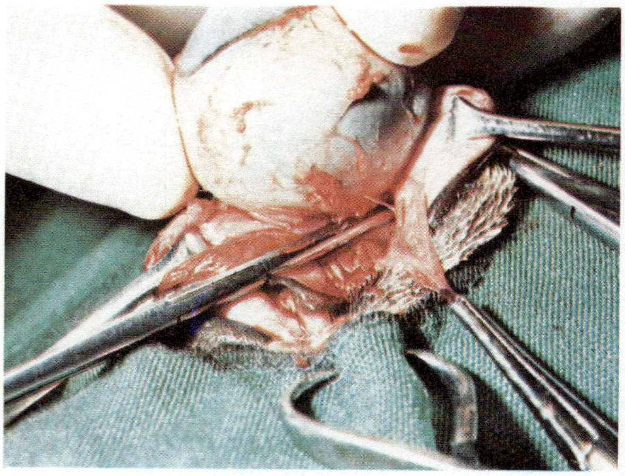

Figure 14—After the retractor bulbi muscle was dissected from the globe, the optic nerve with its vessels was exposed. A mosquito forceps was used to clamp the optic nerve.

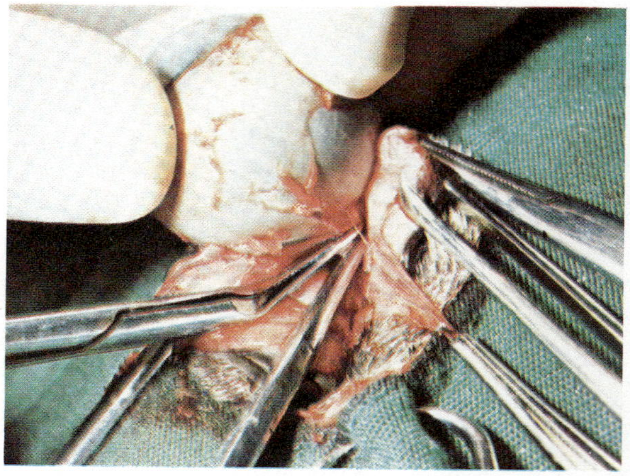

Figure 15—Small scissors were used to sever the optic nerve from the globe.

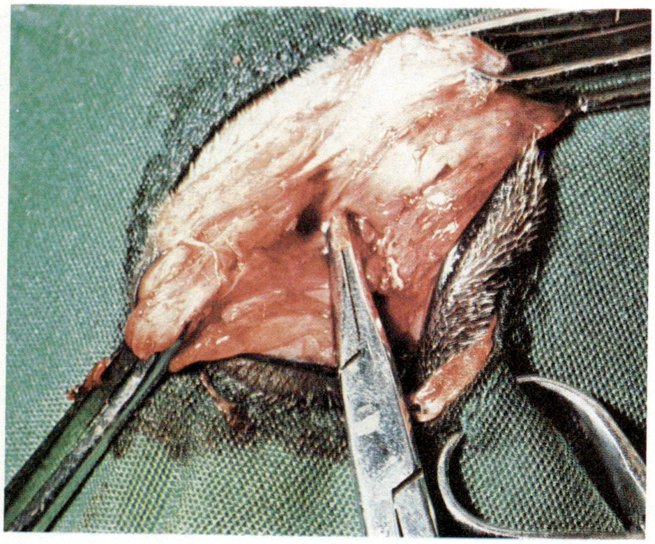

Figure 16—Appearance of the orbit after removal of the globe.

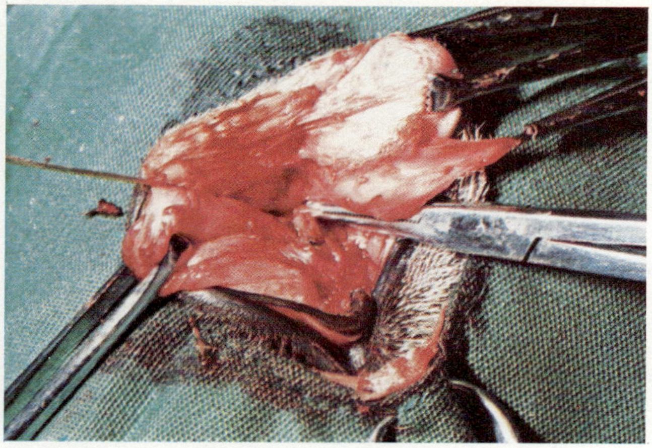

Figure 17—4-0 chromic gut was used to ligate the optic nerve and its vessels.

Figure 18—A second mosquito forceps was used to grasp the tip of the optic nerve before release of the forceps used initially to clamp the nerve and vessels. This allows the surgeon to check the integrity of the ligature before finally releasing the nerve.

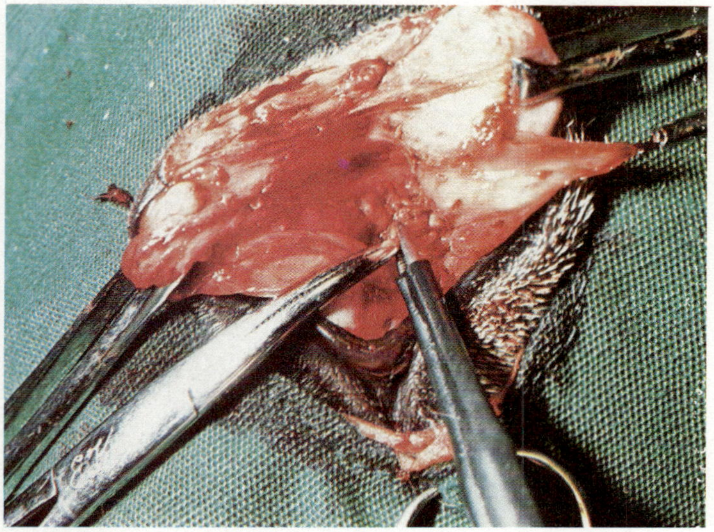

Figure 19—Appearance of the orbit after the second forceps was released. The stump and ligature should be kept in view for a few moments until it is apparent that no hemorrhaging will occur.

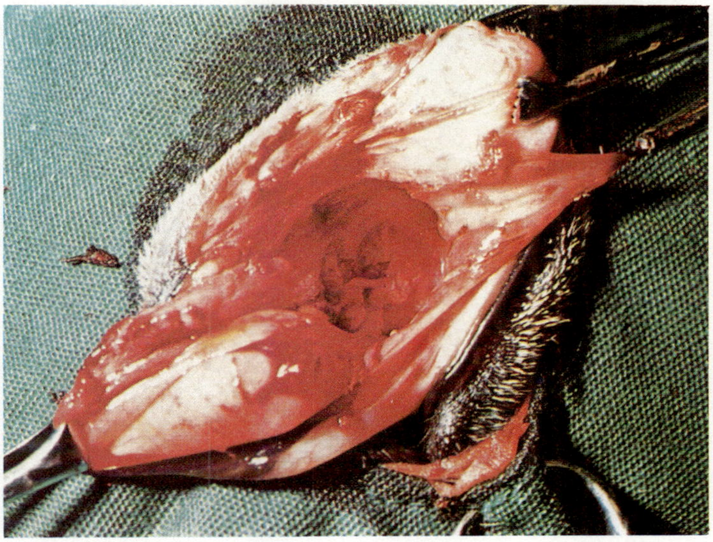

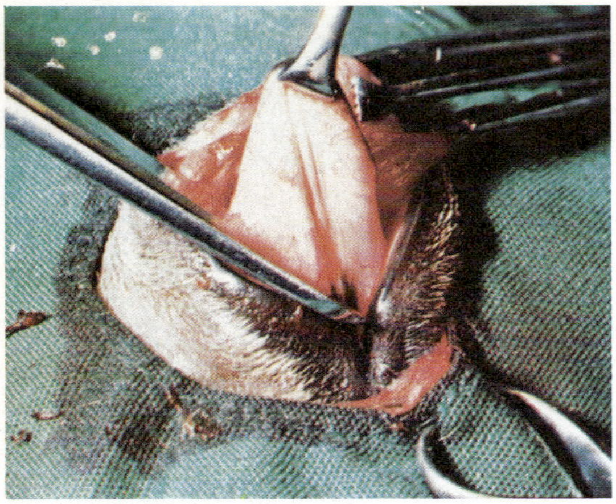

Figure 20—The cartilaginous border of the membrane nictitans was grasped with Allis tissue forceps and the nictitans removed by cutting along its base. Hemorrhage was controlled by pressure and electrocautery.

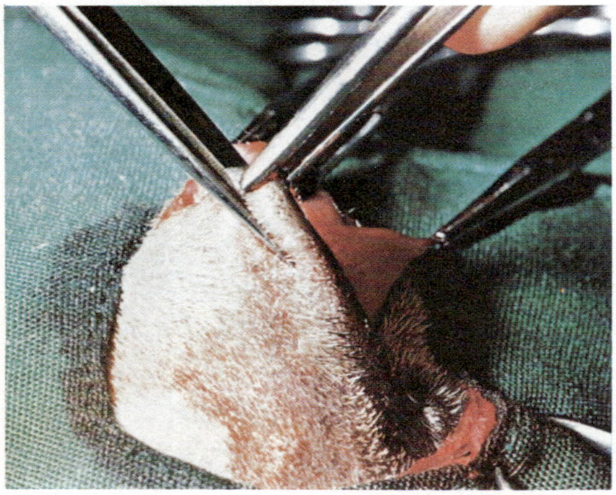

Figure 21—The lower lid was grasped with forceps and ¼ inch of the lid margin was removed with scissors. The excision was continued around the medial canthus to include the caruncle.

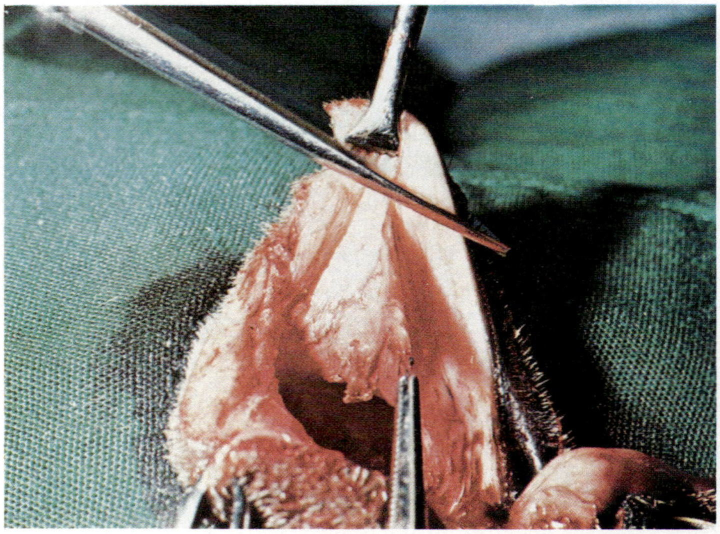

Figure 22—The margin of the upper eyelid was removed in the same manner as the margin of the lower lid.

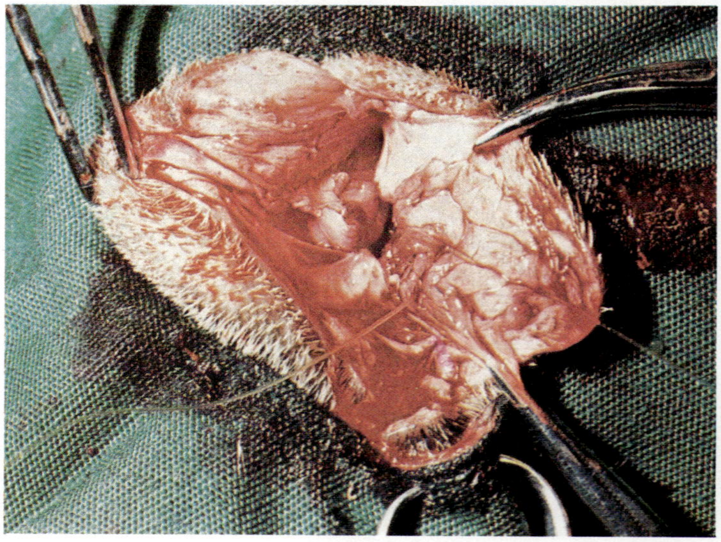

Figure 23—A purse-string suture of 4-0 chromic gut was used to appose the cut edges of the conjunctiva within the orbit.

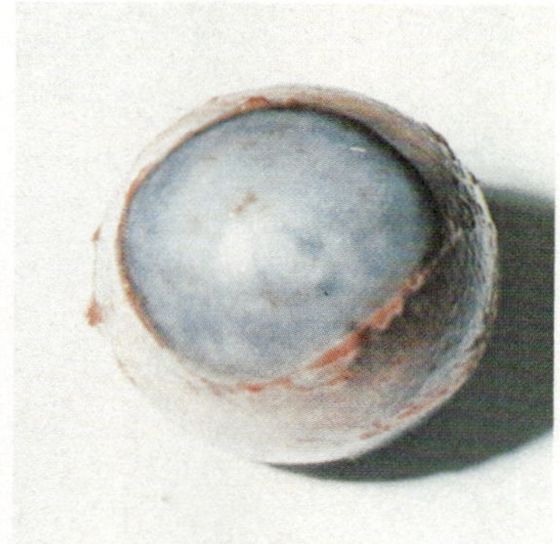

Figure 24—Appearance of the globe soon after its removal.

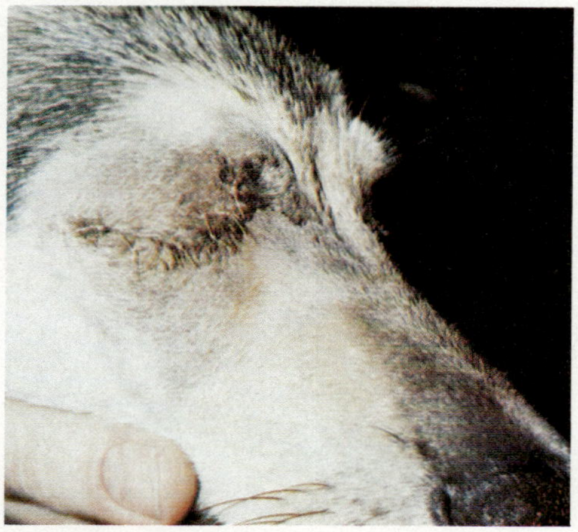

Figure 25—The eyelids were closed with a simple interrupted suture pattern of 2-0 Vetafil® (S. Jackson).

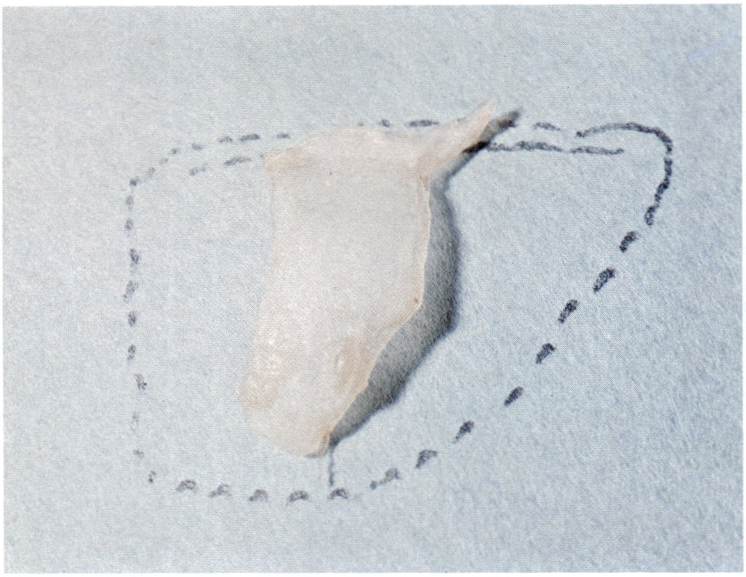

Figure 1
Broken lines depict the membrana nictitans in relation to the cartilaginous plate.

correction of *EVERSION OF THE MEMBRANA NICTITANS* in the dog

Eugene L. Kuhns, DVM, MS
Wyoming Animal Hospital, Inc.
2754 Burlingame SW
Wyoming, Michigan 49509

EVERSION of the membrana nictitans is considered a congenital or acquired anomaly found primarily in the larger breeds of dogs.[1-2]

Both the inner (bulbar) and outer (palpebral) surfaces of the membrana nictitans are covered with epithelium. A cartilaginous structure shaped like a T lies between these two epithelial surfaces. Figure 1 shows an actual cartilaginous plate in relation to the remainder of the membrane. Outward scrolling (eversion) of the cartilaginous plate exposes the inner surface of the membrane, thus frequently leading to chronic follicular conjunctivitis.

The membrana nictitans should never be removed because of this condition. The technique described here was used to remove the aseptic cartilage of an everted membrane nictitans (*Figure 2*) from the right eye of a 1½-year-old, male Saint Bernard mix.

After induction of general anesthesia with thiamylal sodium (Surital® —Parke-Davis), anesthesia was maintained with methoxyflurane (Metofane™—Pitman-Moore) in a closed system. The cul-de-sac was irrigated with 15% Betadine® solution (Purdue Frederick) and rinsed with physiological saline solution. An antibiotic ophthalmic ointment (1% chloramphenicol) was applied to the eye to protect the cornea. The eyelids and adjacent tissues were scrubbed and draped for surgery. A Park-Guyton eye speculum was used to retract the eyelids.

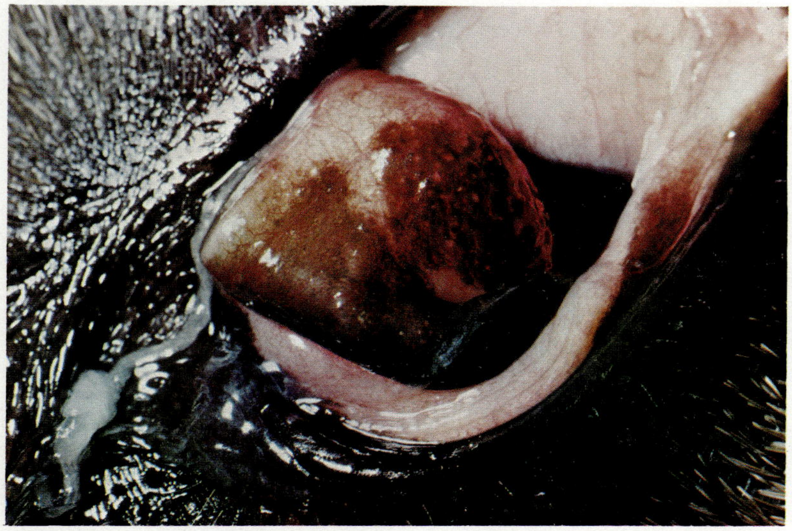

Figure 2—This everted membrana nictitans was repaired by removing the cartilage.

Figure 3 (*below*)—The free edge of the membrana nictitans was grasped with Allis tissue forceps and held taut while the index finger of the same hand firmly supported the nictitans. An incision along the edge of the inner surface of the membrana nictitans was made with a No. 15 Bard-Parker surgical blade.

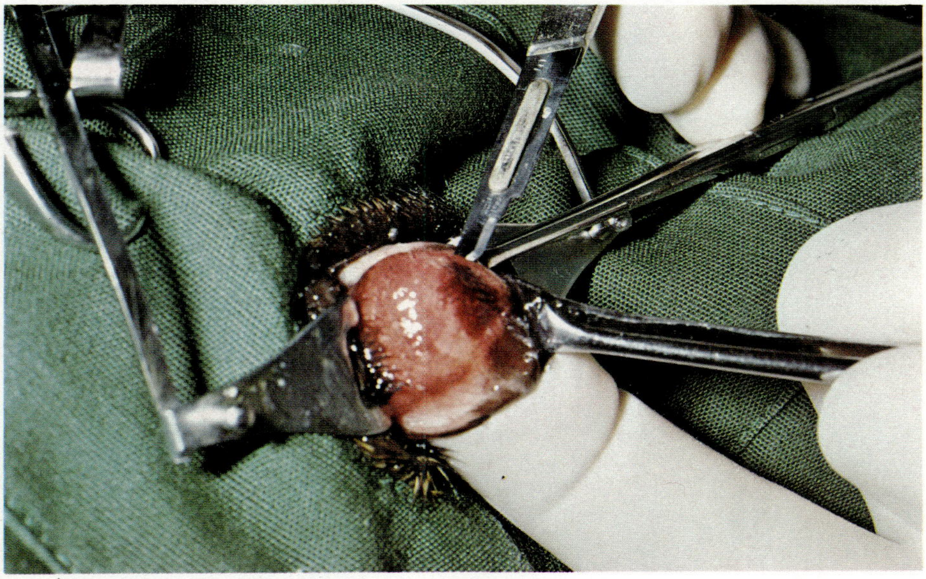

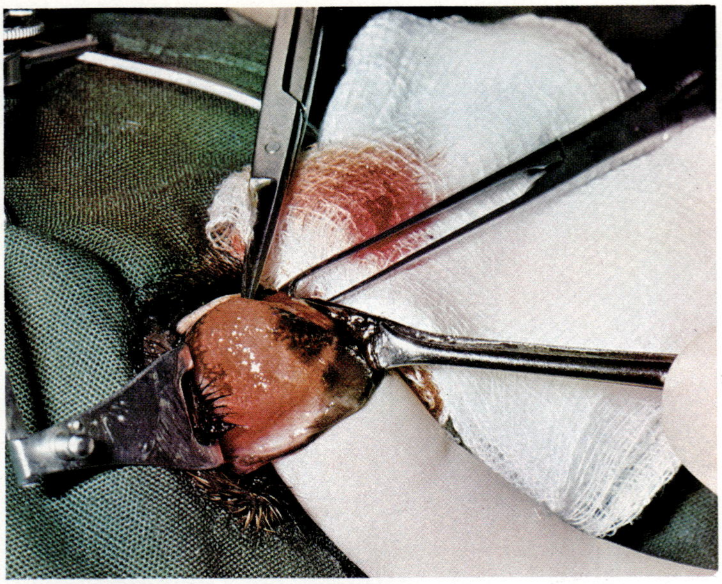

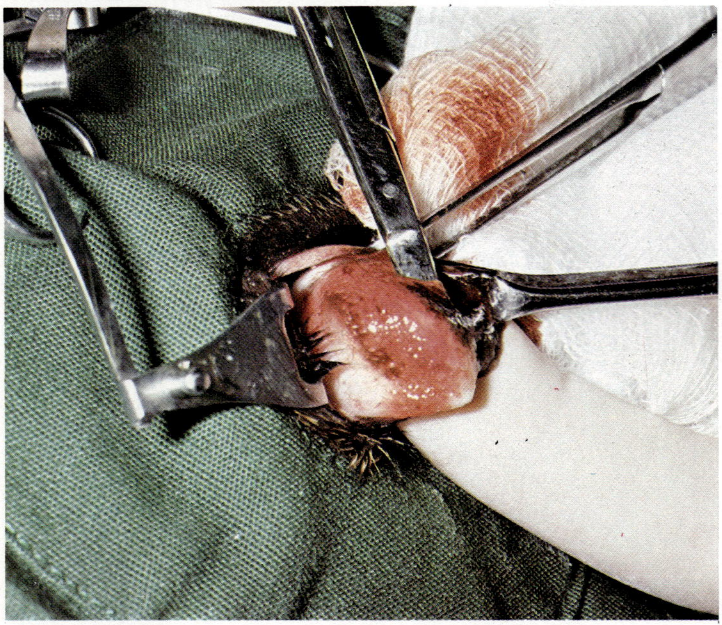

Figures 4 & 5
Small scissors were introduced into the incision. By blunt dissection, the inner surface, which contained the epithelial surface, the glans nictitans, and the shaft of the cartilaginous plate, was freed from the underlying tissue.

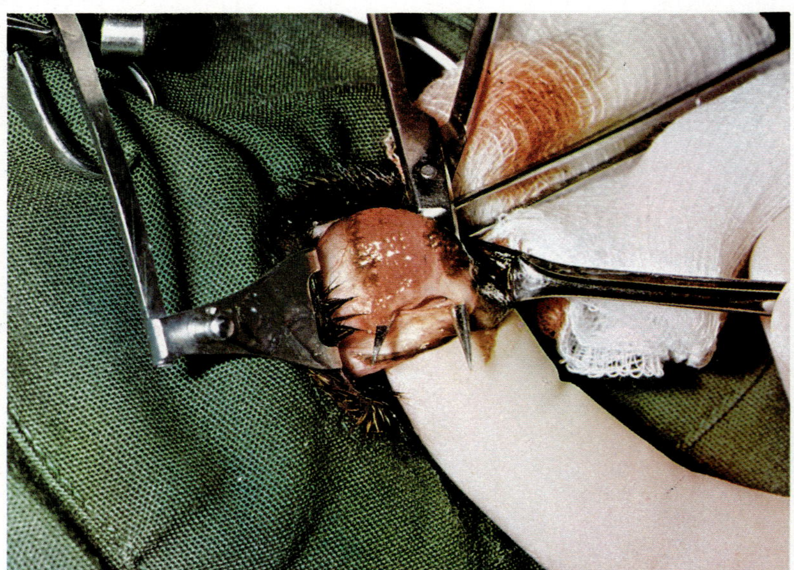

Figure 6—Blunt dissection continued until the scissors emerged from the opposite edge and the inner surface and cartilage were free except for the base and the portion attached to the free end of the membrana nictitans.

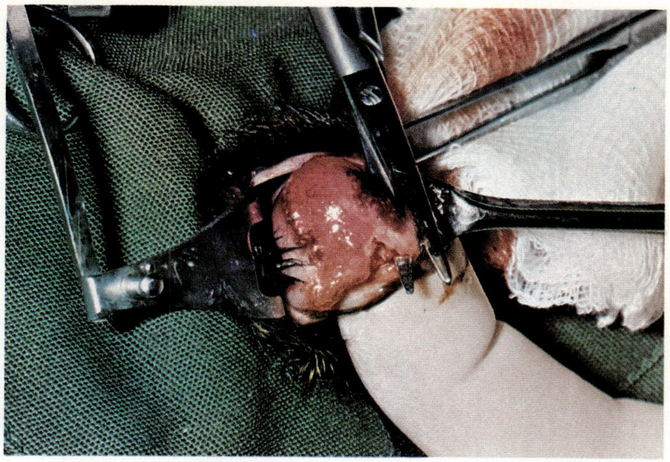

Figures 7 & 8
The portion contiguous with the free border of the membrana nictitans was detached with scissors.

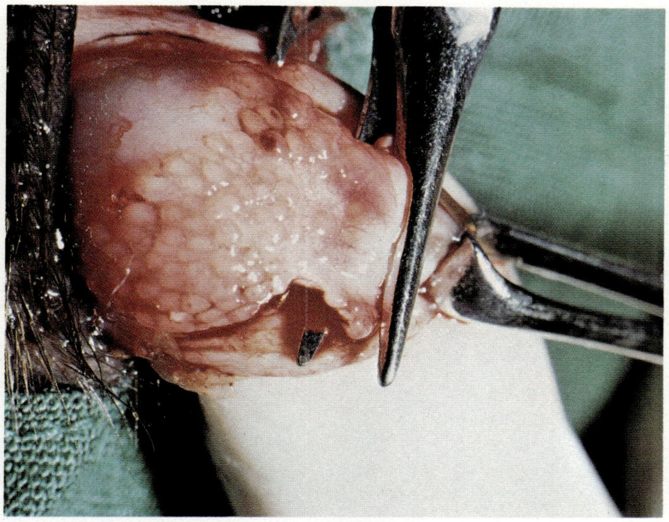

Figures 9 & 10—With another pair of Allis tissue forceps, the freed tissue was elevated so it could be more easily dissected to the base.

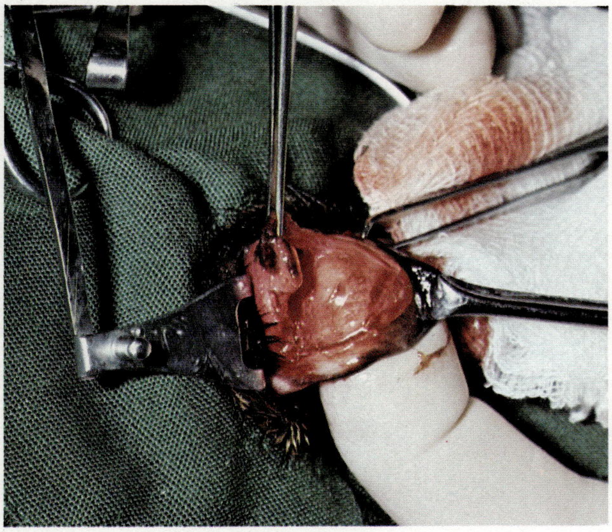

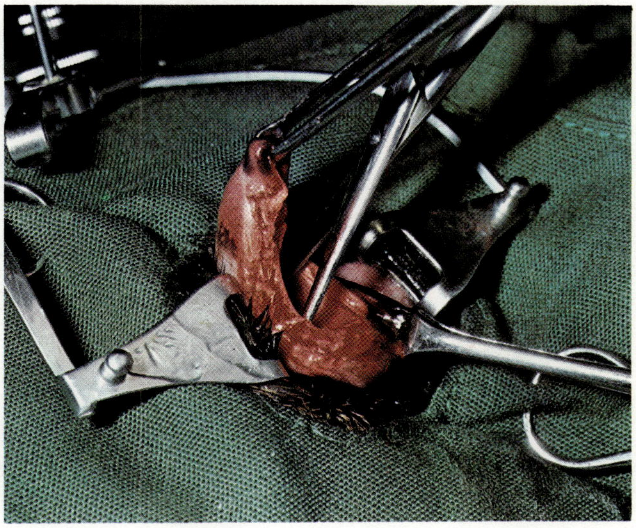

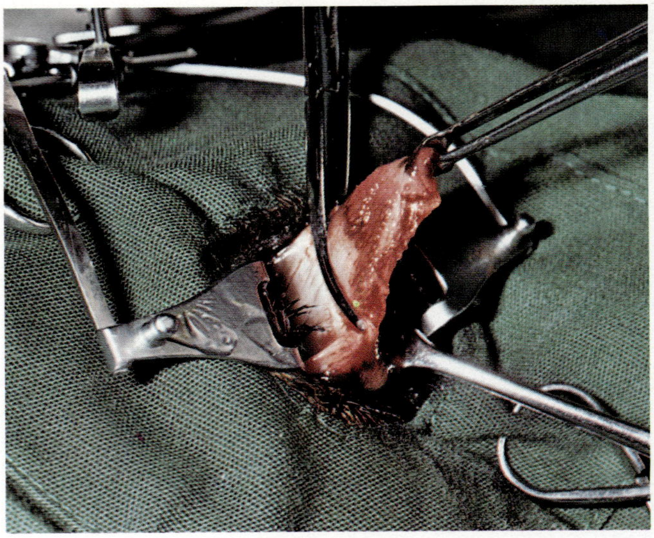

Figures 11, 12 & 13
Dissected tissue containing the inner conjunctival surface, the glans nictitans, and the cartilage was clamped with mosquito forceps and removed with scissors.

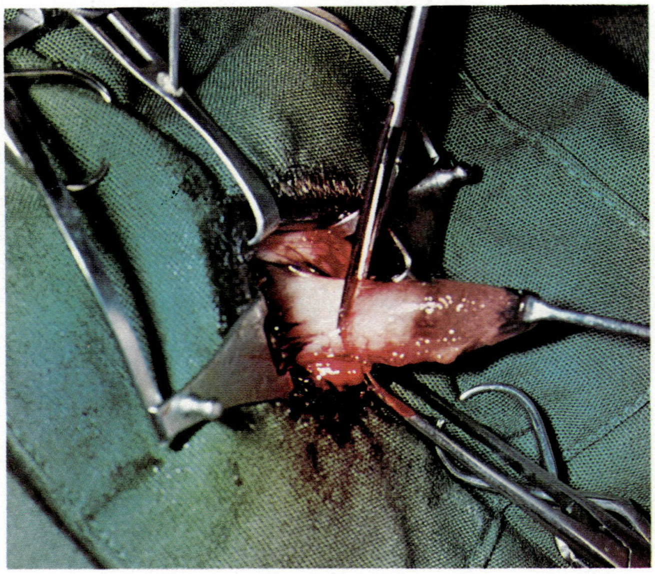

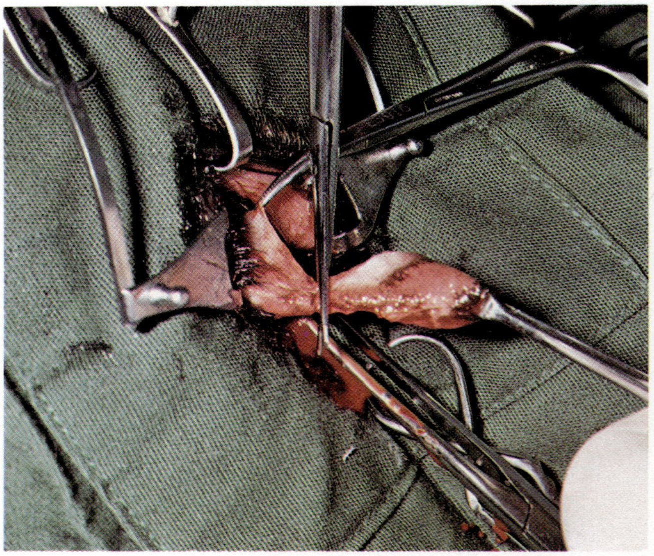

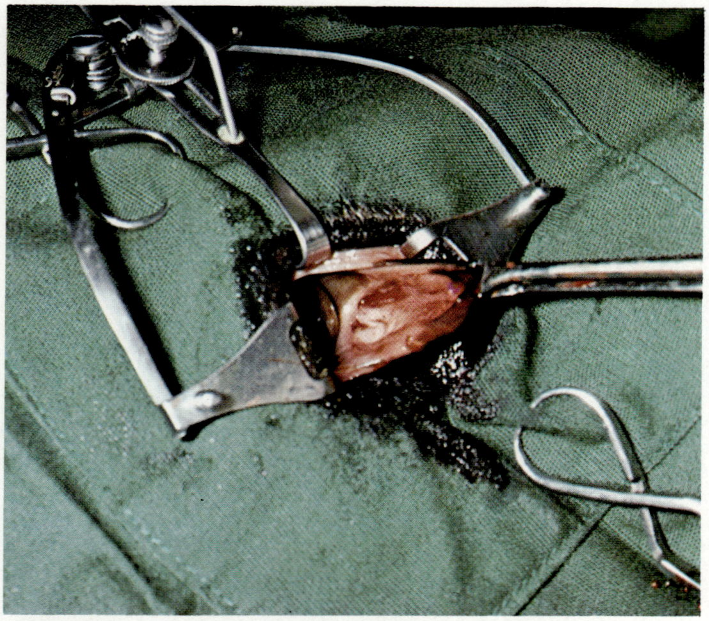

Figure 14—Appearance of the inner surface of the membrana nictitans with dissected tissue removed. The narrow, light band at the base represents the cut edge.

Figure 15—With delicate scissors, the cross-bar of the cartilaginous T was dissected from the inner surface of the free border of the nictitating membrane. Do not inadvertently cut through the full thickness of the nictitans at this point. If it should occur, the rent may be repaired with a single 6-0 gut suture in a manner that does not allow the knot to contact the cornea.

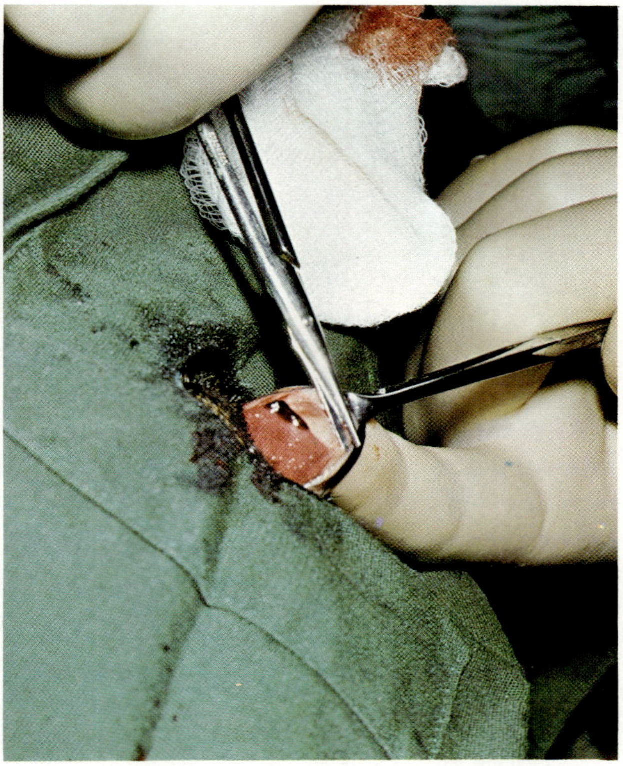

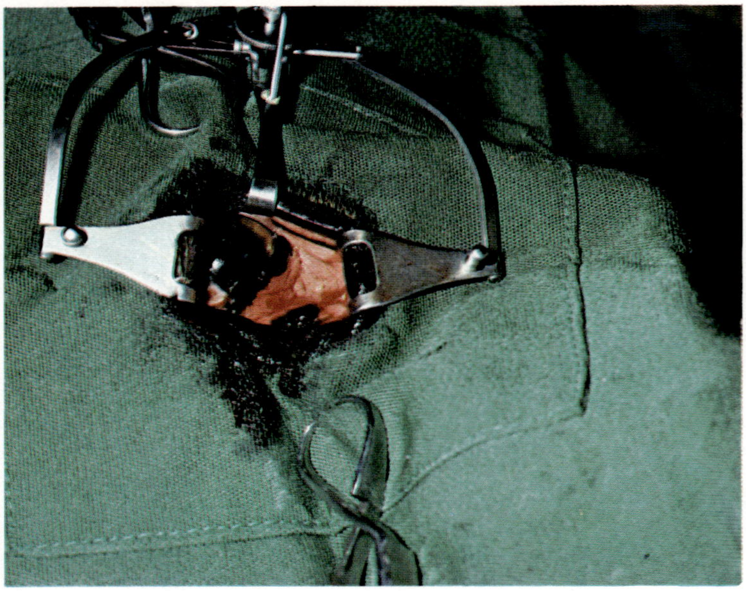

Figure 16—The membrana nictitans has been returned to its natural position with the deformed cartilage removed.

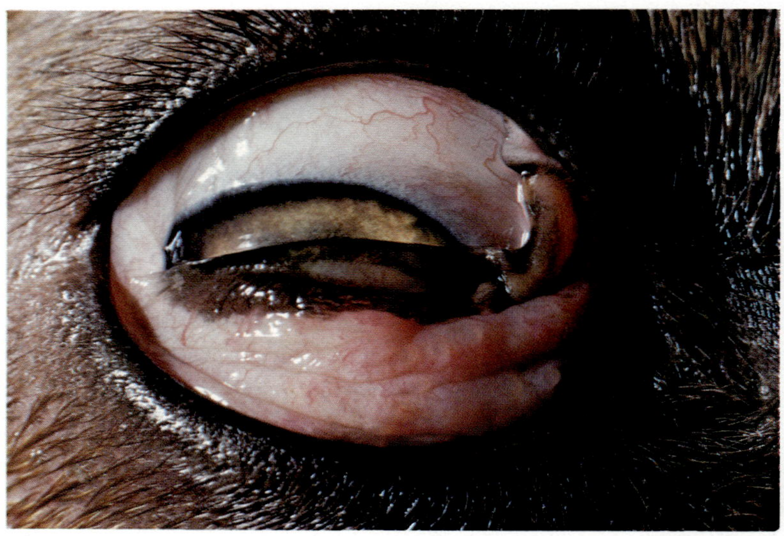

Figure 17—The membrana nictitans four weeks after removal of the cartilage.

After surgery, 1% chloramphenicol ophthalmic ointment was applied topically, four times daily for seven days.

ACKNOWLEDGEMENT

Gratitude is expressed to Patty Feldon, Certified Animal Technician, for her assistance with the photography.

REFERENCES

1. Jensen, J.E.: *Steroscopic Atlas of Clinical Ophthalmology of Domestic Animals.* The C.V. Mosby Co., St. Louis, Mo. 1971; p. 27.
2. Magrane, W.G.: *Canine Ophthalmology*, 2nd ed. Lea & Febiger, Philadelphia, Pa., 1971; p. 66.

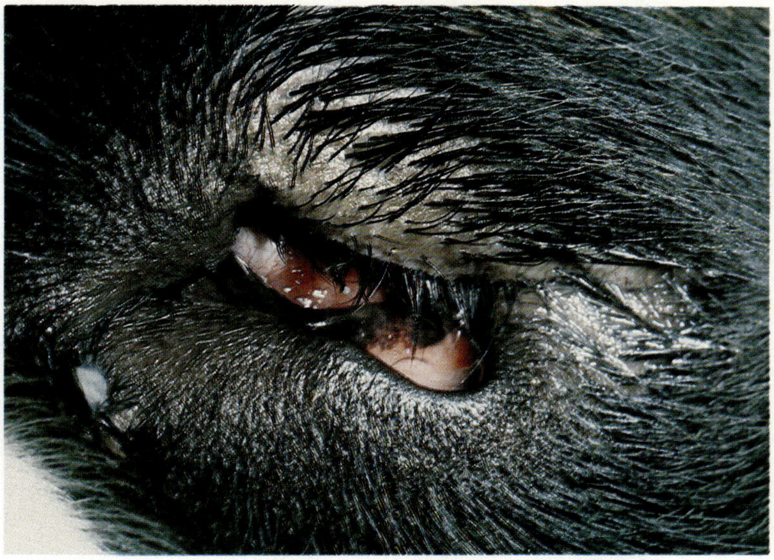

Figure 1—Congenital malformation of the palpebral fissure with resultant abnormal conformation of the eyelids in the left eye of a 10-month-old St. Bernard dog. The condition is related to inadequate support of the lateral canthus. Note the oval shape of the palpebral fissure and the ectropic notching of the central upper and lower eyelids. Entropion with associated corneal irritation is observed medially and laterally.

a suture technique for *LATERAL CANTHOPLASTY*

Robert L. Peiffer, Jr., DVM
Department of Ophthalmology
College of Medicine
University of North Carolina
Chapel Hill, North Carolina 27514

CONGENITAL MALFORMATION of the palpebral fissure related to the absence of support of the lateral canthus is often seen in giant breeds of dogs, notably the St. Bernard. Normal support of the lateral canthus is provided by the lateral canthal ligament (a condensation of the tarsus), and the retractor anguli oculi muscle (a division of the frontalis muscle). These structures, by virtue of their attachments to the temporal fascia, draw the lateral canthus of the palpebral fissure posteriorally.[1] Incompetency of these supporting structures results in characteristic malformation of the palpebral fissure and abnormal conformation of the eyelids.

Diagnosis is based on the owner's reported observations, history, and the characteristic bilateral signs. Trichiasis associated with the abnormal conformation of the lids results in corneal irritation characterized by epiphora, blepharospasm, and frequently an ulcerative or nonulcerative keratitis. The palpebral fissure is oval or round rather than almond-shaped. Medial and lateral entropion and central ectropion of both the upper and lower eyelids is usually present (*Figure 1*). Application of digital pressure temporally at the lateral canthus restores normal palpebral fissure and conformation of the eyelids.

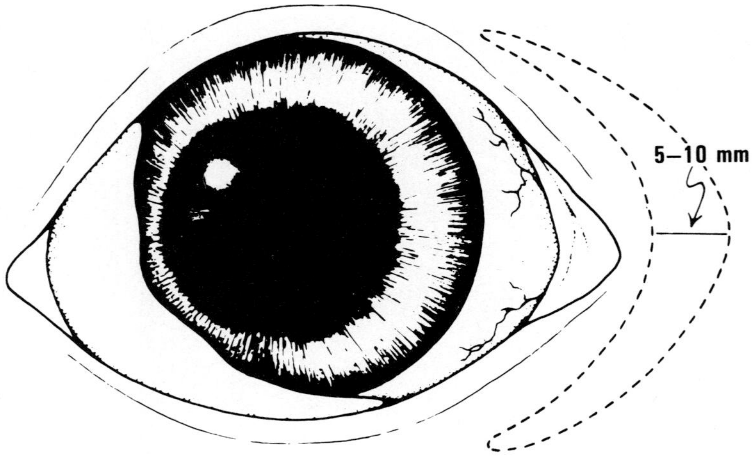

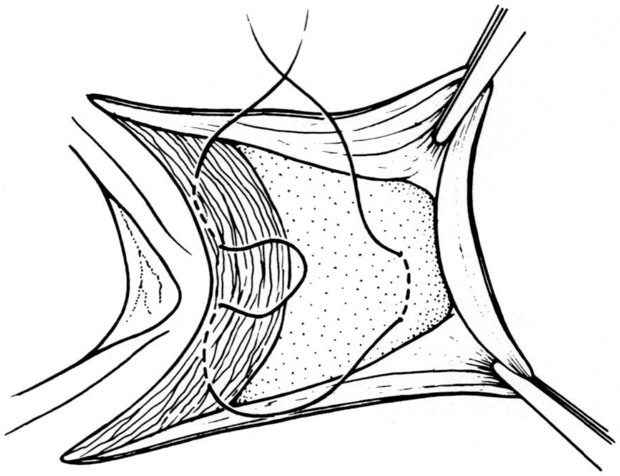

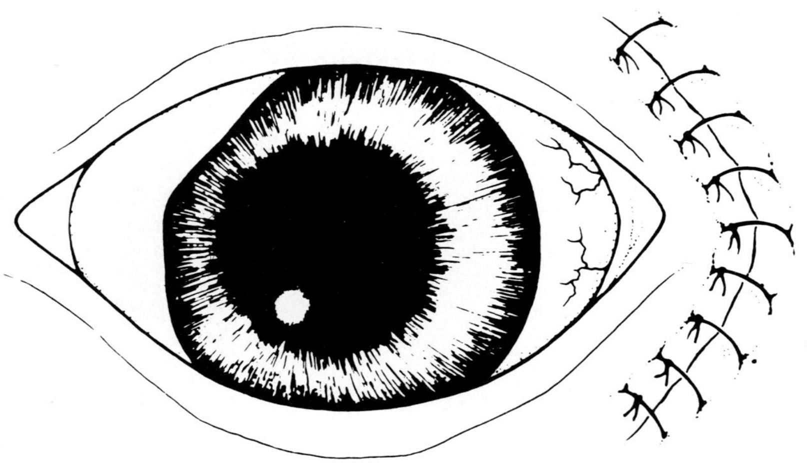

Figure 2 (*above left*)—The initial skin incisions form a crescent around the lateral canthus.

Figure 3 (*above*)—The incised crescent of skin is undermined temporally and excised. The nonabsorbable suture is placed in the periosteum of the dorsal zygomatic arch and the canthal tarsus of the upper and lower eyelids.

Figure 4 (*left*)—The incision is closed with 4-0 silk in a simple interrupted pattern.

Treatment is surgical. Described techniques include an arrowhead-shaped excision at the lateral canthus[2] and the use of pedicles of orbicularis oculi muscle as a replacement for the structures that support the lateral canthus.[3] A technique which utilizes a nonabsorbable suture to provide support for the lateral canthus was devised to incorporate the desirable features of each of these techniques and minimize their disadvantages.

Surgical Technique

With the patient under general anesthesia the eyelids and 5 cm of peripalpebral skin are clipped, scrubbed with 0.5% povidone iodine (Betadine® —Purdue Frederick) and draped in routine fashion.

An elliptical incision is made through the skin, extending from the temporal one-third of the upper eyelid, around the canthus, and along the temporal one-third of the lower eyelid approximately 3 to 5 mm from the margins of the eyelids and canthus. A second elliptical incision is made temporal to and joining the ends of the first incision; it is widest (about 10 mm) at the canthus (*Figure 2*).

The demarcated crescent of tissue is excised by elevation at one end with a small rat-toothed forceps and sharp dissection with a straight strabismus scissors. By blunt and sharp dissection, the skin temporal to the area of excision is separated from the underlying connective tissue for a distance of 2 to 3 cm over the palpable zygomatic arch.

A large half-circle needle is used to pass 2-0 nonabsorbable suture material from dorsal to ventral through the soft tissue to the underlying periosteum of the dorsal zygomatic arch. The suture is passed at the location where it will restore normal configuration to the eyelids and palpebral fissure. This site is identified by grasping the lateral canthus with a forceps and exerting temporal traction.

The suture is inserted through the lower lid, then the upper lid at the canthus. It passes through the orbicularis oculi muscle and the tarsus. Observation of the needle as it passes through the tarsus beneath the palpebral conjunctiva assures its proper placement without perforating the surface of the conjunctiva (*Figure 3*).

As the suture ends are tied, normal conformation of the eyelids and palpebral fissure is restored.

The skin incision is closed with simple interrupted sutures of 4-0 silk (*Figure 4*).

The animal is discharged on the first postoperative day and sutures are removed in 10 to 14 days (*Figure 5*).

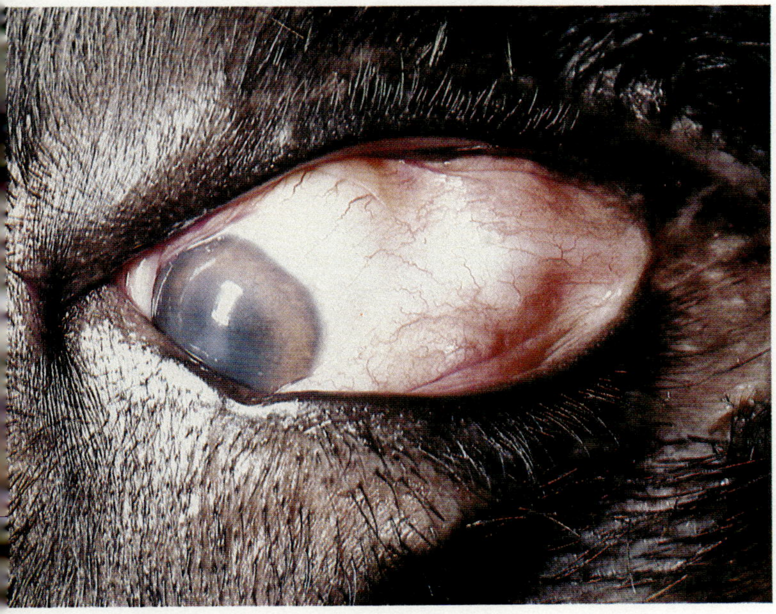

Figure 5—The same eye shown in Figure 1 when skin sutures were removed two weeks after surgery.

Clinical Results

This procedure has been performed on 6 St. Bernards (12 eyes) that demonstrated the stated diagnostic criteria. Results in terms of relief of blepharospasm and corneal irritation were good in all cases.

In one eye, dehiscence of the suture line in the skin occurred on the fourth postoperative day. This was perhaps related to the patient's rubbing of the area. The defect was allowed to heal by secondary intention with satisfactory results. Postoperative edema, discomfort, and fibrosis were minimal in all 12 eyes.

Discussion

In my hands, results with the arrowhead technique[2] have been inconsistent because the reconstructed palpebral fissure is unsupported by rigid structures. Lateral canthoplasty,[3] although providing rigid support for the canthus, is a relatively extensive procedure and may be accompanied by severe postoperative edema and fibrosis.

The technique described in this paper is simple to perform and tissue reaction is minimal. Postoperative medication and restraint are not often necessary. Proper placement of the suture in the periosteum and tarsus (tissues of good suture-holding strength) is the critical point of the technique. Residual entropion may be corrected using a modified Hotz-Celsus technique. Secondary corneal disease must be considered and managed as indicated.

An enlarged palpebral fissure, with exposure of the bulbar conjunctiva of the lateral canthus, may be present after the corrective surgery has been performed. If this defect is cosmetically unacceptable, it may be corrected by trimming and suturing the temporal margins of the eyelids as a secondary procedure.

ACKNOWLEDGMENT

The author gratefully acknowledges the assistance of Michael Schink, medical illustrator, College of Veterinary Medicine, University of Minnesota, in providing the line drawings.

REFERENCES

1. Miller, M.E. *et al*: *Anatomy of the Dog*. W.B. Saunders, Philadelphia, Pa., 1965.
2. Jensen, H.E.: *Ophthalmic Surgery of Domestic Animals*. C.E Mosby, St. Louis, Mo., 1973.
3. Wyman, M.: Lateral Canthoplasty. *JAAHA* 7:196-201; 1971.

Small Animal Surgery

DENTAL

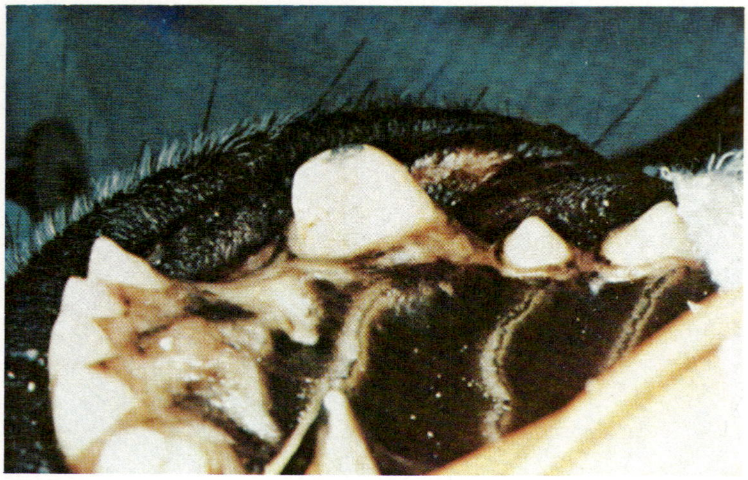

Figure 1 — Short clinical crown of the maxillary tooth in a German Shepherd military patrol dog. Root canal therapy had been performed.

Dowel and core preparation, and full gold coverage of maxillary canine teeth in a German Shepherd

Craig J. Hamilton, BS, DDS
USAMEDDACJ
APO San Francisco, California 96331

Robert L. Ridgway, BS, DVM
447-38-2780
Box 21, Madigan Army Medical Center
Tacoma, Washington 98431

THE PATIENT in the case reported here was a German Shepherd military patrol dog. When the animal was presented for restoration of the maxillary canine teeth, root canal therapy had been completed.

The clinical crowns (that portion of the tooth clinically visible) of the treated teeth were relatively short (*Figure 1*). This presented a problem in restoration of the teeth because of the great occlusal stresses exerted on the canine teeth during mastication and training sessions. For this reason, use of standard gold crowns was deemed unwise, and the decision was made to fabricate gold-dowel prostheses.

The dog was premedicated with 0.02 mg atropine sulfate/lb given subcutaneously. Anesthesia was induced by intravenous administration of 3% thiamylal sodium (Surital® —Parke-Davis). An endotracheal tube was passed and anesthesia maintained with oxygen and methoxyflurane (Metofane™—Pitman-Moore) in an open system.

To open the root canal and remove all gutta percha instilled for root canel therapy, a standard, belt-driven, slow-speed dental engine and handpiece with tapered diamond and stone points was used. The canal was re-entered and penetrated to a depth of approximately 1.5 cm (*Figures 2 & 3*). The core to receive the dowel was made to accommodate as large a dowel as possible, without perforating the root of the tooth. Because a dowel with

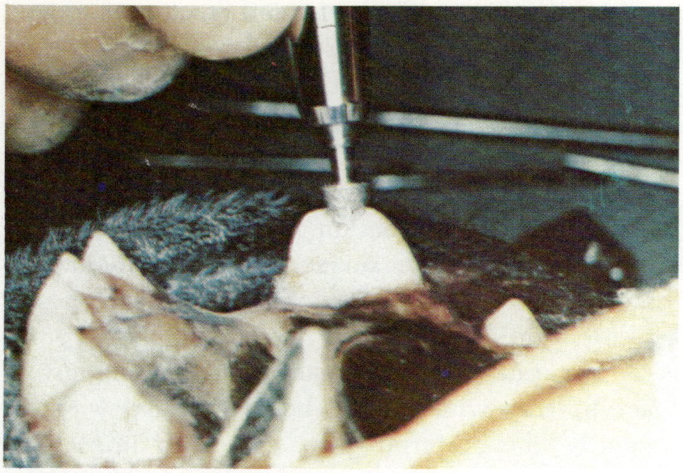

Figure 2—The root canal is entered and a dowel core shaped with tapered diamond and stone points.

Figure 3—Using a tapered diamond point, a retention groove is formed along the lingual surface of the crown.

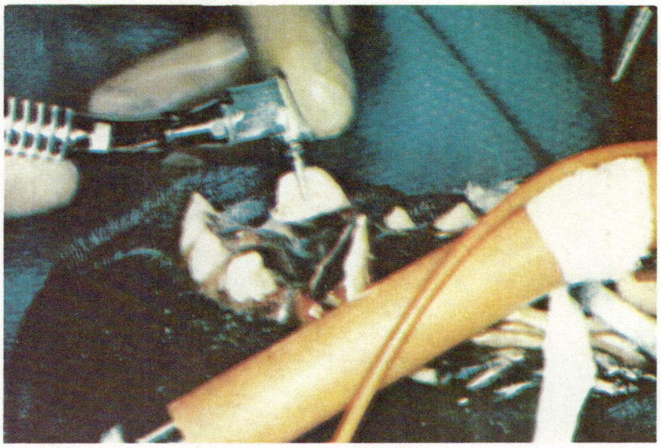

large circumference has a greated surface area, the cement bond is greated when the prothesis is affixed.

It is important that the core be free of any undercut areas, to that impression material can be removed without breaking and the completed case will "draw" (*Figure 4*). From a strictly mechanical point of view, it is also advantageous for the intraradicular portion of the dowl to be at least as long as the clinical crown (*Figure 4*).

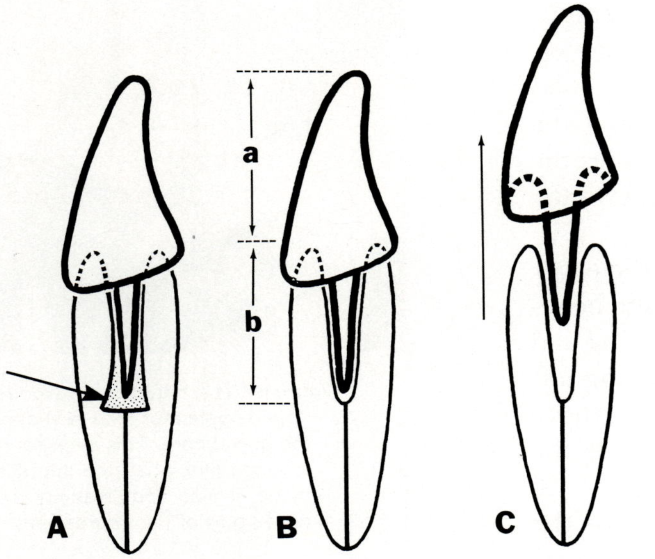

Figure 4—A: an improperly prepared dowel core showing undercutting (*arrow*). B: a properly prepared core. If the tooth structure is adequate, distance **b** should be at least equal to distance **a**. C: "drawing" action of a properly constructed core and prosthesis.

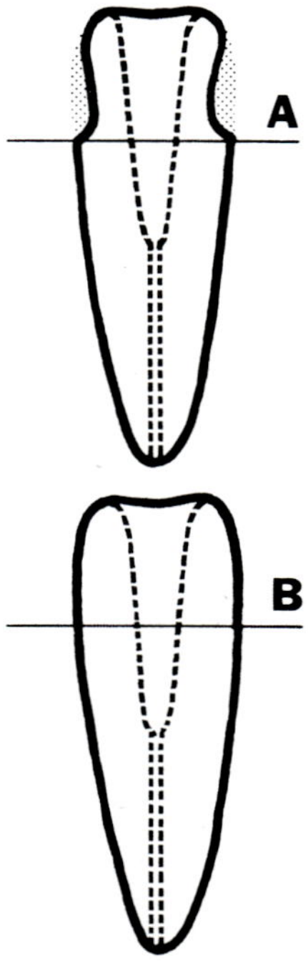

Figure 5—A: an improperly prepared crown showing undercutting. B: a properly prepared crown which will permit making a mold and casting a prosthesis that will fit snugly against the crown.

After preparation of the core, the clinical crown was made ready to accept the prosthesis. This was done with tapered diamonds and stones, again avoiding undercutting (*Figure* 5) and establishing a fine margin for the crown. (The margin is that point where the prosthesis joins the tooth structure.) All margins were kept above the gingiva to aid self-cleaning action.

In this particular case, because of the meager gingivo-incisal length of the clinical crowns to be restored, and because of the tremendous shearing and torquing forces which were anticipated being applied to the finished prothesis, a retention groove was cautiously placed during preparation of the crown.

The retention groove is simply provided on the facial or lingual surface of the crown prep by gently laying a tapered diamond along the apical-incisal axis of the crown. The retention groove, of course, must "draw" with the preparation and be free of any undercuts. Hence, the use of a tapered diamond or stone for placement.

Although the retention groove is small, it is easily impressioned in detail, and greatly enhances the mechanical retention of the cast crown by providing a greater surface area of cementation and, at the same time, a mechanical lock which resists rotational forces.

The next step was fabrication of a custom acrylic tray which could be used to carry to the mouth, the material with which an impression mold of the crown and dental arch would be made. The quadrant of the maxilla from which the impression was to be made was covered with several layers of wetted asbestos sheets 1 mm thick. These created in the tray a recess which would subsequently receive the impression material. After the acrylic had been mixed and allowed to polymerize to an elastic state, it was spread and shaped over the quadrant.

Portions of the tray around the canine tooth were molded directly to adjacent tooth surfaces so that an adequate void would be maintained in the tray. The tray was held in place in this fashion until polymerization was complete (*Figure* 7).

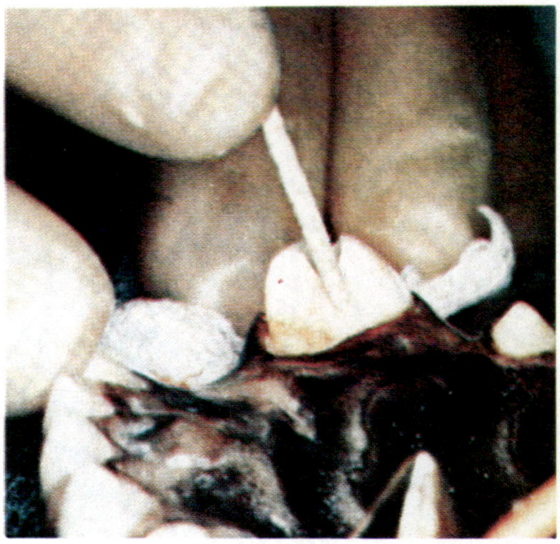

Figure 6—The handle of a wooden, cotton-tipped applicator stick is shaped to fit into the dowel core. This stick serves as a reference point when the impression tray is made; it also adds stability to the fragile dowel part of the impression.

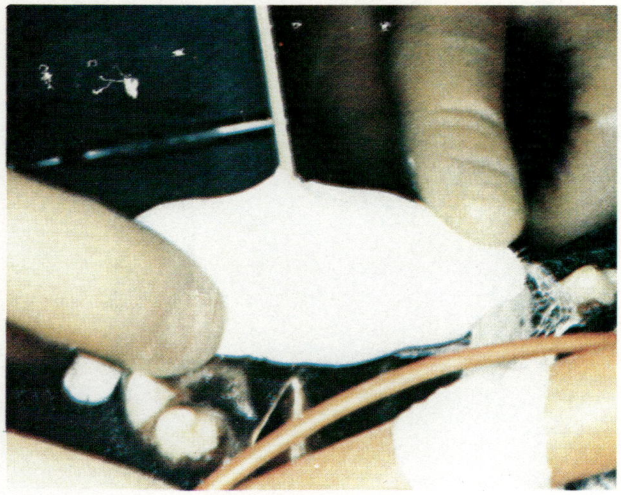

Figure 7—An impression tray for the maxillary left quadrant is custom-made of acrylic. This tray will hold the impression material from which the mold is made.

When fabricating a custom acrylic tray, the asbestos liner is separated from it after the tray is removed. Consequently, a void is left between the tooth to be impressioned and the impression tray itself because of those tray parts serving as occlusal stops which are butted directly to adjacent tooth surfaces, as stated above.

The handle of a wooden cotton-tipped applicator stick, which had previously been shaped to fit partially into the core, was then inserted gently into the core (*Figure 6*). With the tray in place, this preshaped wooden peg was attached to the tray in its appropriate position. It would serve as a reference point when the hardened tray bearing the impression material was later replaced over the quadrant. When the impression was taken, this stick would also lend stability to the rather fragile dowel portion of the impression by providing a surface to which the impression material within the core itself could adhere.

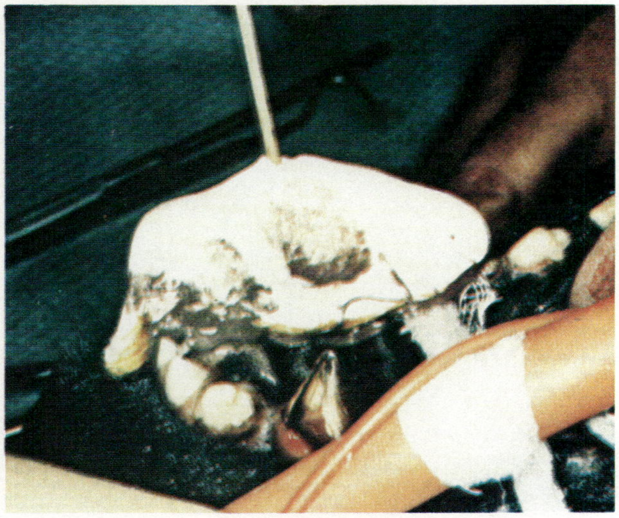

Figure 8—A polysulfide, rubber-base impression material has been poured into the tray and the tray repositioned over the maxillary left quadrant.

To make the mold, a polysulfide, rubber-base impression material (Kerr Co., Romulus, Mich.) was used. This material was put into the tray and the tray positioned in the mouth as the occlusal stops and wooden stick dictated (*Figure 8*). After the material had set, the tray with impression intact, was removed (*Figure 9*).

Figure 9—Appearance of the inner surface of the mold after the impression has been made.

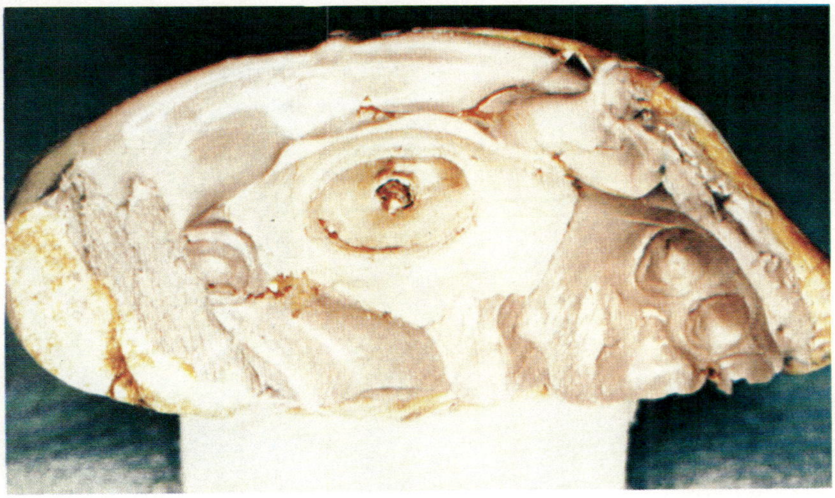

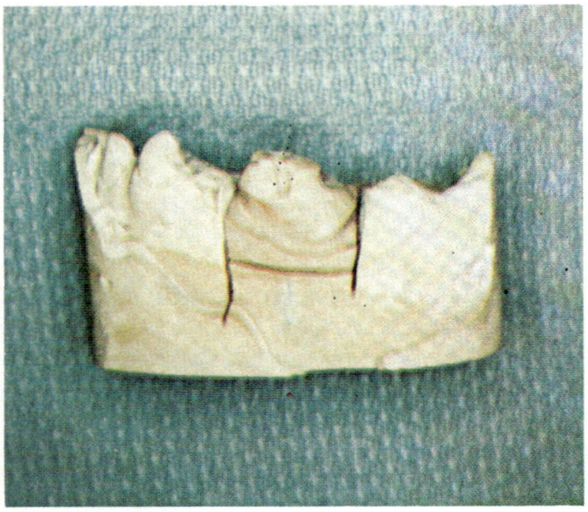

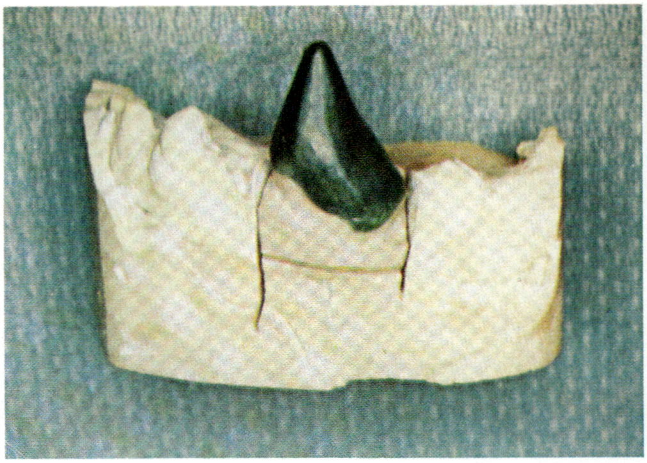

Figure 10 *(upper left)*—A model of the maxillary left quadrant made by pouring dental stone into the impression mold.

Figure 11 *(above)*—A pattern for the prosthesis, carved in wax, is made to approximate, as closely as possible, the normal configuration of the tooth. The pattern is fitted to the stone model before the prosthesis is cast.

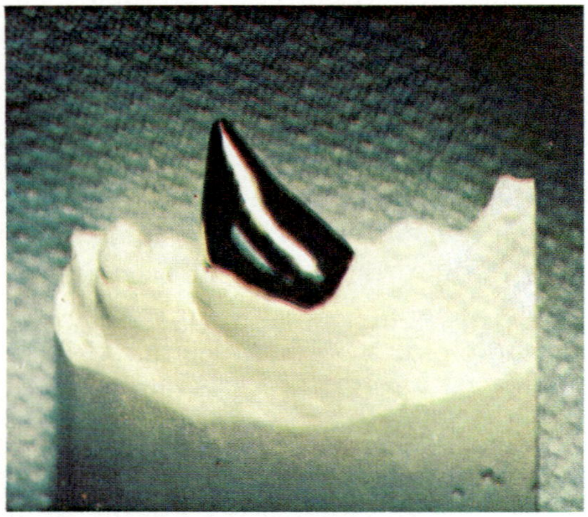

Figure 12 *(left)*—The wax pattern has been cast in gold and the polished and finished casting seated on the stone model to assure proper fit.

Figure 13—The finished gold casting ready for cementing to the crown. Note the fragile dowel portion.

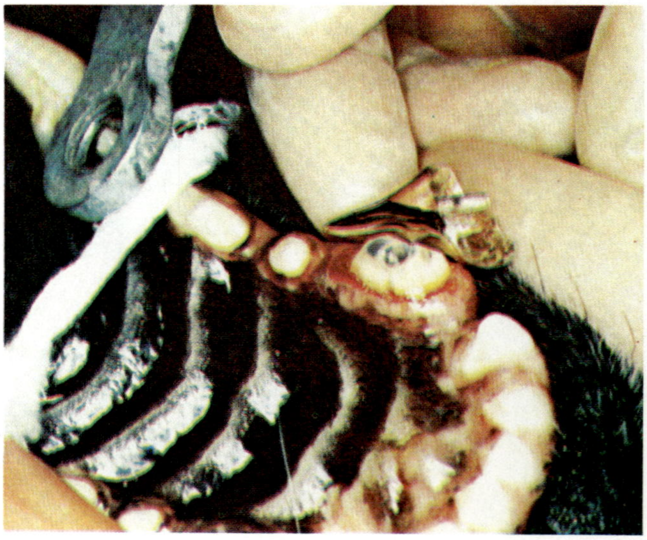

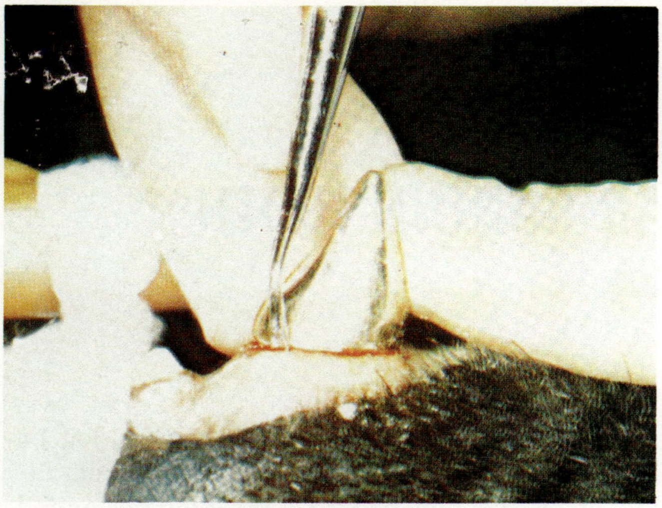

Figure 14—The prosthesis has been cemented to the crown. Excess cement is removed from the subgingival sulcus.

Figures 15 & 16—Completed restoration of both maxillary canine teeth.

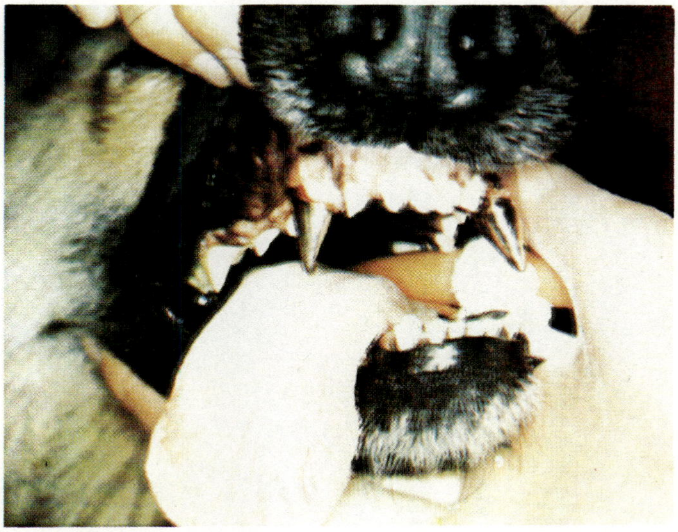

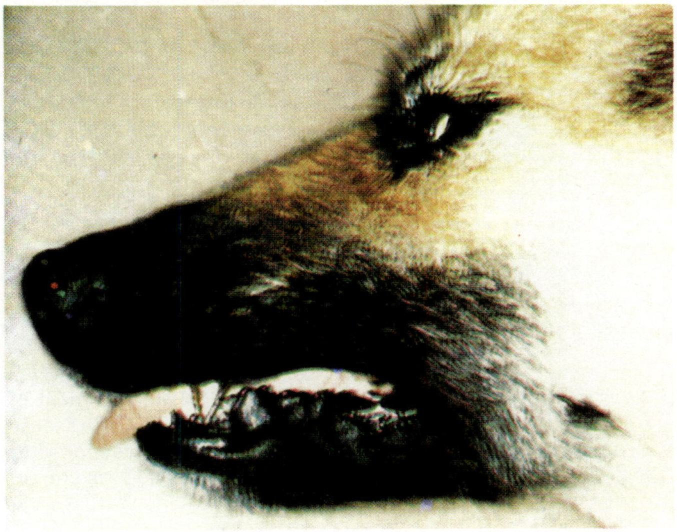

A model of the dental arch and tooth to be reconstructed (*Figure 10*) was obtained by pouring dental stone into the impression mold. A pattern for the dowel and prosthesis was carved from wax, reproducing as closely was possible the normal con- figuration of the maxillary canine tooth (*Figure 11*). The wax pattern was then adapted to the stone model.

Using standard procedures[1] the wax pattern was cast in gold. The rough casting was finished and polished with sandpaper discs, rubber wheels, tripoli, and rouge. It was then adjusted on the stone model in preparation for final seating in the patient's mouth (*Figure 12*).

The prosthesis was cemented with zinc phosphate, and tapped firmly into place with a mallet until the resonance of the maxilla indicated that the dowel and crown were solidly abutting tooth structure. The prosthesis was held firmly in place until the cement had completely hardened. Any cement along the gingiva was removed with a tartar hook (*Figure 14*) to prevent postoperative pericoronal gingival inflammation.

Figures 15 and 16 show the completed prosthesis in the patient's mouth.

ACKNOWLEDGMENT

Gratitude is expressed to Maj. E.G. Peck, Kansas ARNG, for providing the drawings.

REFERENCE

1. Tylman and Tylman: *Theory and Practice of Crown and Bridge Prosthodontics.* C.V. Mosby Co., St. Louis, Mo., 1965.

use of an inclined plane for correction of ECTOPIC MANDIBULAR CANINE TOOTH in a dog

Robert E. Kind, DVM
Conejo Valley Veterinary Clinic
1850 Thousand Oaks Blvd.
Thousand Oaks, California 91360
Richard A. Mays, DDS
Thousand Oaks, California 91360

CORRECTION of malaligned teeth in the dog has been achieved by a variety of techniques, including use of an inclined plane.[1-5] We describe and illustrate the technique because of its simplicity, the short time required for treatment, and the excellent toleration of the inclined plane by the patient.

Case Report

A 6-month-old male Irish Setter was presented because of a left lower canine tooth which was erupting in linguoversion, resulting in traumatic penetration of the hard palate (*Figures 1 & 2*). The owner requested some method of correction other than extraction of the tooth. After consultation

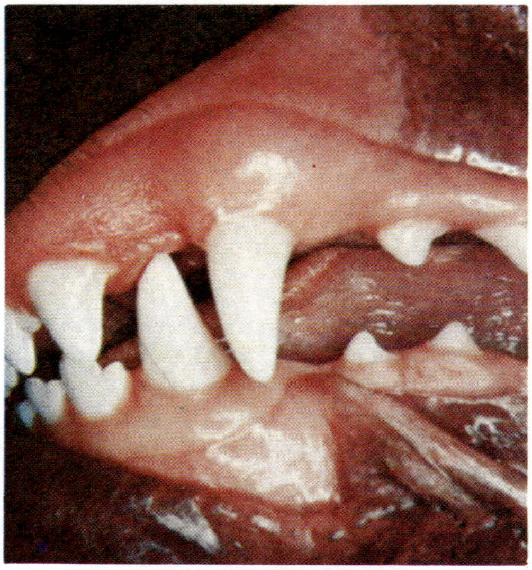

Figure 1—The malaligned mandibular canine tooth contacts the hard palate.

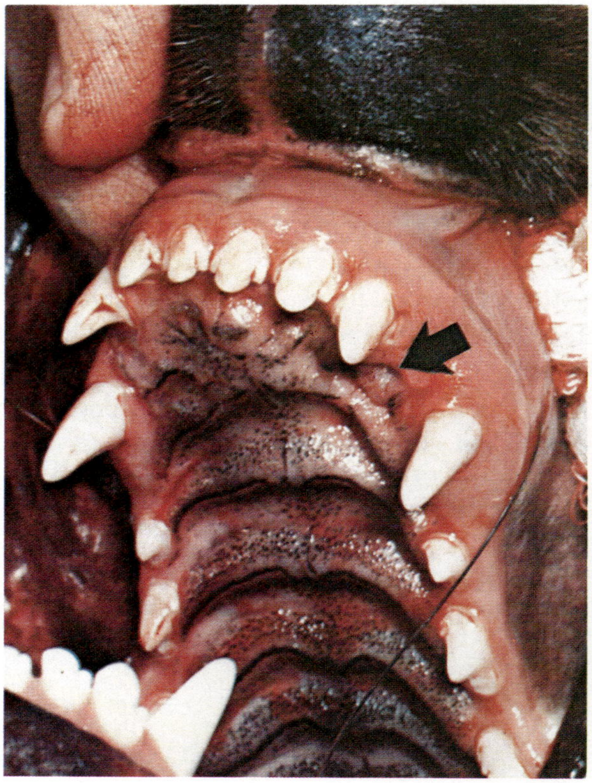

Figure 2—Traumatic penetration (*arrow*) of the hard palate caused by malalignment of the mandibular canine tooth. The wire seen in this photograph is being positioned for retention of the device later installed to correct the malalignment.

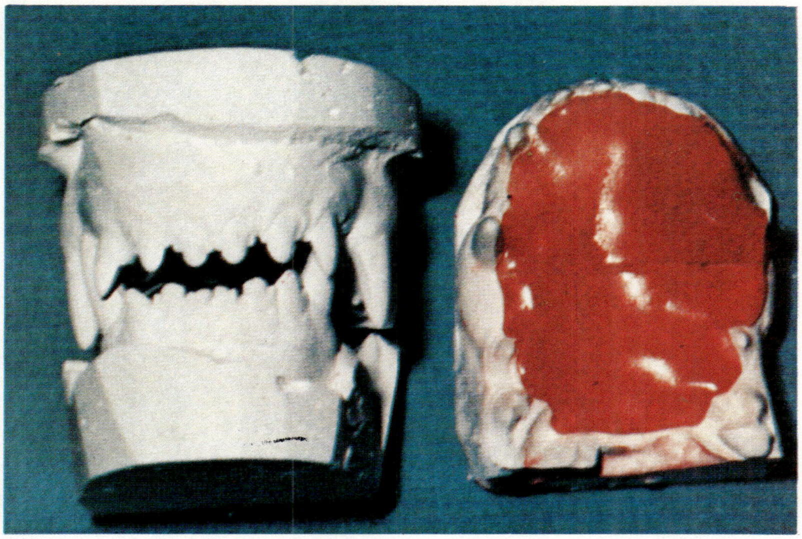

Figure 3—Plaster models (*left*) of the upper and lower teeth show malocclusion. At the right in the photo, the inclined plane is shown being fitted to the working model of the maxilla.

with Donald L. Ross, D.V.M., M.S., Houston, Texas, the decision was made to use an inclined plane for correcting the defect.

The dog was anesthetized with sodium thiamylal, followed by intubation and maintenance of anesthesia with halothane and nitrous oxide.

Impressions were made of the upper and lower teeth using standard dental impression trays and caulk jeltrate (Alginate® —Dentsply International, Inc.), an impression material obtained from a local dental supply house. After the impressions were made, models (*Figure 3*) were cast from plaster (Hydrocal® U.S. Gypsum) purchased from a supplier of building materials.

The orthodontic device was fashioned from methyl methacrylate (Unitek Corp.), an acrylic resin. This device was designed to extend over the hard palate distal to the second premolars. An inclined plane of approximately 45 degrees was carved into the lingual surface of the device between the maxillary canine tooth and third incisor (*Figure 4*). A groove was made on this surface and along the sides of the device to provide partial protection and stability for the wire that would subsequently be used to hold the device in the dog's mouth. The device was so designed that when the dog's tooth would contact the inclined plane, thus moving the canine tooth buccally.

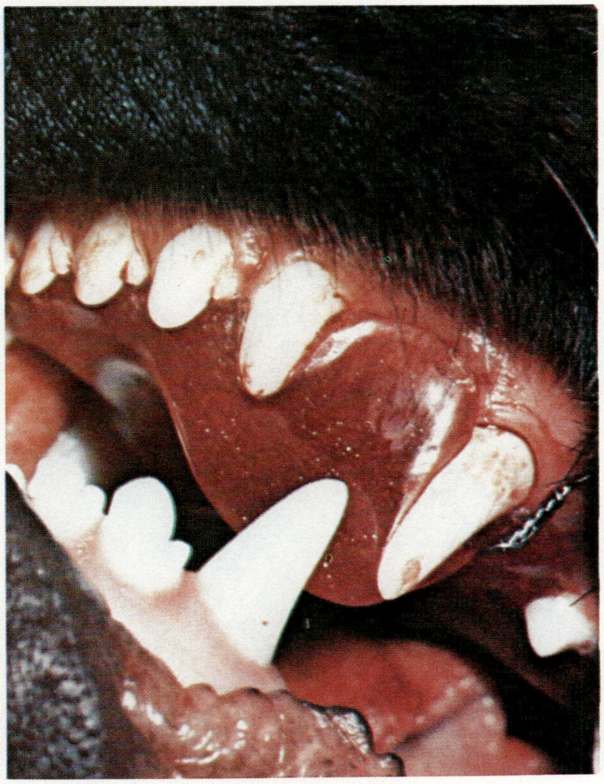

Figure 4—When the device is properly designed and fitted to the mouth, the lower canine tooth is brought into contact with the inclined plane as the mouth is closed. This contact pushes the tooth in a buccal direction.

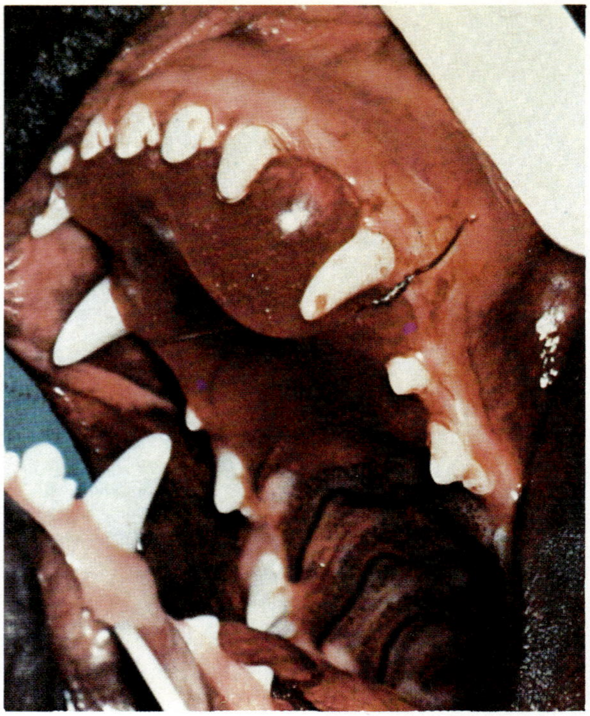

Figure 5—The device is affixed to the maxilla by means of a 26-gauge wire that encircles the maxilla immediately behind the canine teeth. A groove along the lingual surface and sides of the device helps protect and stabilize the wire.

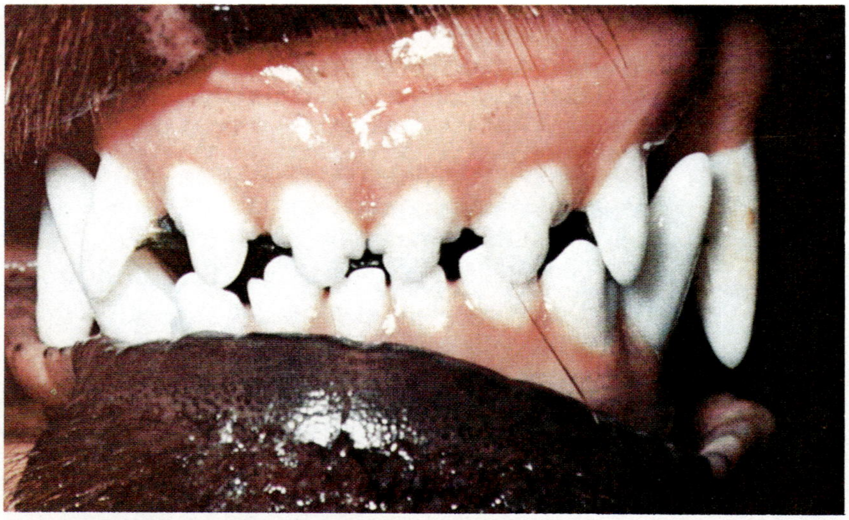

Figure 6—Occlusion of the teeth after the device was removed (10 days after it was installed).

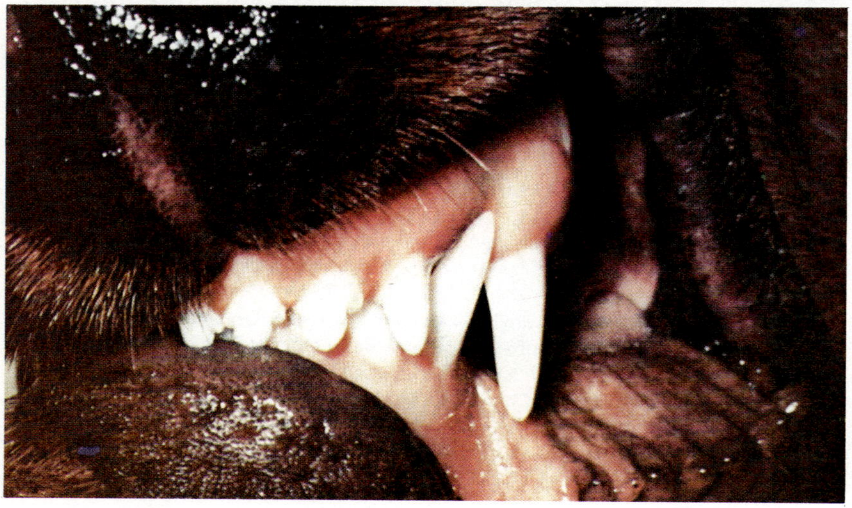

Figure 7—Two weeks after removal of the device the mouth is functionally and cosmetically normal.

When the inclined plane had been completed, the dog was again anesthetized and the device was seated in the upper arcade. The device was affixed immediately behind the canine teeth by encircling the maxilla with 26-gauge stainless steel wire affixed to a 3/8 curved cutting-edge needle. The procedure entailed inserting one end of the wire at the midline on the dorsum of the nose. Following the contour of the maxilla subcutaneously, that end of the wire emerged behind an upper canine tooth. The other end of the wire was then directed through the same opening at midline on the dorsum of the nose and directed subcutaneously to emerge behind the upper canine tooth on the opposite side of the maxilla. Thus the wire was visible only where it passed through the mucosa in the vestibule. The ends of the wire were twisted together behind the left canine tooth to affix the device (*Figure 5*).

Postoperatively, the dog was given 250 mg ampicillin t.i.d. as a prophylactic measure.

Results

During the first eight hours after the device was installed, some hypersalivation was noted by the owner, but this effect proved to be only temporary.

When the dog was examined 10 days after surgery, the malaligned tooth had moved buccally into a more normal position and the device was removed (*Figure 6*). Two weeks later the tooth had drifted into contact with the buccal tissue. In addition, the tooth had erupted upward, which prevented recurrence of any movement toward the tongue (*Figure 7*).

Use of the inclined plane in an orthodontic device resulted in a cosmetically normal mouth in this dog.

REFERENCES

1. Ross, D.L.: Therapeutics of Veterinary Dentistry. *Proc. 40th Annual AAHA Meeting;* 1973.
2. Roe, B.C.; Hall, B.D.: Correction of Malaligned Canine Teeth in a Dog. *JAVMA 146* (10):1066-1068; May 15, 1965.
3. Albrecht, D.T.: Surgical Positioning of Maloccluded Teeth in the Canine. *Small Anim. Clin. 1*:373-376; Dec. 1961.
4. Annis, J.R.: Dental Surgery in *Canine Surgery*, 2nd Archibald ed. American Veterinary Publications, Santa Barbara, Calif., 1974; p. 317.
5. Braber, T.M.: Anterior Cross-Bite; in *Orthodontic Textbook*. W.B. Saunders Co., Philadelphia, Pa., 1963; pp. 656-663.

DENTAL PROSTHESIS
used to crown a canine tooth

Ralph S. Wilhelm. DVM
Robert M. Salisbury, DMD
Bryon B. Emswiller, DVM
450 Northlake Boulevard
Lake Park, Florida 33404

A 1-YEAR-OLD Shepherd-type dog of mixed breeding was presented to the clinic because of an erosion in the permanent left maxillary canine tooth (*Figure 1*). In this paper we describe restoration of the tooth with procedures and materials used routinely in human dentistry.

While still at the veterinary clinic the dog was given an intramuscular injection of atropine sulfate at a dosage of 0.05 mg/kg. Anesthesia was induced with Nembutal® (Abbott) given at the rate of 4.5 mg/kg to effect. The dog was then transported to the dental clinic.

The crowning process consisted of the following steps:

1. Removing all decay from the eroded tooth
2. Applying a medicated base to the surface of the cleaned cavity
3. Filling the defect with a composite resin
4. Making the impression mold of the maxilla
5. Casting the impression mold in plaster
6. Modeling the prosthesis in wax and casting it in metal
7. Applying the metal prosthesis to the eroded tooth

Removal of Decay

Using a high-speed air turbine with a diamond bur and a water spray as a coolant, necrotic material was removed from the eroded tooth. All affected surfaces were drilled down to relatively healthy tissue. Remaining necrotic tissue was removed with hand excavators.

The surfaces of the cavity must be prepared in this way to ensure that the cavity will retain the maximum amount of filler material. The greater the bulk of the filler material, the stronger the base that can be placed, and therefore the greater the support for the prosthesis.

Application of the Medicated Base

After all decayed tissue had been removed, calcium hydroxide (Dycal® — L. D. Caulk, Milford, Del.), a medicated base, was applied with a ball-point applicator in a thin layer over the entire cavity. Dycal consists of a base and a catalyst. When they are mixed, they form a solid compound in about two and one-half minutes.

The layer of Dycal, which actually attaches itself to the tooth, serves several important functions: (1) It provides a solid foundation on which the prosthesis will rest. (2) It helps maintain the vitality of the underlying pulp. (3) It neutralizes acid formed by the filler used in the next layer.

Final Filling of the Defect

The material used to fill the cavity is called a *composite* or *reinforced* resin. We used Adaptic® (Johnson & Johnson), a two-component product. One of the components is the filler particles which are bulk-enhancing agents. The other is a bonding agent which attaches the filler to the tooth. When the two components are mixed in equal parts, the mixture remains workable and can be used for filling for one and one-half minutes. Hardening time is approximately five minutes. With this material the tooth was sufficiently restored to permit the prosthetic crown to be anchored to it (*Figure 2*).

Making the Impression Mold

After the cavity was filled, the bite was checked to determine the amount of clearance available for the crown. At this stage, resin filler could still be added or removed if necessary.

An impression of the eroded tooth and surrounding teeth and maxilla was taken using an elastic impression compound (Xantopren® — Unitek Corp., Monrovia, Calif.). To make the impression, the elastic material was put into an impression tray, the tray was placed in the dog's mouth and the dog's mouth was held closed over the tray until the impression material had set.

Materials for making the impression are essentially liquid polymers, usually with a polysulfide or

Figure 1—Erosion in the left maxillary canine tooth of a 1-year-old Shepherd-type dog.

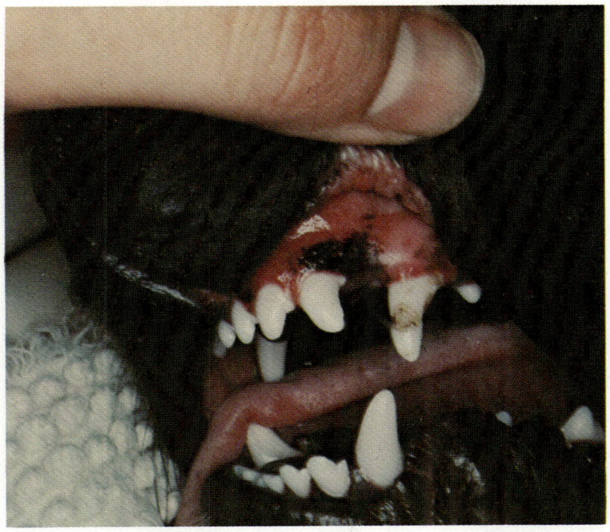

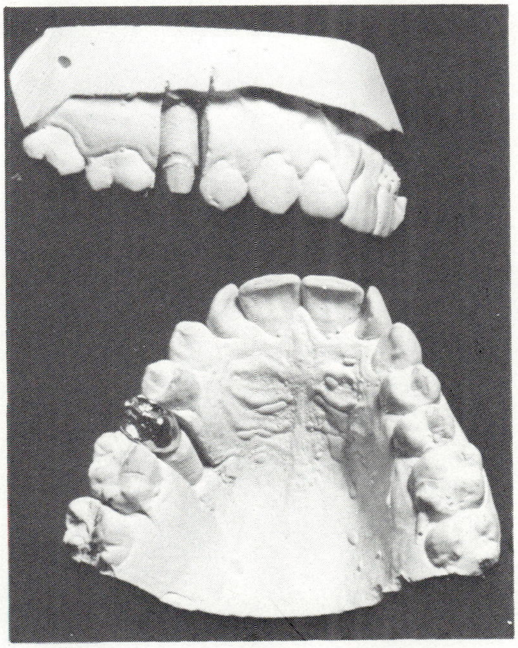

Figure 4—A casting taken from the impression mold shown in Figure 3. A prosthetic crown has been modelled over the tooth to be restored.

Figure 2—Appearance of the tooth after the decayed tissue was removed and a filler implanted.

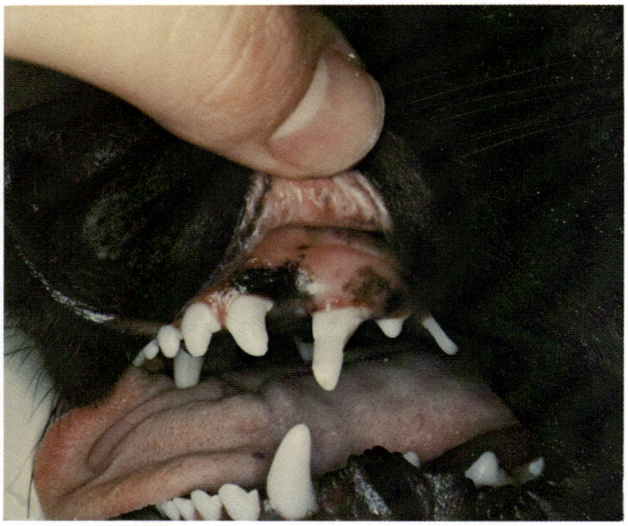

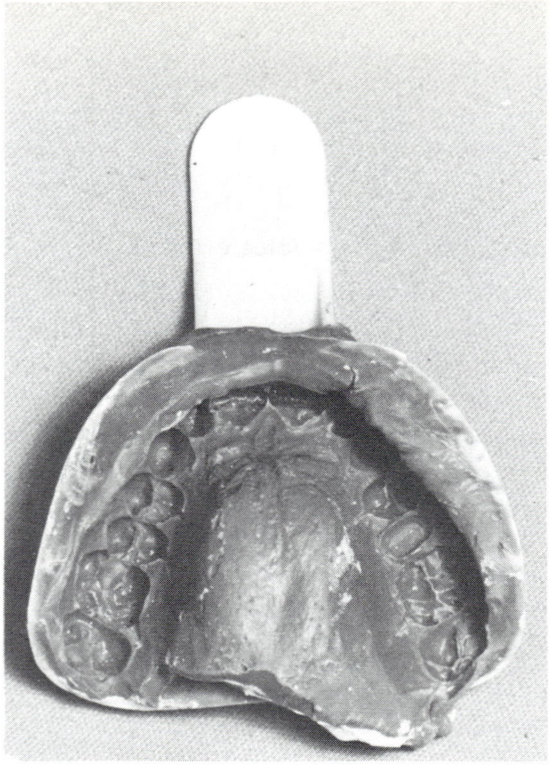

Figure 3—An impression tray bearing the impression mold of a human maxilla. The same type of impression materials are used in canine dentistry.

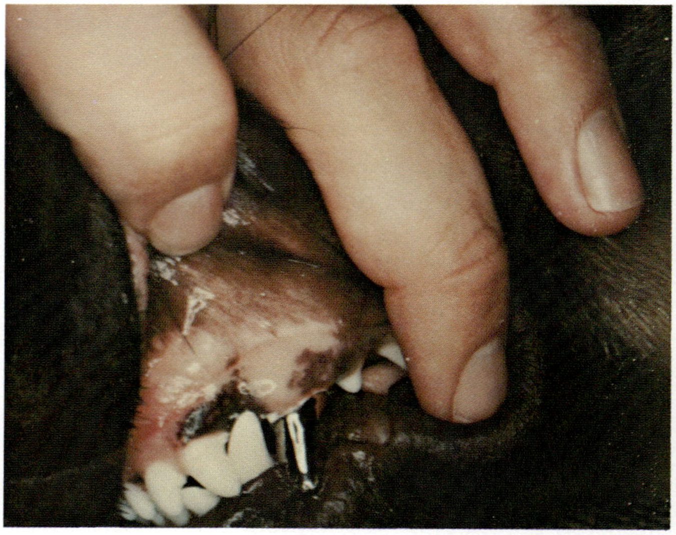

Figure 6—The bite is checked for proper occlusion after the prosthetic crown is applied.

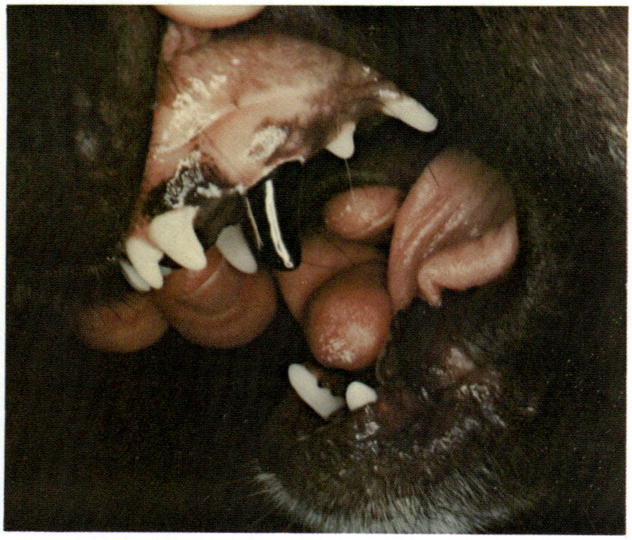

Figure 5—The titanium prosthesis affixed to the eroded canine tooth seen in Figure 1.

silicone base. When mixed with a catalyst at room temperature, the compounds convert to solid rubber. Setting time depends on type of polymer used, amount of catalyst, and room temperature.

Completing the Metal Prosthesis

After the impression was taken, the impression mold was sent in the impression tray to a dental laboratory (*Figure 3*). From this impression mold a plaster casting was made (*Figure 4*). Using the plaster casting as a base, a dental technician then modelled a wax prosthesis. This wax model was put into a device which replaced the wax with molten titanium, thus forming a metal prosthesis.

Application of the Prosthetic Crown

When returned from the dental laboratory, the finished titanium prosthesis was applied over the dog's eroded tooth and the bite was evaluated (*Figures 5 & 6*). If the prosthesis had needed correction to improve the bite, the alterations could have been made at this time with the diamond bur or with hand excavators.

The crown was permanently affixed to the tooth with polycarboxylate cement (Durelon® — Premier, Norristown, Pa.). A thin layer of this cement was applied to both the bonding surface of the tooth and the prosthesis. To achieve a proper bond, all surfaces receiving the cement must be clean, dry, and free of extraneous proteinaceous material. After the prosthesis was affixed in proper position over the tooth, the dog was restrained manually for 15 minutes while the cement hardened.

Polycarboxylate cements consist of zinc oxide powder, magnesium oxide, and approximately 40% liquid polyacrylic acid. The liquid and powder components are mixed to form a paste which hardens into a solid mass. The cement reaches 75% of its total bonding capacity in approximately 15 minutes, and 90% in 60 minutes. These cements have the capacity to chelate to calcium in a tooth, thus forming a bond. They also bond through a process of cross-linking to other metals. They do not bond well with dental porcelain or any amalgam with a low metallic content.

Comment

Dental prostheses are uncommon in veterinary medicine. In selected cases, with the use of materials and techniques employed in human dentistry, these prosthetics can be used in veterinary medicine with good results. In the case described here the prosthesis was well accepted by the dog and the tooth functioned normally.

BIBLIOGRAPHY

Asgar, K.: Elastic Impression Materials. *Dental Clinics of North America 15*:81-98; Jan. 1971.

Gilmore, H.W.: Restoration Materials and Cavity Preparation Design. *Dental Clinics of North America 15*:99-114; Jan. 1971.

Woelfel, J.B.: Newer Materials and Techniques in Prosthetic Resin Materials. *Dental Clinics of North America 15*:455-486; Apr. 1971.

ROOT CANAL THERAPY in dogs

L.D. Rubin, VMD
D.C. Maplesden, DVM, PhD
Rhawnhurst Animal Hospital
7905 Bustleton Avenue
Philadelphia, Pennsylvania 19152

R. R. Singer, DDS
8118 Old York Road
Elkins Park, Pennsylvania 19117

ROOT CANAL THERAPY provides an alternative to extracting teeth that have abscessed. Usually the abscess is the result of decay or trauma.

If the pulp of a tooth dies, a space is left in the tooth. This space (the pulp cavity) is a perfect breeding ground for bacteria because it is warm, moist, and dark. Therefore, systematic enlarging and cleansing of this canal, followed by thorough filling and sealing, represents the treatment of choice in most instances.

Frequently, the canine teeth of dogs are traumatized so that they fracture, exposing the pulp. If this occurs in a watchdog or police dog, maintaining the tooth is especially important. Considering the expense of training such dogs, retention and restoration of their teeth is economically sound. This paper deals with root canal therapy of canine teeth, but the described procedure can be adapted to any of the other teeth.

After trauma, the condition of a tooth may vary from little or no exposure of the pulp, to severe infection that has almost destroyed the pulp. Often a tooth is worn to the degree that the canal is exposed, but infection, if any, is minimal (*Figure 1*).

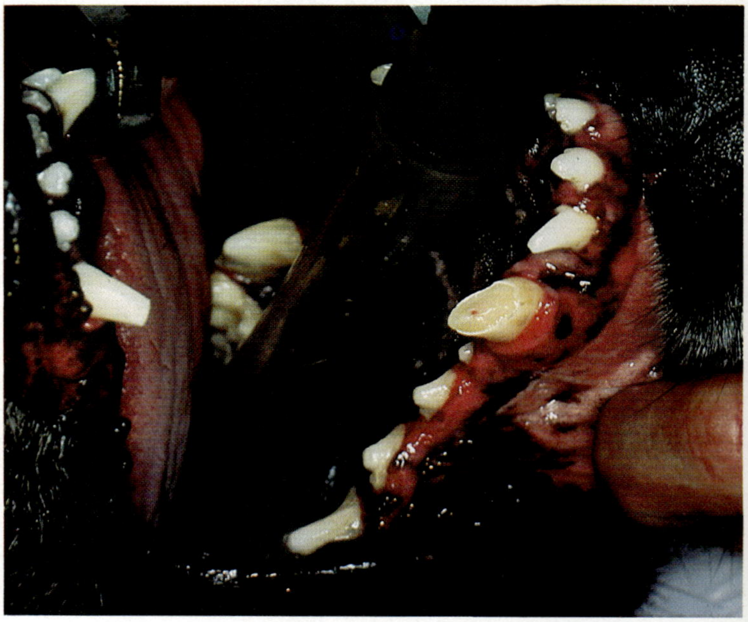

Figure 1
A canine tooth with the root canal exposed.

Special instruments are required for evacuating the root canal and mechanically preparing it for filling. The objective of evacuation is to free the canal of all soft and decayed tissue and create a cavity large enough to permit introduction of filling material (*e.g.*, gutta-percha and amalgam).

Control of infection is of major importance in root canal therapy. Thus, the use of sterile instruments is imperative. Contaminated instruments must be sterilized before they are reused. Normally, as root canal instruments are used, they are sterilized by dipping in a

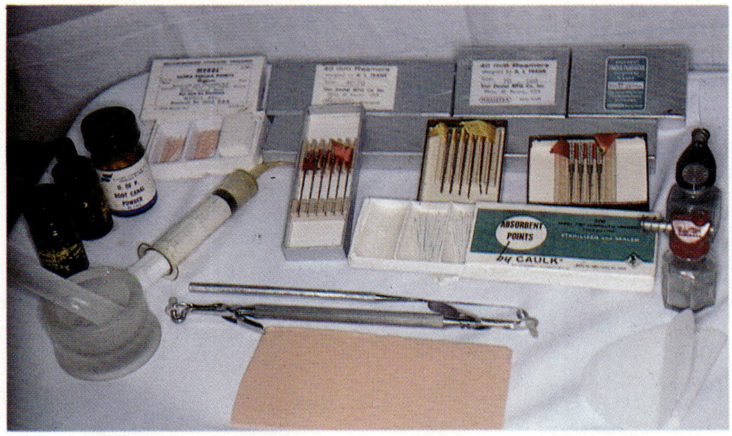

Figure 2
Equipment needed for root canal therapy.

Equipment and Supplies

All necessary instruments and supplies (*Figure 2*) should be laid out in the sequence in which they are to be used. The following are needed:

- Drill, burs and grinding wheel
- Reamers
- Irrigation syringe
- Sodium hypochlorite solution (Clorox®)
- Absorbent points
- Root canal powder and cement
- Gutta-percha sheet
- Glass slab
- Gutta-percha points
- Finger pluggers
- Amalgam
- Mortar and pestle
- Gauze filter
- Amalgam carrier
- Miscellaneous dental instruments (amalgam compactor, tooth scalers)

hot bead (heated dry granular salt) for about five seconds. The gutta-percha points should be sterilized; this can be done by dipping them in a Clorox® solution.

Gutta-percha points of sufficient size for the teeth of large dogs are not available commercially. They must be hand-made. The procedure is as follows:

A sheet of gutta-percha about 3/16″ thick is slightly heated with a thermocautery unit or a hot plate. From this sheet is cut a strip about 1/8″ wide and 2″ long. This strip is heated until it begins to sag slightly. It is then rolled on a glass plate[1] while a microscope slide is used to form it into a cylinder having a diameter about the same as that of a size 100 reamer (approximately 1 mm). Gradually, one end of the cylinder is tapered to a point. If the strip of gutta-percha becomes too hot, it will stick to the glass plate. While the strip is rolled it will cool and become firmer so that in order to finish creating a point, reheating the strip may be necessary.

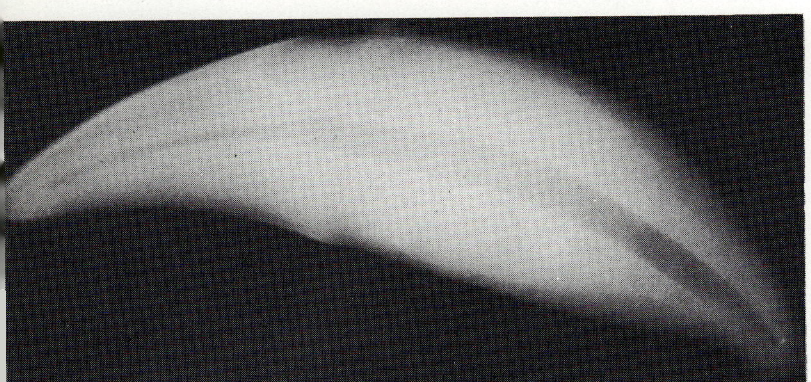

Figure 3 — Radiograph of a canine tooth showing the curved root canal.

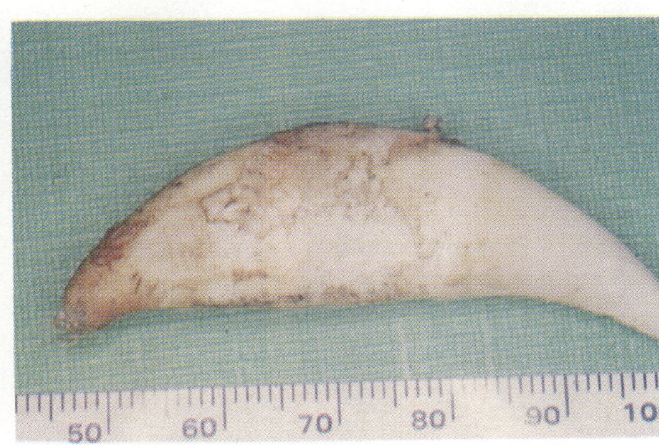

Figure 4 — A canine tooth from a German Shepherd. The canal in this breed is about 50 mm.

Figure 5 — A reamer is inserted fully into the root canal.

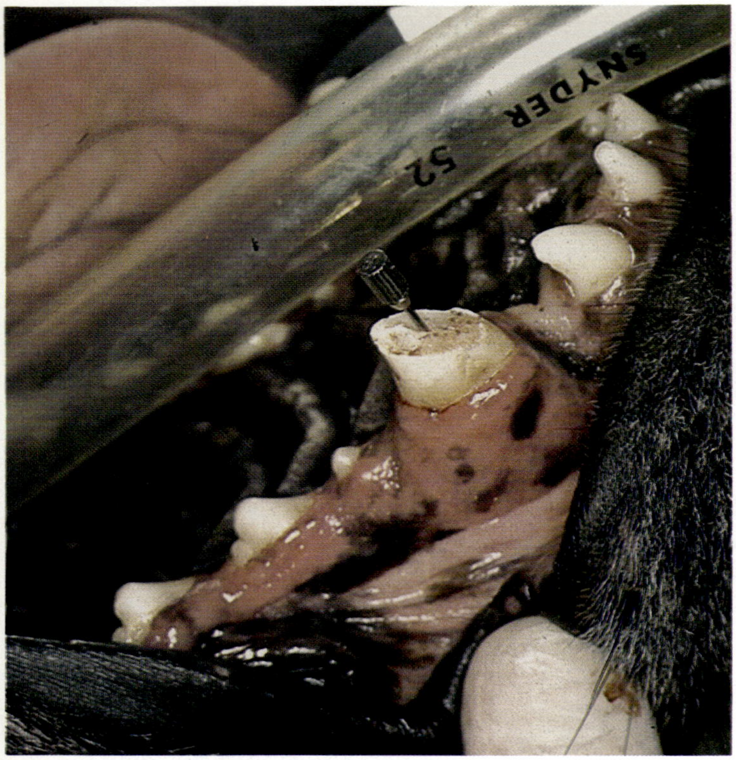

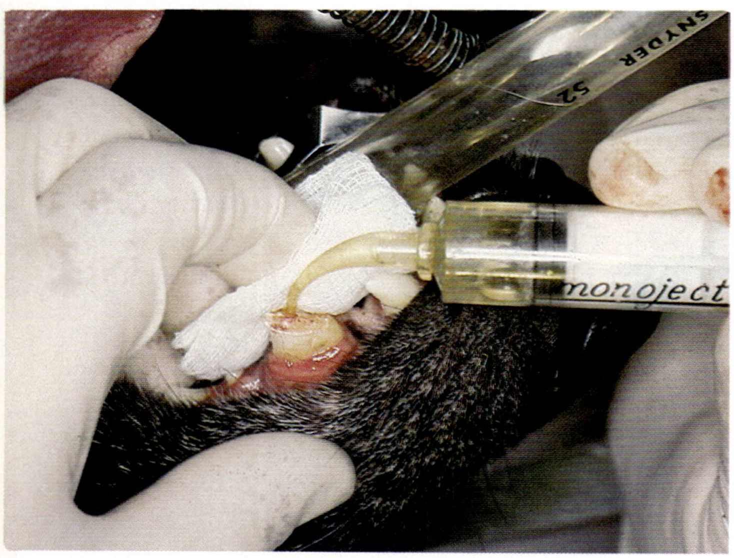

Figure 6 — Flushing the root canal with sodium hypochlorite solution during the reaming operation.

Procedure

If the tooth has been broken or has uneven edges, it should be smoothed with a grinding wheel before the root canal procedure begins.

The exposed root canal is cut into with a round dental bur, care being taken to enlarge the opening on a slight diagonal toward the rear of the tooth, thus creating an oval opening. This is especially important because the root canal of a dog's canine tooth is curved (*Figure 3*) and the oval opening provides easier access to the entire canal.

The canal of an intact canine tooth in the German Shepherd dog is approximately 50 mm long (*Figure 4*). Thus, long reamers must be used. The length of the root canal can be determined by x-ray (*Figure 3*).

Reamers are side-cutting files that work best in straight root canals. For use with canine teeth in the dog, they must be bent to an appropriate curve. The designated size of a reamer indicates its diameter; size 40 is 0.4 mm in diameter, size 45 is 0.45 mm in diameter, etc.

The reamer is used as a vertical file to enlarge and smooth the canal. It is inserted as deeply as possible; its tip should reach the end of the root canal (*Figure 5*). Excessive tension on the reamer must be avoided because removal of a broken reamer from deep within the canal is almost impossible.

When reaming has progressed until the first reamer moves freely in the canal, the reamer of the next larger size should be introduced. The sizes of the reamers increase in increments of 5 from size 40 through size 60. After size 60, the increase is in increments of 10. It is important not to skip a reamer of any size while reaming, because an overlarge reamer may bind, increasing the risk of its breaking. Use of a reamer that binds should be discontinued and the next smaller size should be used until it moves easily in the canal. When the canal is clean, it should accommodate a size 90 or 100 reamer, and only hard tissue residue should be seen on the last reamer used.

Figure 7 — The evacuated root canal is dried with absorbent points.

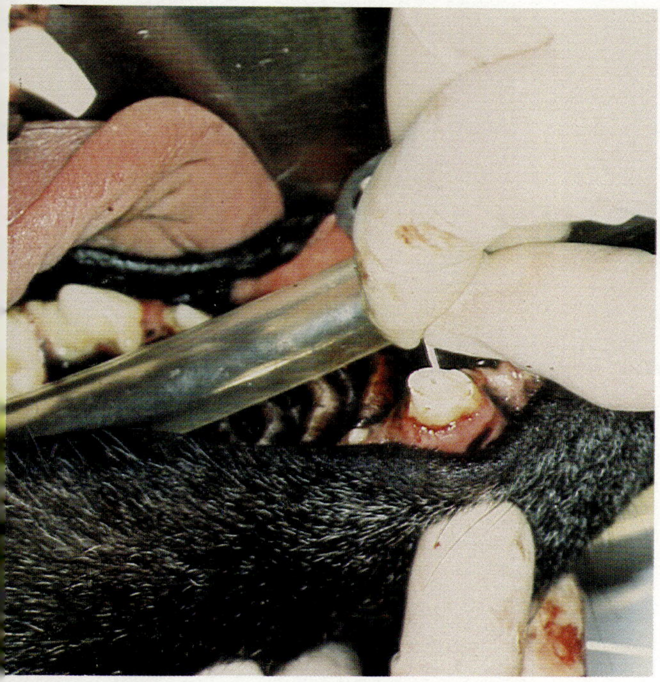

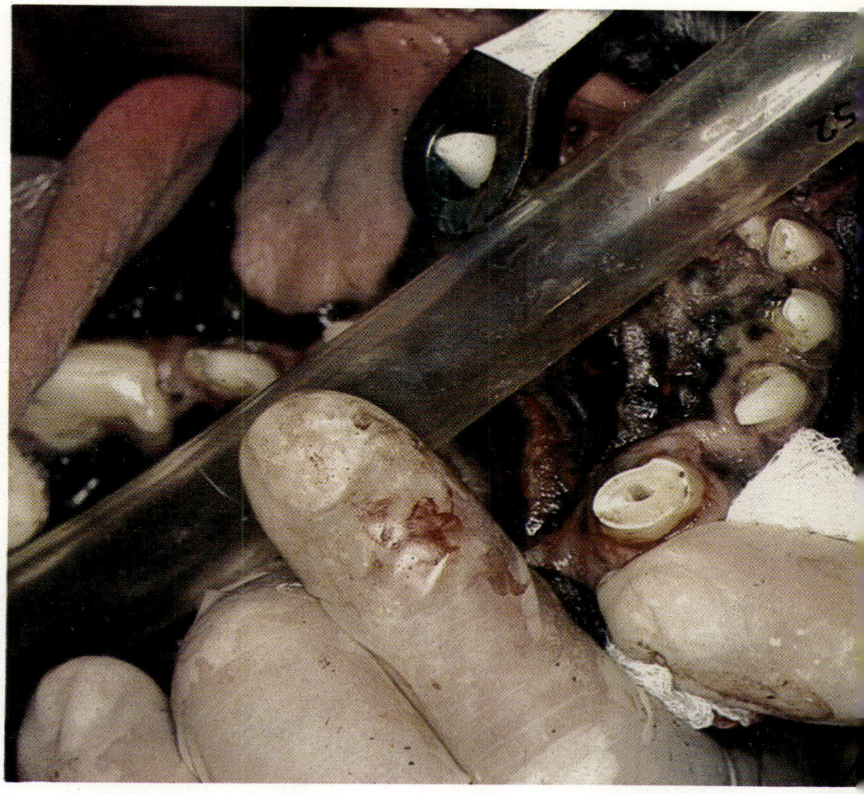

Figure 8 — The root canal is fully prepared for plugging.

In order to clear the canal and increase lubrication, the canal should be frequently flushed with sodium hypochlorite solution during the reaming operation (*Figure 6*). Keeping the canal moist during the reaming process enhances debridement and helps keep the reamer from breaking.

When the canal has been completely reamed out, it is given a final flush with sodium hypochlorite. Then, the debris is blown out with a dry sterile syringe as the source of air. After the canal has been dried with absorbent points (*Figure 7*) it is ready for plugging with gutta-percha points (*Figure 8*).

To prepare the cement that bonds the gutta-percha points to the canal, the contents of one capsule of root canal powder (zinc oxide, resin, bismuth subcarbonate and barium sulfate) are poured onto the glass slab. The powder and cement (eugenol, Canada balsam) are then mixed with a spatula to form a smooth, thick paste.

The large handmade gutta-percha point is rolled in the paste and inserted into the root canal (*Figure 9*). Any excess gutta-percha is cut off with a heated sharp dental instrument and the gutta-percha point is pushed down with a finger plugger (*Figure 10*). Insertion of a medium gutta-percha point (or points) follows. Like the large point, the medium points are rolled in the cement, inserted in the canal (*Figure 11*), and tamped down with the finger plugger. This procedure is repeated with small gutta-percha points until no more points can be driven into the canal with the finger pluggers. Proper packing of the canal with the points should eliminate all air pockets. Excess gutta-percha at the opening into the canal is trimmed away with the heated dental instrument (*Figure 12*).

So that the tooth will hold the amalgam, the canal is cut back about 1 mm under the opening with an undercutting bur (square shoulder). The amalgam is made of two charges of silver alloy from the proportioner and two charges of mercury (*i.e.*, a 1:1 ratio). They are mix-

Figure 9 — A gutta-percha point is inserted into the prepared root canal.

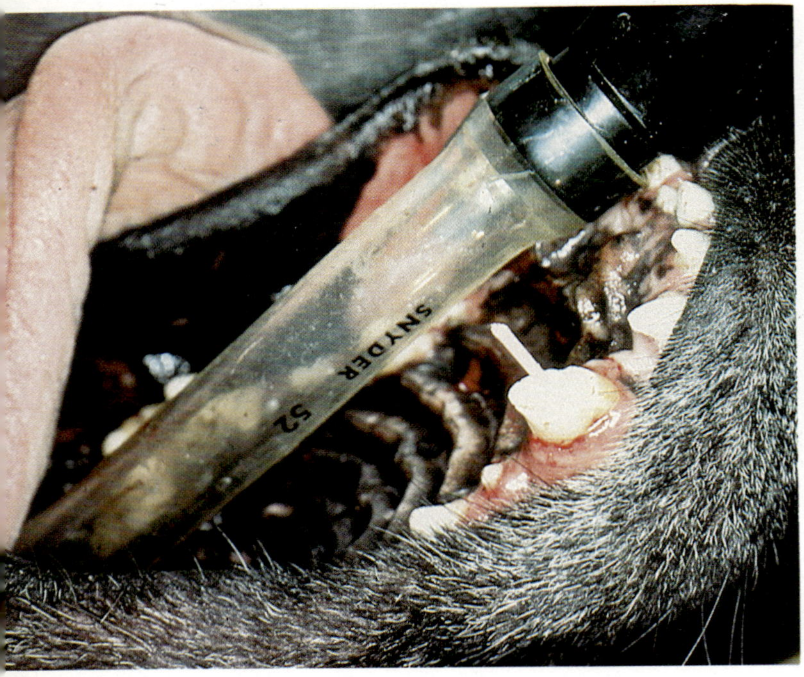

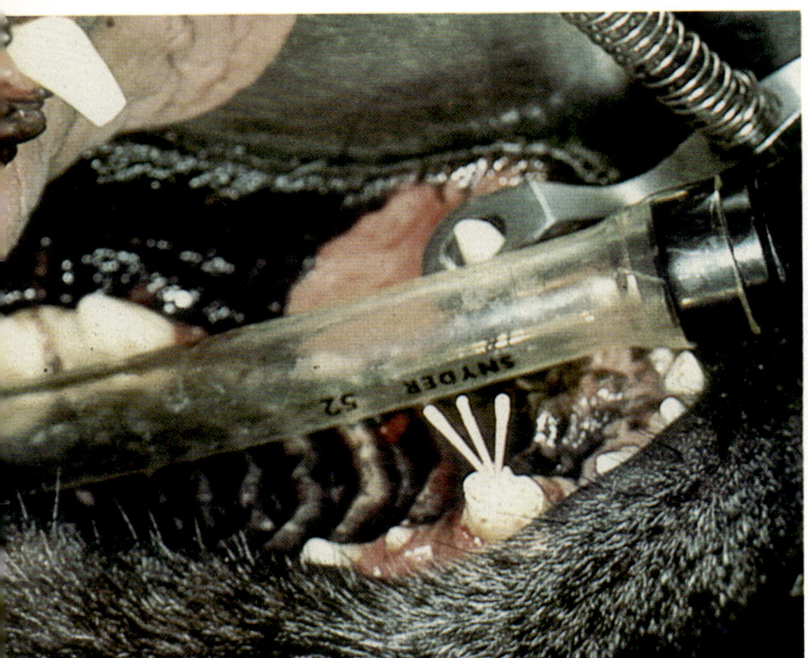

Figure 11 — Smaller points are inserted to fill the canal completely.

Figure 10 — A gutta-percha point is packed into the canal with a finger plugger.

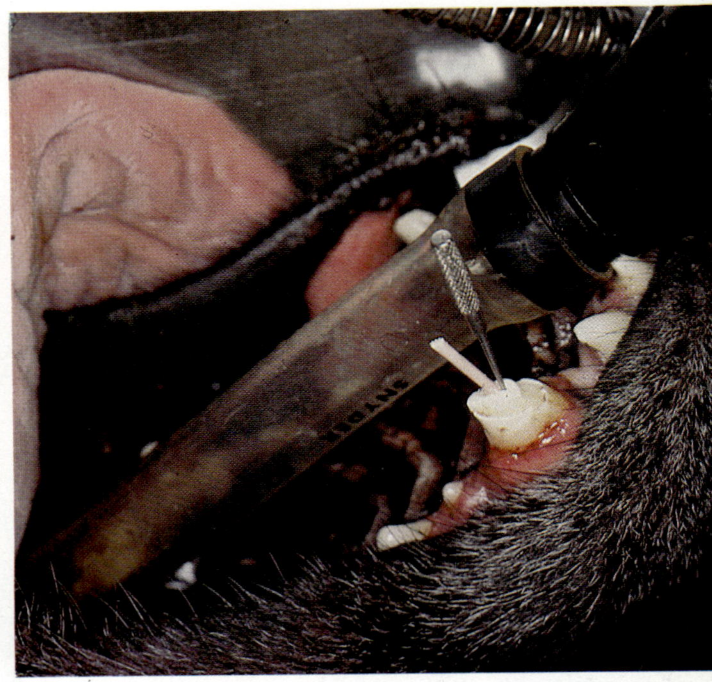

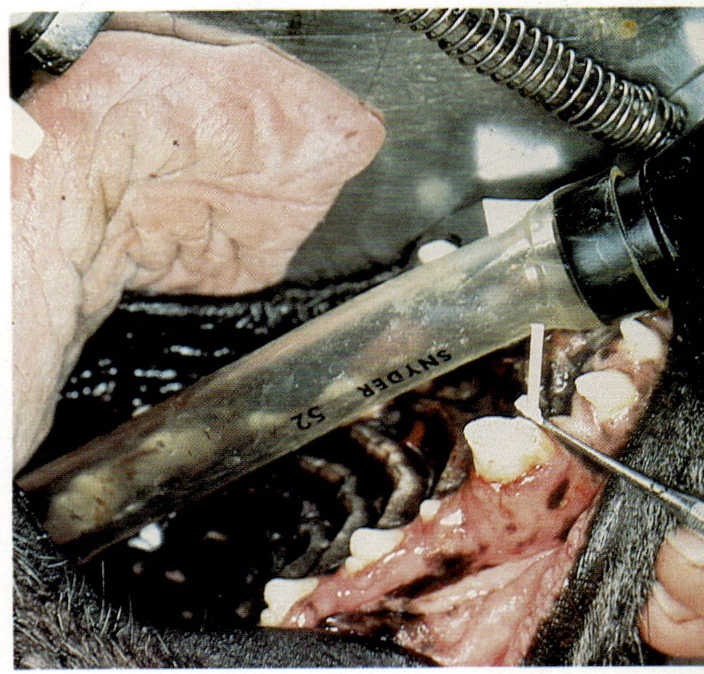

Figure 12 — Excess gutta-percha is trimmed off with a heated dental instrument.

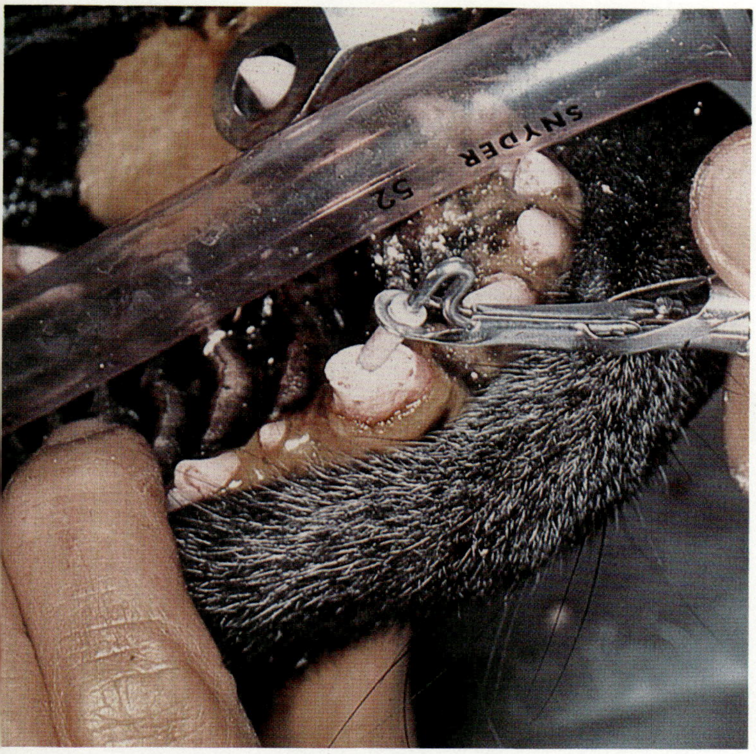

Figure 13
The tooth is filled using an amalgam carrier.

ed with reasonable pressure in a mortar and pestle until all of the silver is picked up by the mercury.

The mixed amalgam is squeezed through several layers of gauze or a special gauze filter to remove the excess mercury. It is then loaded into the amalgam carrier and the tooth is filled (*Figure 13*). The filling must be packed tightly. To complete the procedure, the filling is smoothed off with a dental instrument.

The owner should be instructed to make sure the dog does not chew on any hard objects for a week.

Comments

During the past five years we have performed this procedure on a number of dogs from the Philadelphia Police Department. After the root canal therapy, all of these dogs have been able to perform their duties, including attack work, without any apparent dental discomfort.

REFERENCE

1. Pickard, H.M.: *A Manual of Operative Dentistry* (4th Ed.). Oxford University Press, Ely House, London, W.I., England; 1976.

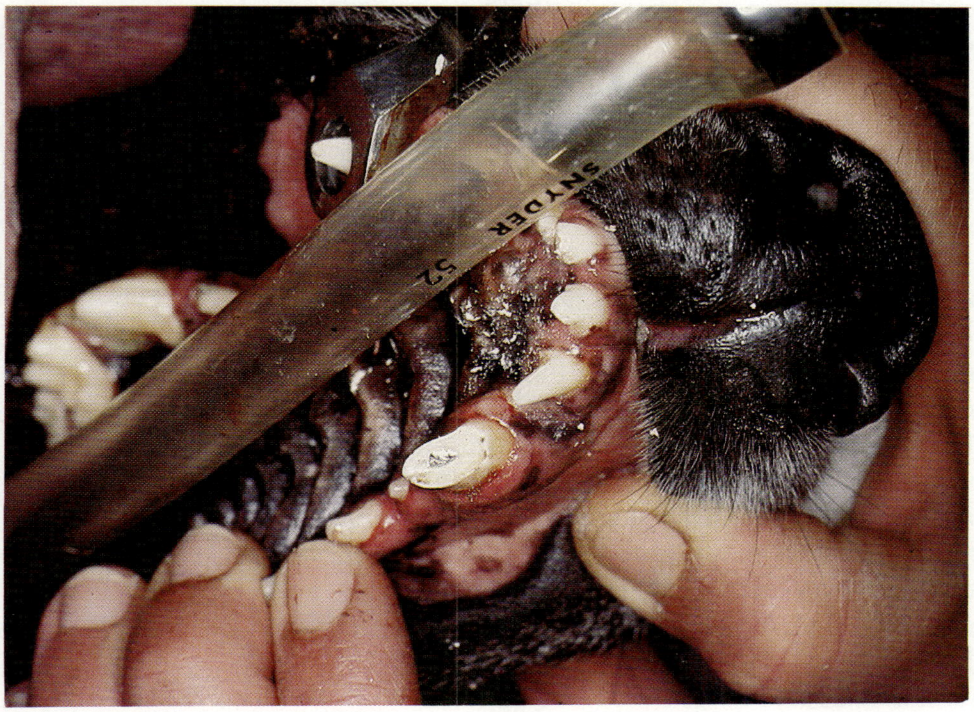

Figure 14
The completed procedure after the filling has been smoothed off.

aesthetic restoration of a FRACTURED ANTERIOR TOOTH in a dog

R.N. Peterson, DVM
Highland Park Veterinary Hospital
3129 South Winston
Tulsa, Oklahoma 74135
J.R. Wightman, DDS, MS
4134 South Harvard
Tulsa, Oklahoma 74135

Root canal therapy and cosmetic restoration of a fractured anterior tooth in a dog were performed in a single procedure. A threaded pin was anchored in the coronal portion of the root canal to reinforce the prosthesis. Considerable anatomic accuracy was possible in restoring the tooth because the restorative material used can be sculpted and shaped indefinitely until it has been exposed to ultraviolet light. The appearance of the restored tooth is quite natural.

Choice of treatment for a dental fracture secondary to trauma in a dog is often a dilemma. Extracting the tooth usually prevents infection and discomfort, but there are both functional and aesthetic drawbacks to the loss of the tooth. Although mastication is not usually impaired by the loss of one tooth, the dog's appearance may be marred. In some cases, appearance is of major concern. For example, the owner of a show dog with a damaged tooth might prefer cosmetic restoration rather than extraction of the tooth.

Restoration of function to canine teeth in sentry and hunting dogs has been reported to be of primary importance.[1-4] Often dental extraction has been performed to avert infection and subsequent pain.[5,6] In some cases full cast-metal crowns have been used to restore the function of a canine tooth after root canal therapy.[2,4] However, published reports have focused primarily on restoring function of the tooth. Apparently improvements have been confined to form, since the resulting restoration has been a shiny metal tooth that may be functional but is not cosmetically pleasing. Restoration of damaged teeth using porcelain fused to metal might offer an aesthetic improvement without significantly increasing the difficulty in constructing the prosthesis. This technique is widely used in human dentistry.

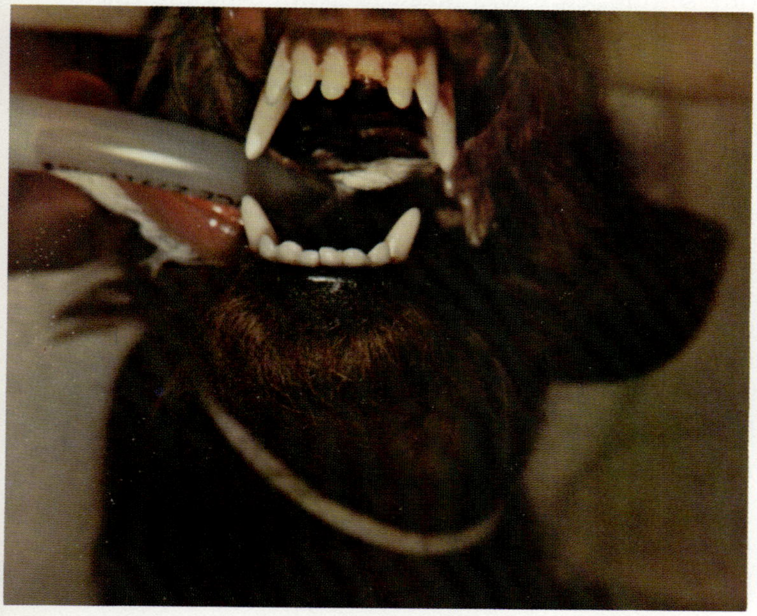

Figure 1—The reinforcing pin has been anchored in the filled root canal of the fractured maxillary incisor tooth.

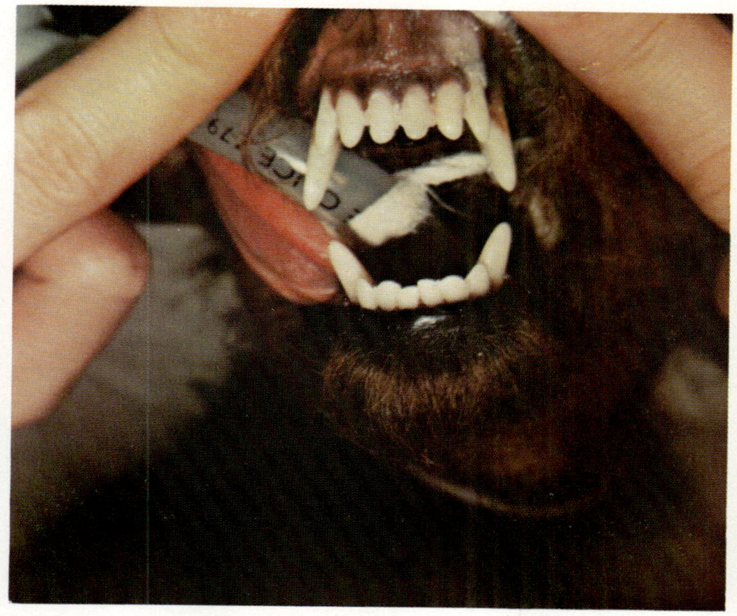

Figure 2—Completed cosmetic restoration of the fractured tooth.

Reinforcing pins and restoration materials that can be polymerized with ultraviolet light have also been used successfully to repair dental fractures in man. In this report we describe use of these methods to repair a fractured tooth in a dog. Such methods can be used to restore the appearance of any fractured tooth not subjected to great stress. Thus, these methods are contraindicated in repairing the canine cuspid or any posterior tooth.

Case Report

A 2½-year-old Wirehaired Dachshund was presented because of a transverse fracture of the upper left central incisor. The cause of the fracture was unknown. After a 12-hour fast, the animal was anesthetized with thiamylal sodium (Surital® —Parke-Davis). An endotracheal tube was passed and anesthesia was maintained with methoxyflurane (Metofane® —Pitman-Moore) and oxygen.

Materials

The following materials were used:

- A RetenPin™threaded reinforcing pin with self-shearing handle (Star Dental Manufacturing Co., Inc., Conshohocken, Pa. 19528).
- Nuva-Fil® restorative kit (L.D. Caulk Co., Div. of Dentsply International, Inc., Milford, Del. 19963) containing 50% phosphoric acid etching solution, Nuva-Seal® preactivated lacquer, Nuva-Fil preactivated restorative material, and applicator tools.
- A portable slow-speed electric dental drill (Golden-West Dental, Inc., Garden Grove, Calif. 92642) with a slow-speed friction-grip contra-angle (Midwest American Dental Co., 901 W. Oakton St., Des Plains, Ill. 60018) and assorted friction-grip diamond burs.
- A Nuva-Lite® ultraviolet gun (3600 Ángstrom units—L.D. Caulk Co.).

Procedure

Root canal therapy was performed using a sterile technique and soft filling material. The fractured edges of the incisor were examined for weakness and bevelled slightly with a diamond bur to prevent a butt junction between the tooth and the restorative material. To create a retentive area, a horizontal undercut groove was made in the remaining part of the tooth on the labial and lingual surfaces, between the bevelled edge and the gingiva.

While firm pressure was applied to the threaded RetenPin, it was twisted into the small root canal until the threads gripped firmly. This resulted in self-shearing of the handle on the pin, leaving a reinforcing post protruding from the opening of the root canal (*Figure 1*).

The exposed surface of the tooth was bathed with 50% phosphoric acid for one minute, then rinsed with water and lightly dried with a cotton pledget and air. This resulted in a dull, etched appearance.

A thick layer of Nuva-Seal preactivated lacquer was brushed on the pin and over the etched area with a short-bristle brush. The lacquer was then exposed to the Nuva-Lite gun for 20 seconds.

The Nuva-Fil restorative material was chosen in a color that matched the dog's teeth. This thick paste was carefully applied with a small plastic spatula in increments 2 mm thick to restore the form of the tooth. To assure adequate retention, a thin layer of restorative material was extended to the gingiva on the labial side of the tooth and into the horizontal groove on the lingual side. Each successive increment was polymerized by exposure to the Nuva-Lite for 20 seconds. To prevent premature setting, care was taken to avoid exposing the Nuva-Fil material to daylight.

The piece of the tooth that was broken off had been saved. It served as a model for forming the prosthesis and was invaluable as an aid to achieving anatomic accuracy. Diamond burs were used in the dental drill to complete the shaping of the prosthesis and to carve anatomic grooves in it.

After the endotracheal tube was removed, the dog's jaws were closed to check for malocclusion of the restored tooth. A final coating of Nuva-Seal was brushed over the restoration and polymerized by the Nuva-Lite for 20 seconds on both the labial and the lingual surfaces.

The total operating time for this procedure was approximately 50 minutes. The result was a very natural-appearing tooth (*Figure 2*).

REFERENCES

1. Sick, E.; Deyoung, D.W.: Apicoectomy and Root Canal Therapy of Canine Teeth in the Dog. *I.S.U. Vet. 36*(2):67-69; 1974.
2. Wiest, L.M., Jr.; Sweeney, E.J.: Restoration of a Fractured Canine Tooth in a Dog. *JAVMA 164*(6):601-602; March 15, 1974.
3. Wilhelm, R.S. *et al*: Dental Prosthesis Used to Crown a Canine Tooth. *VM/SAC 73*(3):299-302; March 1978.
4. Wynne, W.P.D. *et al*: Restoration of a Fractured Tooth in a Dog. *JAVMA 162*(5):396-397; March 1, 1973.
5. Rubin, L.D. *et al*: Root Canal Therapy in Dogs. *VM/SAC 73*(5):593-598; May 1978.
6. Sanco, R.E.; Kelly, J.H.: Root Canal Filling of a Non-Vital Tooth. *VM/SAC 67*(4):382-385; April 1972.

INDEX